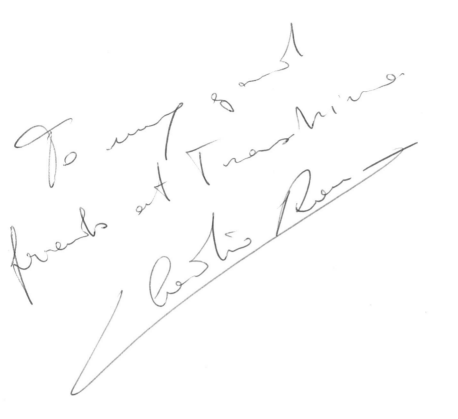

D1737559

Hemodialysis Vascular Access and Peritoneal Dialysis Access

....

Contributions to Nephrology

Vol. 142

Series Editor

Claudio Ronco   *Vicenza*

KARGER

Hemodialysis Vascular Access and Peritoneal Dialysis Access

Volume Editors

Claudio Ronco   *Vicenza*
Nathan W. Levin   *New York, N.Y.*

131 figures, 24 in color, and 24 tables, 2004

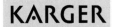
Basel · Freiburg · Paris · London · New York ·
Bangalore · Bangkok · Singapore · Tokyo · Sydney

Contributions to Nephrology

(Founded 1975 by Geoffrey M. Berlyne)

· ·

Claudio Ronco
Department of Nephrology
St. Bortolo Hospital
I–36100 Vicenza (Italy)

Nathan W. Levin
Renal Research Institute
207 East 94th Street, Suite 303
New York, NY 10128 (USA)

Library of Congress Cataloging-in-Publication Data

(CIP-Code is available from the Library of Congress on request)

Bibliographic Indices. This publication is listed in bibliographic services, including Current Contents® and Index Medians.

© Copyright 2004 by S. Karger AG, P.O. Box, CH–4009 Basel (Switzerland)
www.karger.com
Printed in Switzerland on acid-free paper by Reinhardt Druck, Basel
ISSN 0302–5144
ISBN 3–8055–7651–X

Contents

Foreword

Recent developments in hemodialysis techniques have spurred new interest in the field of the vascular access for renal replacement therapies. In particular, the progressive aging of the dialytic population, the high prevalence of diabetes and the demand for increased dialysis efficiency have all pushed the research towards new solutions to access the patient circulation. The program of creating and maintaining a reliable vascular access in hemodialysis patients is today seen as a multidisciplinary task that may include the collaboration of nephrologists, surgeons and interventional radiologists. New techniques have been made available to measure access flow and to perform continuous noninvasive measurements of access recirculation. New biomaterials are today available with improved biocompatibility and surface characteristics and all these new technological issues require a complete and detailed discussion and evaluation.

Finally, the management of complications and the continuous maintenance and care of the access represent one of the most important challenges in the field of hemodialysis.

On the other side of the problem, peritoneal dialysis is emerging as an important renal replacement therapy for a wide spectrum of patients. The field of peritoneal dialysis is also evolving and new devices providing access to the peritoneal cavity have recently been made available. In this setting, the care of the access together with the management of complications represent a further challenge for the clinician. Furthermore, the care of the exit site represents an important aspect of the maintenance of the access and it should be considered as part of the standard access care. Newer techniques of peritoneal dialysis are becoming popular such as continuous flow peritoneal dialysis. In this setting, special catheters are required to provide the flows necessary to perform the programmed treatment schedule.

Based on all these considerations, we felt it was important to generate a book covering all the important issues in the field as well as describing the available technology and methods available today. The book indeed represents an important project and a significant educational effort. We think that a book on this subject will constitute an important contribution in the field of hemodialysis and peritoneal dialysis and is particularly suited for the series *Contributions to Nephrology*.

The book is intended to represent a practical tool for physicians and nurses involved in the management and care of end-stage renal disease patients as well as a reference textbook for medical students, residents and fellows.

Claudio Ronco
Nathan W. Levin

....

Preface

The recent accidental death of Belding Scribner on June 19, 2003 has high-lighted the old adage that precedent claims are rarely correct. The original idea of a bypass to maintain the patency of indwelling arterial and venous catheters was developed by Nils Alwall in 1948 and published in 1949 [1]. In his first animal experiments in rabbits, the carotid artery and jugular vein were cannulated with siliconized glass tubes and patency was maintained with a curved siliconized glass capillary bypass. Following the success of the animal work, Alwall et al. [2] started treating patients with end-stage renal disease. However, because of local infection and clotting he abandoned the technique in 1949. Thus, the real merit of Scribner's contribution (who recognized Alwall's original claim in the first publication in 1960 at ASAIO [3]) was his determination not to abandon the technique. This intense determination to succeed was evident in his presentation at Evian in September 1960 which I had the honor to hear [4]. Alwall [5] also gave a presentation at Evian on the Swedish experience in long-term dialysis and as a consequence of their work, I started a long-term ESRD dialysis program at the Royal Free Hospital London in 1961. At this time, the Teflon shunt had a life expectancy of weeks and for this reason we developed a femoral vessel puncture technique with a modified Seldinger catheter [6]. Attempts at leaving the catheter in permanently were soon abandoned after fatal embolic and infectious complications [7] and we switched to the shunt developed by Quinton in 1961 where he had developed a flexible siliconized rubber tube to replace the original all Teflon shunt [8]. The silicone Teflon Quinton shunt had a life expectancy of months to years and without this development it is unlikely that there would be more than one million people today living on dialysis. However, in my opinion,

X

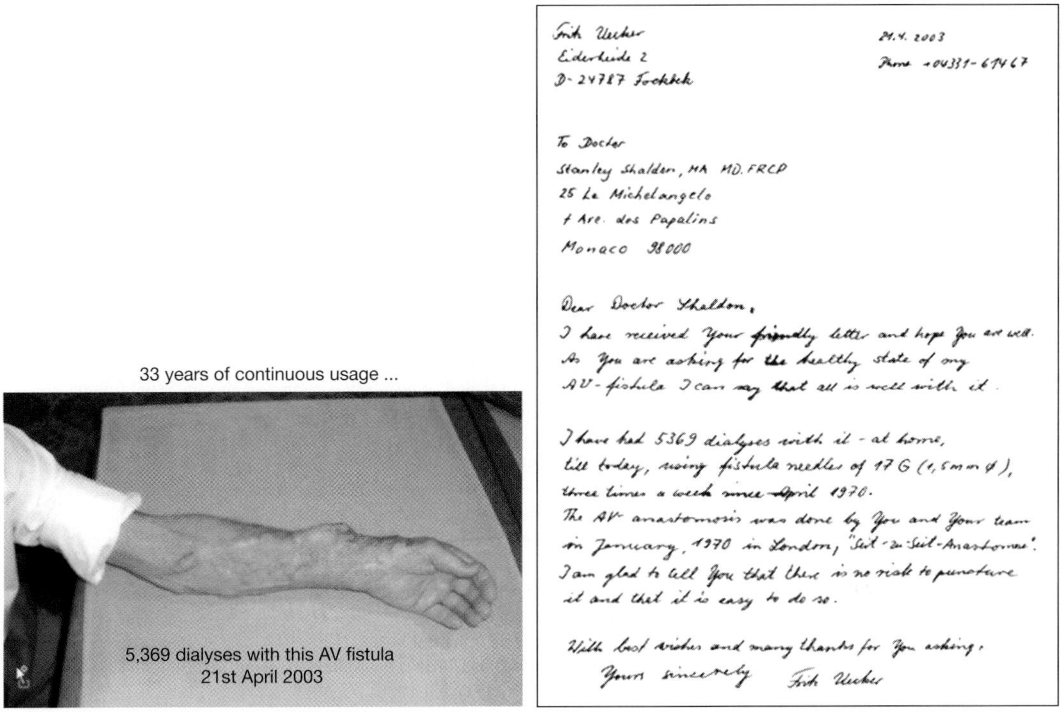

33 years of continuous usage ...

5,369 dialyses with this AV fistula
21st April 2003

a

b

Fig. 1. *a* Radial cephalic fistula (side to side), created by S.S. in January 1970, used continuously since then by F.U. (male, born March 12, 1938), self-puncturing 3–4 × week. *b* Patient's comments.

the definitive access site had to await the development from New York by Cimino and Brescia working at the VA hospital in the Bronx. In 1962 [9], they had attempted to perform regular dialysis with a simple venipuncture and pointed out the advantages of this technique over the indwelling Scribner shunt or our repeated femoral vessel puncture technique. It only required the contribution of Appel, the surgeon of the group, to construct the AV fistula for their argumentation of 1962 to become a reality 4 years later [10]. Today, I have no doubt that the only acceptable long-term approach to hemodialysis is via a venipuncture of a fistularized vein resulting from a surgically created arteriovenous fistula. My personal anectodal belief is based upon the 33 1/2-year survival of a radiocephalic fistula I created in January 1970 that has been punctured more than 5,300 times by the patient himself (3–4 × week) (fig. 1).

Hemodialysis Vascular Access and Peritoneal Dialysis Access edited by C. Ronco and N.W. Levin admirably fulfils its objective as an instructive teaching book. The 27 individual contributions cover completely the fields of vascular and peritoneal access. I feel certain that it will establish itself as a leader in the access field.

References

1   Alwall N, Bergsten B, Gedda P, Norvitt L, Steins AM: On the artificial kidney. IV. The technique in animal experiments. Acta Med Scand 1949;132:392.
2   Alwall N, Norvitt L, Steins AM: The artificial kidney. VII. Clinical experiences of dialytic treatment of uraemia. Acta Med Scand 1949;132:587.
3   Quinton W, Dillard D, Scribner BH: Cannulation of blood vessels for prolonged hemodialysis. Trans Am Soc Artif Intern Organs 1960;6:104–109.
4   Scribner BH: Continuous hemodialysis as a method of preventing uremia in chronic renal failure. Proceedings of the 1st International Congress of Nephrology, Evian, 1960.
5   Alwall N: Fifteen hundred treatments with the artificial kidney (dialysis, ultrafiltration) 1946–1960. Proceedings of the 1st International Congress of Nephrology, Evian, 1960.
6   Shaldon S, Chiandussi L, Higgs B: Haemodialysis by percutaneous catheterization of the femoral artery and vein with regional heparinisation. Lancet 1961;ii:857–859.
7   Shaldon S, Baillod R, Compty C, Oakley J, Sevitt L: Eighteen months experience with a nurse patient operated chronic dialysis unit. Proc Eur Dial Transplant Assoc 1964;1:233–242.
8   Quinton WE, Dillard DH, Cole JJ, Scribner BH: Eight months experience with silastic-teflon bypass cannulas. Trans Am Soc Artif Intern Organs 1962;7:236–243.
9   Cimino JE, Brescia JB: Simple venipuncture for hemodialysis. N Engl J Med 1962;267:608–609.
10   Cimino JE, Brescia JB, Appel K, Hurwich BH: Chronic hemodialysis using venipuncture and a surgically created arteriovenous fistula. N Engl J Med 1966;275:1089.

Stanley Shaldon MA, MD, FRCP
25 Le Michelangelo
7 Avenue des Papalins
Monaco 98000
Tel. +37 79 20 56 166
Fax +37 79 20 59 026
E-Mail stanley_shaldon@monaco 377.com

Ronco C, Levin NW (eds): Hemodialysis Vascular Access and Peritoneal Dialysis Access.
Contrib Nephrol. Basel, Karger, 2004, vol 142, pp 1–13

....

History and Evolution of the Vascular Access for Hemodialysis

M. Bonello[a], N.W. Levin[b], C. Ronco[a]

[a] Department of Nephrology, St. Bortolo Hospital, Vicenza, Italy;
[b] Renal Research Institute and Beth Israel Medical Center, New York, N.Y., USA

One day in the early 1940s, Dr. Alwall from Lund entered his living room and asked his wife whether in her opinion blood could be washed. She answered that theoretically everything could be washed and this probably started the adventure of clinical dialysis. Nevertheless, very little credit is given to Dr. Alwall; however, without his important contribution dialysis would probably have died in its early stages since the experiments of Scribner and Kolff were not encouraging at the beginning. Dialysis, used as a substitute therapy for patients suffering from chronic renal failure, was introduced in the early 1960s in Seattle, Wash. when Scribner and his collaborators worked out a technique for long-term vascular access and designed a complete device for preparing the dialysis solution [1]. Again, the important contribution of Dr. Alwall should be acknowledged. Long-term vascular access was obtained by inserting a rigid Teflon tube into both the radial artery and one of the forearm veins [2] (fig. 1). The dialysate was prepared in a container and refrigerated to avoid bacterial contamination. A pump forced the dialysate into the filter in the opposite direction of the bloodstream [3]. The Kiil kidney [4] was used as a dialyzer. It was composed of two sheets of plastic material cut into thin tubes which were covered with sheets made of Cuprophan. During each dialysis session these sheets formed two separate bags into which the blood was pumped by the patient's blood pressure. The same pressure permitted the blood to return into the patient's bloodstream, prior to heating through the venous line immersed in a receptacle containing heated water [5].

The first dialysis center was set up in Seattle, Wash. where patients were initially dialyzed once a week and subsequently twice a week. In the following

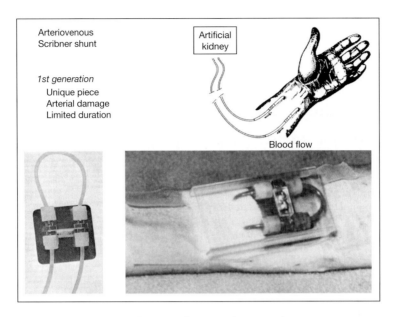

Within the figure:

Arteriovenous
Scribner shunt

Artificial
kidney

1st generation
Unique piece
Arterial damage
Limited duration

Blood flow

Fig. 1. First generation of Scribner arteriovenous shunts.

years considerable improvements were made in the materials used, in the procedures and in the dialysis techniques. Since the very beginning, however, the problem of the vascular access was considered the most important aspect to perform a chronic renal replacement therapy through an extracorporeal blood purification.

The most important innovations took in fact place in the area of the vascular access in the early years of dialysis. The external shunt was created using a softer material known as silastic [6, 7] (fig. 2). In those years, sodium acetate was used instead of bicarbonate as a buffer [8]. The solution-containing acetate was found to be self-sterilizing, therefore reducing the risk of bacterial contamination of the dialysis liquid. Besides a method of preparing of the dialysis liquid, centralized for several patients, was devised [9].

The dialysis program introduced by the Scribner team for chronic patients was adopted by many other hospitals in the USA and in Europe and soon it became clear that more dialysis sites and larger economic resources were necessary for chronic patients. Almost contemporarily (1963–1964) dialysis programs with limited assistance and home dialysis became more widespread in Europe and in the USA [10, 11]. On the basis of the Seattle model of dialysis machines created in the early 1960s, single apparatuses fitted with balanced systems of water/concentrate using hydraulic or electric pumps were introduced.

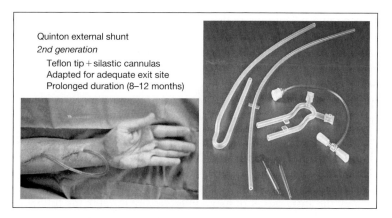

Fig. 2. Second and later generations of external arteriovenous shunts.

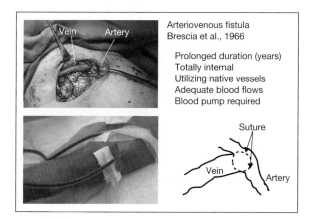

Fig. 3. Arteriovenous fistula as proposed by Brescia et al. [12]. The vein is connected to an artery and it can be used later for needle insertion with easy access.

In the mean time, in 1966 Brescia et al. [12] proposed the possibility of surgically creating an internal arteriovenous fistula on the forearm where the vein was made easily accessible for percutaneous puncture due to the enlargement and increased flow secondary to the connection with an artery. This long-lasting vascular access was less prone to traumas and thrombosis than the external shunt and it was completely internal with no risks of infection (fig. 3). In the span of 10 years the use of the arteriovenous fistula as a vascular access replaced the external shunt and currently represents the first choice of vascular access for intermittent hemodialysis at least in Europe. The development of hemodialysis programs for chronic patients in the early 1960s soon produced brilliant results so that Scribner (in a conference during the 1966 EDTA conference) was able to proclaim the following: '…Dialysis for chronic renal failure is no longer experimental. The results speak for themselves. …The problem logistically of organizing dialysis for all who need it is now the real challenge.'

Other important contributions in the 1960s were the percutaneous cannulation of the femoral artery and vein proposed by Shaldon et al. [13] in 1961 and the semipermanent catheter applied to the thigh vessels proposed by Rae et al. [14] and Thomas [15]. In the mean time, the hollow fiber hemodialyzer was introduced into the clinical routine of dialysis by Gotch et al. [16] in collaboration with Cordis Dow, and higher blood flows started to be explored for an increased efficiency.

In conclusion, the early stages of hemodialysis went through the following evolution as far as vascular access was concerned: intermittent hemodialysis was developed starting from 1960 when the Scribner team in Seattle, Wash. projected a series of external shunts to be applied between the forearm veins and the radial artery. The first samples were manufactured in rigid Teflon and therefore had the characteristic of transmitting the pulse wave of the artery. The problem with this first vascular access was the damage of the intima, the susceptibility to infections, the consequent thrombosis and a very limited life span [17, 18]. Some years later (1962–1964) the Seattle team produced a new generation of external shunts consisting of a soft cannula made from silastic, prefolded to favor the cutaneous exit on which a Teflon vessel tip of 3–4 cm was assembled and which remained inside the vessels [19].

Various types of silastic shunts were introduced later (the Ramirez shunt [20], the Buselmeier shunt [21]; fig. 2), but all of them were susceptible to thrombosis and had a short life span (6–8 months). In 1969 shunts which could be left in the thigh vessels were introduced: the Allen-Brown and Thomas shunts [15]. These vascular accesses were afterwards abandoned (at the end of the1970s) because of infection. In 1966 Brescia et al. [12] proposed an internal arteriovenous fistula on the native vessels, thus eliminating the cutaneous emergencies and ensuring good blood flow; the use of the arteriovenous fistula has, however, immediately raised the problem of providing the dialysis system with a pump capable of guaranteeing a constant blood flow to the filter, in the absence of an arteriovenous gradient such as that present in the shunts [22–25].

Starting from the 1970s the arteriovenous fistula gradually replaced the external shunts that were indeed abandoned by the beginning of the 1980s.

Already in 1969 Rae et al. [14] had introduced the use of the autologous or homologous saphena for the creation of permanent vascular access. Moreover, since the early 1970s biological and nonbiological materials were introduced to create internal arteriovenous fistulas. Grafts, bovine carotid arteries, human umbilical veins and synthetic materials were used (fig. 4–6).

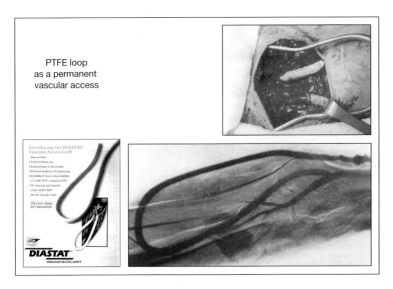

Fig. 4. Prosthetic graft made of PTFE. This allows a connection of an artery and a vein with the possibility of a subsequent direct puncture.

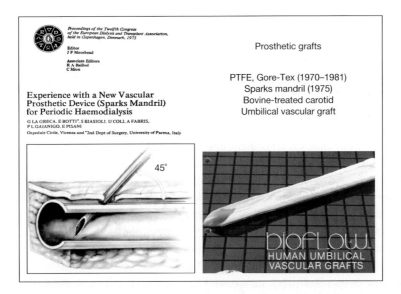

Fig. 5. Other prosthetic materials used for vascular grafts were human umbilical vessels and other synthetic materials.

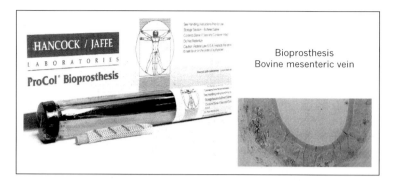

Fig. 6. Grafts were also made of bovine mesenteric veins.

The use of saphena veins removed from patients suffering from varicose veins reached a certain popularity in the 1970s and 1980s and in some cases is still in use. In favor of this technique are the low costs, the relative ease of preparation and conservation of the veins and the low antigenicity. In various publications the efficient functioning of the graft varies from 20 to 60% after 2 years; fibrosis and stenosis of the vessels caused by the continuous puncture may compromise the life of the vascular access.

The most common synthetic material used at present is polytetrafluoroethylene (PTFE). It was introduced in 1973 by the Kolff group [26]. Three years later a modified PTFE (expanded PTFE) [27] was introduced and this then became the most commonly used artificial material for vascular graft in hemodialysis. The PTFE graft was introduced almost contemporarily with other grafts in the 1970s and this really explains its slow development. In the course of the years many attempts were made to modify the structure of vascular grafts in PTFE so as to improve the endothelization on the internal part, the hemostasis after the puncture and the risk of thrombosis which is the primary cause of graft loss.

In 1993 a graft in modified PTFE consisting of a multilayer structure and known as stretch Gore-Tex was introduced by Davidson et al. [28]. The graft made by Gore-Tex, an American company which is among the biggest manufacturers of expanded PTFE, should have (as opposed to the PTFE used so far) better characteristics in terms of compatibility between the graft material and the blood vessels, less tendency to kinking, increased ease to puncture with a good reparation in the area of penetration of the needle. This graft also seems to be utilizable within 48 h from insertion. The initial experience showed that the immediate puncture is possible but not advisable, that the blood flow obtainable is good and that survival is superior to the traditional grafts.

Very recently the Hancock-Jaffe Laboratories have introduced a new bio-graft made from a bovine mesenteric vein treated with glutaraldehyde and

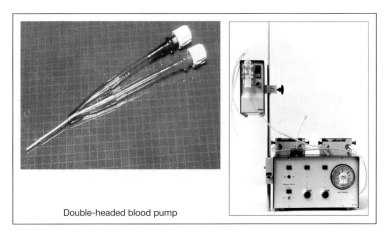

Double-headed blood pump

Fig. 7. Single-needle dialysis made it possible to treat patients with difficult vascular access. For this, double-headed blood pumps had to be utilized.

gamma radiations [29]. Also regarding this graft the initial experience is encouraging but like in the preceding case, there is not sufficient medium- to long-term experience to evaluate whether the benefits are effectively consistent.

Vascular access is currently one of the biggest problems of chronic dialysis. In 1972 Kopp et al. [30] proposed a single-needle dialysis with a peristaltic pump which alternatively aspirated and forced in order to achieve the traumatism of a double puncture (fig. 7). The technique was proposed not just for chronic dialysis patients but also for acute patients utilizing a jugular or a femoral catheter as a vascular access. In 1973 for the same reason Van Waeleghem et al. [31] proposed a blood pump with a double head which allowed a better blood flow and less recirculation of the vascular access (fig. 7). In 1980 Uldall et al. [32] designed a double-lumen catheter to place in the subclavia for short- and medium-term treatments. With this type of access the patient undergoes just one puncture of the vessel and the pump with a single head could achieve a good blood flow with reduced recirculation of the vascular access. Since the mid 1980s dialysis machines had blood pumps for single-needle treatments and systems for detecting blood flows and pressures in the blood circuit. At the same time double-lumen catheters with different internal configurations were developed (parallel flux or coaxial flux) (fig. 8). In fact, to facilitate insertion, it is possible to find catheters which are rigid at room temperature and soften once they are inserted. Also different biomaterials are utilized including processes of coating to prevent biofilm formation and infection/thrombosis.

In the last 20 years the wide experience with central catheters has demonstrated that catheters in the subclavian vein often cause stenosis of the subclavia

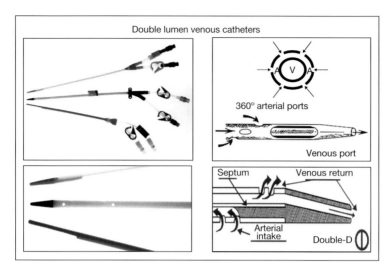

Fig. 8. Different double-lumen venous catheters.

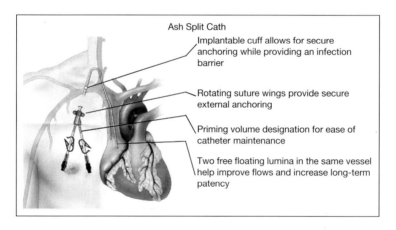

Fig. 9. Evolution of double-lumen catheters include the Ash Split catheter.

and of the superior cava vein with consequent malfunction of the vascular access and important clinical implications [33]. For these reasons it is actually preferable to use silicone catheters in the jugular vein (single Canaud catheter [34], double Tesio catheter [35] and double-lumen Ash catheter [36]; fig. 9); catheters placed in this way have cuffs to fix the catheter and to avoid exogenous infections; the exit site is in the subclavear region and these catheters permit high flux for the dialytic treatment. It is possible to place jugular catheters under echografic guidance so the risk of puncturing the carotid is avoided [37].

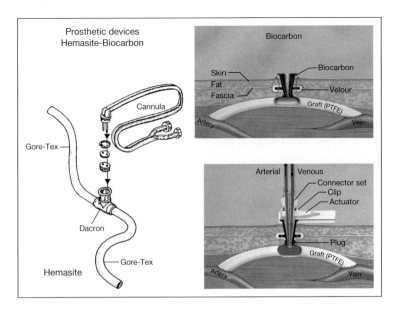

Fig. 10. Different types of needleless vascular access.

At the beginning of the 1980s two types of vascular grafts which did not need a percutaneous puncture were created and commercialized: the CTAD (carbon transcutaneous access device) [38] and the Hemasite [39] (fig. 10). The CTAD produced by Bentley had a device made of biocarbon with a cutaneous exit site, and a polyethylene cap which was in place when it was not in use; a biocarbon device was connected to the blood lines permitting the circulation of the blood for the dialytic treatment. Hemasite had a special device made of titanium surrounded by velvet Dacron with a cutaneous exit site. These percutaneous buttons where assembled on a PTFE graft connected to the patient's artery and vein. This vascular access was used during the 1980s making dialysis a punctureless treatment. However, these buttons were prone to infections which consequently caused thrombosis of the graft, drastically reducing the life time of the vascular access. In addition to this the high costs and the clinical proof that there were few advantages compared to the original vascular access in PTFE gradually reduced its use until it disappeared at the end of the 1980s.

In 1985 the concept of high-flux, efficient hemodialysis [40] was introduced. For this type of dialysis higher blood flows, accurately calibrated blood pumps, low-resistance fistula needles and precise control systems of the ultrafiltration became necessary. The flow of the native arteriovenous fistula and the amount of blood recirculation then started to be taken into consideration.

It could be seen that the flow of an efficiently working fistula amounted to about 700–800 ml/min and that this capacity did not change during dialysis. The hemodynamic impact of the high extracorporeal blood flow turned out to be quite low and well tolerated by the patients [41] and the hemodynamic instability characterized by episodes of low blood pressure during dialysis depends largely on the ultrafiltration rate [42].

Following the development of 'rapid haemodialysis' and of the subsequent need of high blood flow, the fistula needles were also modified. As the needle represented the point of major resistance for the passage of blood towards the filter, shorter needles with an ultrathin wall were produced.

The modern hemodialytic techniques need such high blood flows that make the evaluation of the entity of blood recirculation very important. The most modern dialysis machines are equipped with devices capable of measuring the recirculation. It is possible to use a conductimetric system (differential conductibility after a saline bolus), a thermic system (difference of temperature after thermic bolus) and an ultrasonic-fluximetry system (measurement of the flowmetric dilution and transit time) with excellent and reproducible results.

Moreover, whether we are dealing with a native fistula or artificial or biological grafts, it is possible to evaluate the flow of the vascular access using the ultrasonic flowmetric system during the creation of the access and later, during its chronic utilization, thus monitoring the function over time. All these methods allow for an accurate discrimination of a malfunctioning vascular access and make it possible to implement corrective measures in good time.

In vascular stenosis, positioning an endoluminal stent is a recently introduced and very promising technique, which allows the recovery of dysfunctioning fistulas. It is not unusual that part of an arteriovenous fistula, becomes stenotic because of trauma or because of the numerous punctures. The patient risks to undergo dialysis with an inadequate blood flow; such a condition moreover increases the degree of recirculation of the vascular access. This malfunction can therefore be detected early with repeated recirculation measurements done with on-line techniques. The approach to correct this problem consists of the study of the vascular access function with echo-Doppler and angiography, in the evaluation of recirculation and subsequently the treatment of the stenosis with the transluminal angioplasty [43] and eventually positioning of a stent in the stenotic area [44]. A recent contribution to the problem of vascular access exploits the concept of blood ports implantable under the skin. This approach has been used mostly in oncology for the administration of antitumor therapy [39]. Recently the initial clinical experience with these devices was published and the first results seem to be very encouraging (fig. 11) [45].

In the USA, where two thirds of patients on dialysis have a graft as a vascular access (in Italy less than 20%) many studies are carried out especially

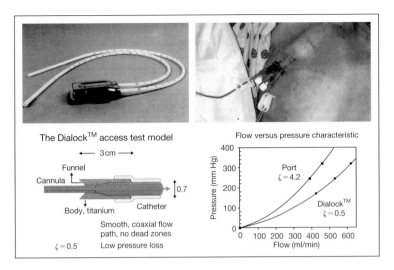

The Dialock™ access test model   Flow versus pressure characteristic

Fig. 11. Example of a recent 'internal blood port'.

to avoid thrombosis in PTFE grafts and eventually to find a graft which is resistant to thrombosis.

Finally we want to emphasize that as far as we are concerned the most efficient, lasting, reliable and low-cost vascular access is the native arterio-venous fistula. Although PTFE was modified it causes the same problems as in the 1970s. It is necessary to find new materials for graft and/or to modify PTFE in order to make it more compliant with the native vessels.

The most important characteristic for vascular access is the flow which must be adequate for extracorporeal treatment even though the population on dialysis is getting older. Some problems are caused by erythropoietin (viscosity), which is widely used and by central venous catheters which determine venous stenosis; the dilatation of the stenosis with transluminal angioplasty and the application of venous stents can resolve this problem.

All these problems will make dialysis more difficult in the future, when a very old population will receive renal replacement therapy. Nevertheless, the evolution of technology will probably help clinicians find new solutions and new strategies.

References

1   Scribner BH, Buri R, Caner JEZ, Hegstrom R, Burnell JM: The treatment of chronic uremia by means of intermittent hemodialysis: A preliminary report. Trans Am Soc Artif Intern Organs 1960;6:114.
2   Quinton WE, Dillard D, Scribner BH: Cannulation of blood vessels for prolonged hemodialysis. Trans Am Soc Artif Intern Organs 1960;6:104.

3   Scribner BH, Caner JEZ, Buri R, Quinton WE: The technique of continuous hemodialysis. Trans Am Soc Artif Intern Organs 1960;6:88.
4   Kiil F, Amundsen B: Development of a parallel flow artificial kidney in plastics. Acta Chir Scand Suppl 1960;253:142–149.
5   Cole JJ, Quinton WE, Williams C, Murray JS, Sherris JC: The pumpless low temperature hemodialysis system. Trans Am Soc Artif Intern Organs 1962;8:209.
6   Quinton WE, Dillard D, Cole JJ, Scribner BH: Possible improvement in the technique of long-term cannulation of blood vessels. Trans Am Soc Artif Intern Organs 1961;7:60.
7   Quinton BH, Dillard DH, Cole JJ, Scribner BH: Eight month's experience with silastic-teflon bypass cannulas. Trans Am Soc Artif Intern Organs 1962;8:236.
8   Mion CM, Hegstrom RM, Boen ST, Scribner BH: Substitution of sodium acetate for bicarbonate in the bath fluid for hemodialysis. Trans Am Soc Artif Intern Organs 1964;10:110–114.
9   Grimsrud L, Cole JJ, Lehman GA, Babb AL, Scribner BH: A central system for the continuous preparation and distribution of hemodialysis fluid. Trans Am Soc Artif Intern Organs 1964;10:107.
10   Shaldon S, Baillod RA, Conty C, Oakley J, Sevitt L: 18 months experience with a nurse-patient operated chronic dialysis unit. Proc Eur Dial Transplant Assoc 1964;1:233.
11   Merril JP, Schupak E, Cameron E, Hampers CL: Hemodialysis in the home. JAMA 1964;190:468.
12   Brescia MJ, Cimino JE, Appel K, Hurwick BJ: Chronic hemodialysis using venipuncture and a surgically created arteriovenous fistula. New Engl J Med 1966;275:1089–1091.
13   Shaldon S, Chiandussi L, Higgs B: Hemodialysis by percutaneous catheterisation of the femoral artery and vein with regional heparinisation. Lancet 1961;ii:857.
14   Rae AI, Baird RM, Gerein AN: Thigh cannula: A femoral saphenous cannula for use in maintenance hemodialysis. Lancet 1969;ii:1402.
15   Thomas GI: A large vessel applique A-V shunt for hemodialysis. Trans Am Soc Artif Intern Organs 1969;15:288.
16   Gotch F, Lipps BJ, Weaver J, Brandes J, Rosin J, Sargent J, Oja P: Chronic dialysis with the hallow fiber artificial kidney (HFAK). Trans Am Soc Artif Intern Organs 1969;15:87.
17   Eschbach IW, Wilson WE, Peoples RW, Wakefield AW, Babb AL, Scribner BH: Unattended overnight home hemodialysis. Trans Am Soc Artif Intern Organs 1966;12:346.
18   Erben J, Kvasnicka J, Bastecky J, Vortel V: Experience with routine use of subclavian vein cannulation in hemodialysis. Proc Eur Dial Transplant Assoc 1969;6:59.
19   Scribner BH, Babb AL: Chronic hemodialysis in Seattle 1960–1966. Part II. Dial Transplant 1982; 11:324.
20   Ramirez O, Swartz C, Onesti G, Mailloux L, Brest AN: The winged in-line shunt. Trans Am Soc Artif Intern Organs 1966;12:220–223.
21   Buselmeier TJ, Kjellstrand CM, Simmons RL, Duncan DA, Von Hartitzsch B, Rattazzi LC, Leonard AS, Najarian JS: A totally new subcutaneous prosthetic arterio-venous shunt. Trans Am Soc Artif Intern Organs 1973;19:25.
22   May J, Tiller D, Johnson J, Stewart J, Sheil AGR: Saphenous vein arterio-venous fistula in regular dialysis treatment. N Engl J Med 1969;280:770.
23   Richie RE, Johnson HK, Walker P, Ginn E: Creation of an arteriovenous fistula utilizing a modified bovine artery graft: Clinical experience in fourteen patients. Proc Dial Transplant Forum 1972;2:86.
24   Dardik H, Ibrahim IM, Dardik I: Arteriovenous fistula constructed with modified human umbilical vein graft. Arch Surg 1976;60:111.
25   Flores L, Dunn I, Frumkin E, Forte R, et al: Dacron arteriovenous shunts for vascular access in hemodialysis. Trans Am Soc Artif Intern Organs 1973;19:33.
26   Volder IGR, Kirkham RL, Kolff WJ: A-V shunts created in new ways. Trans Am Soc Artif Intern Organs 1973;19:38.
27   Baker LD Jr, Johnson JM, Goldfarb D: Expanded polytetrafluoroethylene (PTFE) subcutaneous arteriovenous conduit: An improved vascular access for chronic hemodialysis. Trans Am Soc Artif Intern Organs 1976;22:382.
28   Davidson I, Melone D: Preliminary experience with a new PTFE graft for vascular access for hemodialysis. Part III; in Henry ML, Ferguson RM (eds): Hemodialysis Vascular Access. Chicago, Gore & Associates and Precept Press, 1993, pp 133–136.

29   Bourquelot PD: Procol Bioprosthetic Vascular Grafts for Dialysis Access. Paris, Angio Access Surgery, Jouvenet Medical Centre, 1997.
30   Kopp KF, Gutch CF, Kolff WJ: Single needle dialysis. Trans Am Soc Artif Intern Organs 1972; 18:75.
31   Van Waeleghem JP, Boone L, Ringoir S: New technique on the one needle system during hemodialysis. Eur Dial Transplant Nurses Assoc 1973;1:10.
32   Uldall PR, Woods F, Merchant N, Crichton E, Carter H: A double lumen subclavian cannula (DLSC) for temporary hemodialysis access. Trans Am Soc Artif Intern Organs 1980;26:93.
33   Schillinger F, Schillinger D, Montagnac R, Millent T: Postcatheterization vein stenosis: Comparative angiographic study of 50 subclavian and 50 internal jugular accesses. Nephrol Dial Transplant 1991;6:722.
34   Canaud B, Saumier F, Beraud JJ, Joyeux H, Mio C: La cannulation jugulaire interne avec deux cathéters silastic. Une nouvelle méthode d'access vasculaire pour hémodialyse. Néphrologie 1986;7:57.
35   Tesio F, De Baz H, Panarello G, Calianno G, Quaia P, Raimondi A, Schinella D: Double cannulation of the internal jugular vein for hemodialysis: Indications, techniques and clinical results. Artif Organs 1994;18:301.
36   Mankus RA, Ash SR, Sutton JM: Comparison of blood flow rates and hydraulic resistance between the Mahurkar catheter, the Tesio Twin catheter, and the Ash Split Cath. Am Soc Artif Intern Organs 1998;44:M532.
37   Conz PA, Dissegna D, Rodighiero MP, La Greca G: Cannulation of the internal jugular vein: Comparison of the classic Seldinger technique and an ultrasound guided method. J Nephrol 1997; 6:311.
38   Golding AL, Nissenson AR, Higgins E, Raible D: Carbon transcutaneous access device (CTAD). Trans Am Soc Artif Intern Organs 1980;26:105.
39   Collins AJ, Shapiro FL, Keshaviah PR, Illstrup KM, Andersen RC, et al: Blood access without percutaneous punctures (Hemasite). Trans Am Soc Artif Intern Organs 1981;27:308.
40   Rotellar E, Martinez ME, Plans A, Ferragut A: Hemodialysis: Only six hours once a week. Proc Eur Dial Transplant Assoc 1985;22:312.
41   Ronco C, Fabris A, Chiaramonte S, De Dominicis E, Feriani M, Brendolan A, Bragantini L, Milan M, Dell'Aquila R, La Greca G: Impact of high blood flows on vascular stability in hemodialysis. Nephrol Dial Transplant 1990;1(suppl 5):109–114.
42   Ronco C, Fabris A, Chiaramonte S, De Dominicis E, Feriani M, Brendolan A, Bragantini L, Milan M, Dell'Aquila R, La Greca G: Comparison of four different short hemodialysis techniques. Int J Artif Organs 1988;3:169–174.
43   Beathard G: Percutaneous transvenous angioplasty in the treatment of vascular access stenosis. Kidney Int 1992;42:1390.
44   Guenther RW, Vorwerk D, Bohndorf K, Klose K, Kistler D, Mann H, Sieberth H, El Din A: Venous stenosis in dialysis shunts: Treatment with self-expanding metallic stents. Radiology 1989; 170:401.
45   Levin NW, Yang P, Hatch DA, Dubrow A, Caraiani NS, Ing T, Gandhi VC, Alto A, Davila SM, Prosi FR, Polaschegg HD, Megerman J: Initial results of a new access device for hemodialysis. Technical note. Kidney Int 1998;54:1739.

Claudio Ronco, MD, Director,
Department of Nephrology, St. Bortolo Hospital,
Viale Rodolfi, IT–36100 Vicenza (Italy)
Tel. +39 0444 993869, Fax +39 0444 993949, E-Mail cronco@goldnet.it

Ronco C, Levin NW (eds): Hemodialysis Vascular Access and Peritoneal Dialysis Access.
Contrib Nephrol. Basel, Karger, 2004, vol 142, pp 14–28

....

Epidemiology of Vascular Access for Hemodialysis and Related Practice Patterns

Rajiv Saran[a,b], *Ronald L. Pisoni*[c], *William F. Weitzel*[a]

[a] Division of Nephrology, Department of Internal Medicine and
[b] Kidney Epidemiology and Cost Center, University of Michigan and
[c] University Renal Research and Education Association, Ann Arbor, Mich., USA

The vital importance of vascular access (VA) for optimal delivery of hemodialysis (HD) is well recognized. Timely creation and meticulous maintenance of these 'lifelines' are crucial for the care of HD patients. Clinical practice guidelines [1] have therefore made VA a priority area. According to the 2002 USRDS report [2], the number of HD VA procedures increased by almost 4 times between 1991 and 2000, while costs for these procedures grew from USD 104 million to almost USD 200 million. Over this time, delivery of VA services has moved steadily from the inpatient to the outpatient arena. As a result, the physician and institutional payments have decreased for all types of VA services in the United States. However, VA procedures and complications have been reported previously to account for over 20% of hospitalizations of dialysis patients in the United States and cost about USD 1 billion annually, and therefore remain the single greatest categorical expense for dialysis patient care [3, 4].

This chapter aims to provide a critical overview of the epidemiology of VA utilization as well as an appraisal of recent literature with regard to patterns of practice that have been observed to affect VA outcomes.

VA Practices around the World

The Dialysis Outcomes and Practice Patterns Study (DOPPS) [5] is undoubtedly a rich international resource of epidemiological data pertaining to practice patterns related to VA outcomes worldwide. A brief overview of the study design of this major international effort is therefore pertinent. DOPPS phase I was initiated as an international, prospective observational study of HD practice patterns in 7 countries (France, Germany, Italy, Japan, Spain, the United Kingdom, and the United States). Phase II began in the spring of 2002, and the study has now been expanded to include 5 additional countries (Australia, Belgium, Canada, New Zealand, and Sweden). The published data from the DOPPS thus far is from phase I of the study, for which new patient enrollment ended in 2001, having accumulated demographic and mortality data for >50,000 HD patients, with detailed comorbidity and longitudinal follow-up data for >17,000 HD patients. Details of DOPPS data collection and study design have been published previously [5]. Briefly, nationally representative samples of randomly selected HD facilities were recruited in each country. Facility selection was stratified to provide proportional sampling by geographic region and type of dialysis facility within each country. The DOPPS used uniform data collection instruments translated into the native language of each country to allow for direct comparison of HD practices across countries and dialysis facilities.

VA Use Comparison between Incident and Prevalent HD Patients in the DOPPS

Several prior regional studies supported the existence of substantial differences in VA use between Europe and the United States [6–10]. However, more recently, data from the DOPPS has allowed a comprehensive and broad-based comparison of VA use and survival [11]. A comparison of VA use across 7 countries was based on data from 145 US HD facilities, 101 European facilities and 64 Japanese facilities. These results indicated high use of autogenous arteriovenous fistula (AVF) in >80% of prevalent HD patients in Japan and Europe (country range: 67–93%). In the US, on the other hand, synthetic arteriovenous grafts (AVG) have been the predominant access for 58% of the HD patients with only 24% of US HD patients using an AVF. The high use of AVF in Europe is seen in a variety of patient subgroups. On the other hand, AVF use in the US is less than half that in Europe or Japan even among younger male HD patients without diabetes, peripheral vascular disease, and coronary artery disease. However, preliminary data from phase II of DOPPS indicates that since 1998, the use of AVF has increased among US patients from 24 to 28% of prevalent HD population in 2002. While still far from ideal, this is an encouraging trend [DOPPS; unpubl. data].

Among incident HD patients, 65–67% of new ESRD patients in Japan and Europe initiated HD with an AVF compared with 15% in the US [11, 12]. In contrast, 24% new HD patients in the US compared with only 3% in Europe and Japan used synthetic grafts. These differences in permanent access use remain even after adjustment for patient characteristics and comorbidities, and therefore cannot be ascribed entirely to differences in case mix by country.

Catheter use is very common among new ESRD patients, with 60% of US patients and 31% of HD patients in Europe starting dialysis with a catheter [11, 13]. This could partly be explained by late referral during the course of chronic kidney disease combined with suboptimal access planning during the pre-ESRD period.

VA Practices within the US

In a landmark study, Hirth et al. [14] described substantial geographic variations within the US regarding the use of AVF among new dialysis patients. The prevalence of AVF among incident HD patients ranged from 77% in New England to 15% in the South East in this report. These differences persisted even after adjustment for case mix. Similar results were reported by the HEMO study [15]. The national profile of practice patterns for HD VA in the US was published recently [16]. This data is derived from the Centers for Medicare and Medicaid Service's (CMS), national ESRD Clinical Performance Measures (CPM) project [17]. This initiative has been in place since 1999 and is designed to collect information on clinical practices regarding various core indicators and clinical performance measures including VA in ambulatory HD patients, and has as its chief aim the identification of opportunities for improvement of care for adult, Medicare maintenance dialysis beneficiaries. A total of 8,154 HD patients were sampled; 17% (n = 1,399) were incident. Twenty-eight percent were dialyzed by an AVF, 49% through an AVG and 23% via a percutaneous catheter.

Predictors of Type of VA Placed at Start of HD

Gender
A number of studies have made the observation that women are more likely to receive an AVG than an AVF [14–16, 18, 19], and are indeed more likely to dialyze via a percutaneous catheter [16] owing to higher rates of technical failure associated with using an AVF. It has been hypothesized [3] that this is perhaps because women have smaller caliber blood vessels. A recent

study [20] examined this hypothesis in a prospective manner having utilized routine preoperative sonographic mapping of both arteries and veins in the upper extremities prior to the surgical placement of AVF. While the diameter of the artery used in AVF placement was significantly larger in men versus women, there were no significant differences in venous diameter by gender. Moreover, there were no significant differences between preoperative arterial or venous dimensions in AVF that matured successfully versus those that did not. This raises the possibility that rather than a simple difference in vessel diameter, variations in vascular biology (vascular reactivity, platelet aggregation, vascular remodeling etc.) might provide clues as to the etiopathogenesis of gender differences in initial success of VA placement and VA survival.

Age
Ageing is associated with compromised vasculature owing to both atherosclerosis and arteriolosclerosis. It is therefore plausible that the odds of placement of tunneled percutaneous catheter is higher than the odds of AVG or upper arm AVF as the initial VA with advancing age. A recent report of DOPPS data [11] analyzed patient characteristics associated with AVF versus AVG use in incident and prevalent HD patients in Europe and the United States. AVF use was strongly associated with younger age (adjusted odds ratio for every 10 years older = 0.89; $p < 0.0001$). Similar results have been reported by others [15, 21].

Race
African-American race appears to be a predictor for greater probability of the placement of AVG than AVF, supported by data from the DOPPS as well as the HEMO study [15, 22]. Whether this is a function of late presentation to ESRD or unrelated factors such as diminished availability of suitable vessels for AVF is unclear.

Diabetes
Diabetics are more likely to get AVG than AVF as an initial access when data on prevalent HD patients in both Europe and the US are considered together [11]. In the case of incident HD patients, however, this difference was not statistically significant.

Peripheral Vascular Disease
Presence of peripheral vascular disease was associated with significantly lower odds of AVF versus AVG use among prevalent HD patients in Europe and the US [11]. While the same trend was noted in the case of patients incident to ESRD, it was not statistically significant.

Duration of Predialysis Care

Patient responses to questionnaires in the DOPPS study [11] indicate that a substantially greater proportion of European patients receive longer-term pre-ESRD care, with 69% of European patients seeing a nephrologist for at least 1 year prior to ESRD compared to 44% in the US. The ratio of AVF versus AVG use was significantly higher if patients received nephrologic care >30 days prior to ESRD compared with ≤30 days (adjusted odds ratio = 1.95, p = 0.01).

Type of Physician Placing VA and Use of Surgical Trainees

There is country variation with regard to the type of physician who generally places permanent VA for HD patients. In France, Germany, Spain, the UK and the US, 65–89% of permanent VA were placed by a vascular surgeon per DOPPS data [11]. In contrast, approximately 80% of permanent access placements in Italy were performed by a nephrologist, consistent with another published report from Italy [6]. No consistent relationship was found between the type of surgeon/physician placing permanent VA in a dialysis unit and the odds of AVF versus AVG use, except when the nephrologist was the primary type of physician placing permanent VA (data mostly from Italy, where this practice pattern is most common), when the odds of fistula were significantly higher. Furthermore, surgical trainees perform/assist in placing permanent VA; it has been shown in the DOPPS [11] that this is associated with a lower odds of 0.6 for AVF placement versus AVG.

VA Preferences at Individual Dialysis Facilities

In another DOPPS study, utilizing data from 133 participating US HD facilities only, the investigators found that in addition to a substantial variation in the utilization of AVF versus AVG across regions and facilities, grafts were preferred over fistulae by 21% of medical directors and nearly 40% of nurse managers. Furthermore, patients in facilities in which a preference for grafts was indicated were more than twice as likely to have a graft than a fistula [23]. This data supports the notion that dialysis personnel might actually influence the type of VA created by the surgeon and provides for an approach to altering the practice pattern at a given facility.

Preoperative Sonographic Mapping and the Multidisciplinary Approach

Several recent studies have demonstrated that preoperative sonographic mapping leads to an increase in the proportion of patients dialyzing via AVFs [24–28]. Preoperative vascular mapping changed the procedure performed by the surgeon based on initial history and physical examination in 31% of the cases, half of these being a change from graft to fistula in a recent report [26]. The same group has also shown in a prospective study [29] that a multidisciplinary approach optimized by the utilization of a dedicated VA coordinator can lead to continuous quality improvement and placement of a greater number of AVFs. No association was demonstrable in the DOPPS between presence of access monitoring programs and VA preferences [23].

The Dedicated Surgeon Effect
Konner et al. [30] in Germany have achieved nearly 100% fistula placement rates at their center with a combination of diligent preoperative evaluation, exclusive use of native vessels, utilization of unique surgical approaches, and cumulative experience of a single dedicated operator, in this case, a nephrologist.

VA Type, Patient Morbidity and Mortality

VA complications are known to be responsible for 20% of hospital admissions in dialysis patients at a significant cost to the exchequer [2, 3]. The greatest morbidity and mortality are associated with the use of dialysis catheters, the major risks being infection and thrombosis with resultant bacteremia, sepsis, potential for metastatic infections and endocarditis [31]. In an important study based on the US Renal Data System Dialysis Morbidity and Mortality Wave 1 Study, Dhingra et al. [32] found significantly increased relative risk of mortality with the use of central venous catheters compared to AVG or AVF over a 2-year follow-up period. For both diabetics and nondiabetics, those with AVF had better overall survival than those with AVG, although the comparison in nondiabetics was not statistically significant. The group with central venous catheters had the worst survival after statistical adjustment for various comorbid conditions. Pastan et al. [33] have reported similar results from the southeastern US. Analysis of the DOPPS data reveals higher mortality for those dialyzing with central catheters [13]. In addition to a higher risk of infection, patients dialyzing with catheters have been shown to have lower blood flow rates on dialysis with a resultant significantly lower delivered dose of dialysis [16, 34].

Fistula versus Graft Survival

This topic is controversial because studies comparing AVGs to AVFs often ignore the primary access failure that is much higher in the case of AVF [35, 36]. The recent reports from the DOPPS, however, seem to support the notion that AVFs have a better long-term survival overall [11]. It has, therefore, become increasingly clear that while in the short-term placing an AVF requires a greater investment in time and technique, there may be handsome dividends in the form

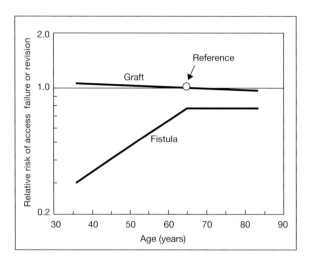

Fig. 1. Cox-adjusted relative risk of failure or revision for an AVF compared with an AVG by patient age. The risk for fistulae, but not for grafts, varies significantly with age of the patient. The difference between the two access types is greatest at younger ages, but then declines because the risk of AVF failure increases with age up to the age of 65 years (RR = 1.40 per 10 years; p < 0.01). Older than 65 years of age, the relative risk for an AVF compared with an AVG is constant (RR = 0.76; p = 0.02) [adapted from 38 with permission of the publisher].

of reduced patient morbidity, fewer interventions, complications and perhaps even lower mortality as discussed above.

Factors Determining VA Survival

Patient Demographics (Unmodifiable)
Age
Woods et al. [37] sought to identify factors that were associated with survival of permanent VA. They found no difference in AVG survival for patients younger or older than 65 years of age, although for both groups, AVG survival was significantly lower than AVF survival overall (fig. 1). AVF survival was better in patients less than 65 years of age. However, even above 65 years of age, AVF were 24% less likely to fail than AVG. These data would support placement of AVF whenever possible despite the age barrier.

Gender
Gender has been shown repeatedly to be associated not only with lower placement rates but also with poorer survival of AVF [38, 39]. The precise reasons for

poor maturation and survival of AVFs in females are unknown and need to be investigated further.

Race

Black race has similarly been associated with lower utilization as well as lower survival in the case of AVF [22, 40]. It is possible that the latter might be due to a more vigorous tissue response to vascular injury in black individuals, akin to a greater predisposition to keloid formation in the skin, leading perhaps to a greater degree of neointimal hyperplasia and fibrosis within the AV anastomosis thereby leading to its earlier occlusion.

Comorbidities

Diabetics and nondiabetics do not show any significant difference in maturation of AVFs, but the presence of peripheral vascular occlusive disease is predictive of poorer AVF survival and lower serum albumin for poorer AVG survival [11, 37, 41]. Whether better control of diabetes or aggressive management of vascular risk factors will lead to better survival of AVF, while a reasonable hypothesis, is at present unproven by clinical studies.

Practice Pattern Related (Modifiable)

Country Differences

Survival of AVF is superior in Europe when compared to the US [11] (fig. 2). Some have argued that these differences are due to lower levels of comorbidity in Europe. However, these results hold true even after adjustment for multiple comorbidities, stratification by continent and accounting for facility clustering. This suggests that there may be other (most likely practice pattern-related) differences between countries that could explain these differences in AVF survival. Whether it is differences in surgical approach, less frequent use of trainees for VA surgery, or differences in the number of experienced staff involved in VA cannulation is not known and merits further investigation.

Site/Type of VA

Radiocephalic AVF has a high primary failure (or nonmaturation) rate compared with upper arm AVF in most reported series [42, 43]. A 1-year patency rate of 76% for forearm AVF compared with 93% for upper arm AVF was reported [44]. Increased utilization of upper arm brachiobasilic transposition AVF has led to a few formal comparisons of access survival between brachiocephalic AVF and brachiobasilic AVF as well as upper arm AVG. The primary failure rates of these two types of upper arm AVF are reportedly similar [43, 45]. When primary failures were included in the study by Oliver et al. [36], the cumulative survival was comparable for both types of upper arm AVF and AVG. However, intervention

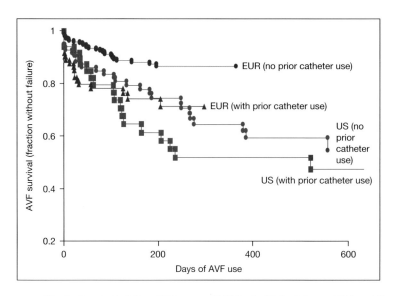

Fig. 2. Survival of first AVF versus AVG in the United States (US) and Europe (EUR) for incident patients using permanent VA at study start (DOPPS). The study was adjusted for differences in age, gender, diabetes, peripheral vascular disease and body mass index. The new HD patients entered DOPPS within 5 days of first-ever dialysis. Access survival obtained by adjusted Cox regression analyses. Prior catheter use lowers the survival of AVF and AVG [adapted from 11 with permission of the publisher].

rates per access year to achieve long-term patency were 2.4 for grafts, 0.7 for brachiobasilic and 0.4 for brachiocephalic AVF.

Prior VA

Prior VA, especially any form of catheter use, has been shown to compromise subsequent AVF/AVG survival in the DOPPS study (see fig. 2) [11].

Multidisciplinary Approach

Involving the key role of an access coordinator has been shown in a prospective study to increase the number of AVF placed at a single institution [29]. It is therefore plausible that in such a program the survival of VA placed will also be enhanced, especially with utilization of preoperative vascular mapping.

Preoperative Sonographic Vascular Mapping

Preoperative sonographic vascular mapping has been shown in a number of studies to increase not only the percentage of AVF but also reduce the percentage of primary fistula failure rates. This subject was recently reviewed [26].

Dedicated/Experienced Surgeons

While this is not proven, single center experiences from Europe suggest that experienced VA surgeons committed to the success of a VA surgery program are vital to the longevity of VA [30].

Interventional Nephrology and Its Role in Access Management

A multidisciplinary approach that includes interventional nephrology utilizing percutaneous approaches to AVG/AVF malfunction is claimed to provide results comparable to surgical approaches [45]. The role of percutaneous dilatation of AVF has been highlighted in a number of recent reports evaluating a prophylactic approach using preoperative fistulography in a randomized prospective fashion [46] as well as treatment of thrombosed AVF [47–49].

VA Monitoring Policy

A separate chapter is devoted entirely to this subject in this issue (pp. 216–227). Whether VA blood flow monitoring reduces access morbidity and cost remains a contentious issue [50, 51].

First Cannulation Times

Timing of first cannulation of VA (especially AVF) is currently not evidence based and could potentially affect VA outcomes. According to the NKF-K/DOQI guidelines [1] a period of at least 2 months should be allowed for adequate maturation of an AVF before first cannulation. In the DOPPS study there is a wide variation with regard to first cannulation times for both AVF and AVG. For instance, 74% of Japanese and 50% European dialysis facilities practice first cannulation of AVF at 1 month or less after AVF creation, in contrast to only 2% of US facilities [DOPPS; unpubl. data]. Two different approaches to looking at the effects of first cannulation time from the DOPPS data reveal consistent results. A patient level (n = 894 newly placed AVF) analysis of first cannulation times and AVF outcomes was published recently [12]. The median time to first cannulation varied greatly between countries: Japan and Italy 25 and 27 days, respectively, Germany 42 days, Spain and France 80 and 86 days, respectively, and the UK and USA 96 and 98 days. No association was found between cannulation ≤28 days versus ≥28 days with patient characteristics of age, gender and 15 classes of comorbid conditions. However, cannulation ≤14 days was associated with a 2.1-fold increase in relative risk of subsequent AVF failure compared to cannulation ≥14 days (p = 0.006). No significant difference in AVF failure was seen with fistulae cannulated in 15–28 days compared to 43–84 days. The study concluded that fistulae should be left to mature for a minimum of 14 days prior to first cannulation. An analysis of data at the dialysis facility level (intent-to-treat, conceptually) rather than patient level (as-treated, conceptually) based on the DOPPS reveals similar results [DOPPS; unpubl. data], thus substantiating the hypotheses that AVF may be amenable to earlier cannulation than hitherto thought possible. If true, the current policy in the US of waiting at least 2 months prior to first cannulation of AVF may be causing excessive reliance on temporary/tunneled catheter access in the interim and is a modifiable practice. However, the final proof can be provided only by a multicenter randomized trial of different first cannulation practices as they relate to VA outcomes.

Blood Flow Rate Practices

Variations in blood flow rate (pump speed) practices on dialysis are not associated with adverse VA outcomes in the DOPPS [DOPPS; unpubl. data].

Drug Use and VA Outcomes

There is renewed interest in the application of pharmacological prophylaxis for improving VA outcomes [52, 53]. Thus far there has been a paucity of randomized clinical trials to improve VA outcomes. Recently, the National Institutes of Health have called for the initiation of randomized clinical trials in this important area. A few clinical trials do exist and deserve mention. Sreedhara et al. [54] demonstrated the potential value of dipyridamole in improving the longevity of AVG in a small placebo-controlled, double-blind, randomized clinical trial. Fish oil has been demonstrated to be of benefit in a study with 24 patients (12 on drug and 12 on placebo) [55]. The primary patency rates at 1 year were 14.9% for the control group and 75.6% in the fish oil-treated group. The vasculoprotective properties of fish oil need to be tested in larger clinical trials in dialysis patients for benefits not restricted to VA outcomes. Low-intensity warfarin was not found effective for the prevention of PTFE graft failure in patients on HD in a multicenter randomized placebo-controlled clinical trial [56]. Observational data from DOPPS supports the use of angiotensin-converting enzyme inhibitors (ACEIs) for AVF (fig. 3) and aspirin as well as calcium channel blockers for AVG [57]. The use of ACEIs was also reported to be of benefit in the case of AVG in a single center retrospective study [58]. These data, based on observational studies, should not substitute for but certainly should point towards priorities for future clinical trials. The newer antiplatelet agents (ticlodipine and clopidogrel) deserve further study in this regard (please see note added in proof). There may also be a role for angiotensin receptor blockade in prolonging VA survival.

Cost Issues

As pointed out earlier, VA-related procedures are increasingly performed as outpatient procedures. However, inpatient treatment is often required for

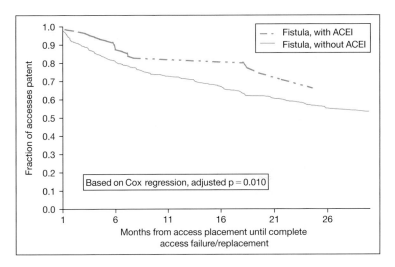

Fig. 3. Secondary (assisted survival) patency for AVF by drug therapy, in this instance ACEI versus no ACEI use. Survival is seen to be significantly higher in those fistulae associated with ACEI use. The Cox regression analyses were adjusted for multiple comorbidities, demographics, and prior permanent VA [adapted from 54 with permission of the publisher].

access-related morbidity such as line sepsis. An estimate of the outpatient VA-related expenditures can be obtained from the website of the ongoing Medicare-sponsored Prospective Payment System Study being carried out at the Kidney Epidemiology and Cost Center in Ann Arbor, Mich. [59]. Between July and December 2000, the expenditures incurred for outpatient VA-related procedures totaled over USD 125 million. A recent cost analysis of patients with ESRD concluded that among patients treated with HD, the cost of VA-related care was lower by more than 5-fold for patients who began the study period with a functioning AVF compared to those treated with a percutaneous catheter or AVG (p < 0.001) [60], further strengthening the argument for AVF as the VA of choice.

Summary and Conclusions

VA serves as a lifeline for HD patients. VA-related expenditures are the largest component of dialysis-related costs. Wide variations in VA practices and outcomes around the world have emerged from analysis of the DOPPS data. Both patient and practice pattern-related factors determine type of VA placed as well as VA outcomes. Type of VA is associated with patient survival after adjustment for case mix. A multidisciplinary approach is crucial for success of any VA program with emphasis on pre-ESRD planning and implementation. AVF should serve as the gold standard. Use of catheters should be minimal, but this will likely remain a challenge for some time. Observational data suggest that earlier cannulation of AVF may not be as deleterious as previously thought. Clinical trials are sorely needed in many aspects of VA management to improve both VA and patient outcomes.

References

1   NKF-K/DOQI Clinical Practice Guidelines for Vascular Access. New York, National Kidney Foundation, 2001, pp 1–98.
2   US Renal Data System: Excerpts from the USRDS 2002 Annual Data Report: Atlas of End-Stage Renal Disease in the United States. Am J Kidney Dis 2003;41(suppl 2):S1–S260.
3   Feldman HI, Kobrin S, Wasserstein A: Hemodialysis vascular access morbidity. J Am Soc Nephrol 1996;7:523–535.
4   Hakim R, Himmelfarb J: Hemodialysis access failure: A call to action. Kidney Int 1998;54: 1029–1040.
5   Young EW, Goodkin DA, Mapes DL, et al: The Dialysis Outcomes and Practice Patterns Study (DOPPS): An international hemodialysis study. Kidney Int 2000;57(suppl 74):S74–S81.
6   Bonucchi D, D'Amelio A, Capelli G, et al: Management of vascular access for dialysis: An Italian survey. Nephrol Dial Transplant 1999;14:2116–2118.
7   Ezzahiri R, Lemson MS, Kitslaar PJ, Leunissen KM, Tordoir JH, et al: Hemodialysis vascular access and fistula surveillance methods in the Netherlands. Nephrol Dial Transplant 1999;14:2110–2115.
8   Besarab A: Vascular access in Europe and the U.S.: Striking contrasts. Contemp Dial Nephrol 1999;20:22–28.
9   Rodriguez JA, Lopez J, Cleries M, et al: Vascular access for hemodialysis – An epidemiological study of the Catalan Renal Registry. Nephrol Dial Transplant 1999;14:1651–1657.
10 Quarello F, Forneris G, Boero R, et al: Vascular access for chronic hemodialysis: Current status and new directions in the Piedmont. Minerva Urol Nefrol 1998;50:9–15.
11 Pisoni RL, Young EW, Dykstra DM, et al: Vascular access use in Europe and the United States: Results from the DOPPS. Kidney Int 2002;61:305–316.
12 Rayner HC, Pisoni RL, Gillespie BW, et al: Creation, cannulation and survival of arteriovenous fistulae: Data from the Dialysis Outcomes and Practice Patterns Study. Kidney Int 2003;63: 323–330.
13 Combe C, Pisoni RL, Port FK, Young EW, Canaud B, Mapes DL, Held PJ: Dialysis Outcomes and Practice Patterns Study: données sur l'utilisation des cathéters veineux centraux en hémodialyse chronique. Néphrologie 2001;22:379–384.
14 Hirth RA, Turenne MN, Woods JD, et al: Predictors of type of vascular access in hemodialysis patients. JAMA 1996;276:1303–1307.
15 Allon M, Ornt D, Schwab S, et al: Factors associated with the prevalence of A-V fistulas in hemodialysis patients in the HEMO study. Kidney Int 2000;58:2178–2185.
16 Reddan D, Klassen P, Frankenfield DL, et al: National profile of practice patterns for hemodialysis vascular access in the United States. J Am Soc Nephrol 2002;13:2117–2124.
17 Centers for Medicare and Medicaid Services. 2002 Annual Report, End Stage Renal Disease Clinical Performance Measures Project. Baltimore, Department of Health and Human Services, Centers for Medicare and Medicaid Services, Center for Beneficiary Choices, 2002.
18 Ifudu OM, Nacey LJ, Homel P, et al: Determinants of type of initial hemodialysis vascular access. Am J Nephrol 1997;17:425–427.
19 Rocco MV, Bleyer AJ, Burkart JM: Utilization of inpatient and outpatient resources for the management of hemodialysis access complications. Am J Kidney Dis 1996;28:250–256.

20   Miller CD, Robbin ML, Allon M: Gender differences in outcomes of arteriovenous fistulas in hemodialysis patients. Kidney Int 2003;63:346–352.

21   Seghal AR, Silver MR, Covinsky KE, Coffin R, Cain JA: Use of standardized ratios to examine variability in hemodialysis vascular access across facilities. Am J Kidney Dis 2000;35:275–281.

22   Saran R, Dykstra DM, Wolfe RA, et al: Fistula use and outcomes among blacks and women in the Dialysis Outcomes and Practice Patterns Study (DOPPS). J Am Soc Nephrol 2002;13:113P.

23   Young EW, Dykstra DM, Goodkin DA, Mapes DL, Wolfe RA, Held PJ: Hemodialysis vascular access preferences and outcomes in the Dialysis Outcomes and Practice Patterns Study (DOPPS). Kidney Int 2002;61:2266–2271.

24   Allon M, Lockhart ME, Lilly RZ, et al: Effect of preoperative sonographic mapping on vascular access outcomes in hemodialysis patients. Kidney Int 2001;60:2013–2020.

25   Silva MB, Hobson RW, Pappas PJ, et al: A strategy for increasing use of autogenous hemodialysis access procedures: Impact of preoperative noninvasive evaluation. J Vasc Surg 1998;27: 302–308.

26   Robbin ML, Gallichio ML, Dierhoi MH, Young CJ, Weber TM, Allon M: US vascular mapping before hemodialysis access placement. Radiology 2000;217:83–88.

27   Aschere E, Gade P, Hingorani A, Gunduz Y, Fodera M, Yorkovich W: Changes in the practice of angioaccess surgery: Impact of dialysis outcomes quality initiative recommendations. J Vasc Surg 2000;31:84–92.

28   Gibson KD, Caps MT, Kohler TR, Hatsukami TS, et al: Assessment of a policy to reduce placement of prosthetic hemodialysis access. Kidney Int 2001;59:2335–2345.

29   Allon M, Bailey R, Ballard R, et al: A multidisciplinary approach to hemodialysis access: Prospective evaluation. Kidney Int 1998;53:473–479.

30   Konner K, Hulbert-Shearon TE, Roys EC, Port FK: Tailoring the initial vascular access for dialysis patients. Kidney Int 2002;62:329–338.

31   Butterfly D, Schwab SJ: The case against chronic venous hemodialysis access. J Am Soc Nephrol 2002;13:2195–2197.

32   Dhingra RK, Young EW, Hulbert-Shearon TE, Leavey SF, Port FK: Type of vascular access and mortality in U.S. hemodialysis patients. Kidney Int 2001;60:1443–1451.

33   Pastan S, Soucie JM, McClellan WM: Vascular access and increased risk of death among hemodialysis patients. Kidney Int 2002;62:620–626.

34   Seghal AR, Snow RJ, Singer ME, et al: Barriers to adequate delivery of dialysis. Am J Kidney Dis 1998;31:593–601.

35   Allon M, Robbin M: Increasing arteriovenous fistulas in hemodialysis patients: Problems and solutions. Kidney Int 2002;62:1109–1124.

36   Oliver MJ, McCann RL, Indridason OS, et al: Comparison of transposed brachiobasilic fistulas to upper arm grafts and brachiocephalic fistulas. Kidney Int 2001;60:1532–1539.

37   Woods JD, Turenne MN, Stawderman RL, et al: Vascular access survival among incident hemodialysis patients in the United States. Am J Kidney Dis 1997;30:50–57.

38   Astor BC, Coresh J, Powe NR, Eustace JA, Klag MJ: Relation between gender and vascular access complications in hemodialysis patients. Am J Kidney Dis 2000;36:1126–1134.

39   Miller CD, Robbin ML, Allon M: Gender differences in the outcomes of arteriovenous fistulas in hemodialysis patients. Kidney Int 2003;63:346–352.

40   Bay WH, Cosio FG, Cleef SSV, Davies EA, Henry ML: Impact of race on the survival of hemodialysis arteriovenous fistulas. J Am Soc Nephrol 1998;9:166A.

41   Miller PE, Carlton D, Deierhoi MH, Redden DT, Allon M: Natural history of arteriovenous grafts in hemodialysis patients. Am J Kidney Dis 2000;36:68–74.

42   Miller PE, Tolwani A, Luscy CP, et al: Predictors of adequacy of arteriovenous fistulas in hemodialysis patients. Kidney Int 1999;56:275–280.

43   Hakaim AG, Nalbandian M, Scott T: Superior maturation and patency of primary brachiocephalic and transposed basilic vein arteriovenous fistulae in patients with diabetes. J Vasc Surg 1998;27: 154–157.

44   Bender MHM, Bruyninckx MA, Gerlag PGG: The brachiocephalic elbow fistula: A useful alternative angioaccess for permanent hemodialysis. J Vasc Surg 1994;20:808–813.

45 Turnel-Rodrigues L, Pengloan J, Bourquelot P: Interventional radiology in hemodialysis fistulae and grafts: A multidisciplinary approach. Cardiovasc Intervent Radiol 2002;25:3–26.

46 Tessitore N, Mansueto G, Bedogna V, et al: A prospective controlled trial on effect of percutaneous transluminal angioplasty on functioning arteriovenous fistula survival. J Am Soc Nephrol 2003; 14:1623–1627.

47 Haage P, Vorwerk D, Wildberger JE, Piroth W, Schurman K, Gunther RW: Percutaneous treatment of thrombosed primary arteriovenous hemodialysis access fistulae. Kidney Int 2000;57:1169–1175.

48 Clark TWI, Hirsch DA, Jindal KJ, Veugelers PJ, LeBlanc J: Outcome and prognostic factors after percutaneous treatment of native hemodialysis fistulas. J Vasc Interv Radiol 2002;13:15–59.

49 Turmel-Rodriguez L, Pengloan J, Rodriguez H, et al: Treatment of failed native arteriovenous fistulae for hemodialysis by interventional radiology. Kidney Int 2000;57:1124–1140.

50 Lumsden AB, MacDonald MJ, Kikeri D, et al: Cost efficacy of duplex surveillance and prophylactic angioplasty of arteriovenous ePTFE grafts. Ann Vasc Surg 1998;12:138–142.

51 McCarley P, Wingard RL, Shyr Y, et al: Vascular access blood flow monitoring reduces access morbidity and costs. Kidney Int 2001;60:1164–1172.

52 Himmelfarb J: Pharmacologic prevention of vascular access stenosis. Curr Opin Nephrol Hypertens 1999;8:569–572.

53 Diskin CJ, Stokes TJ, Pennel A: Pharmacological intervention to prevent hemodialysis vascular access thrombosis. Nephron 1993;64:1–26.

54 Sreedhara R, Himmelfarb J, Lazarus JM, Hakim RM: Anti-platelet therapy in graft thrombosis: Results of a prospective, randomized, double-blind study. Kidney Int 1994;45:1477–1483.

55 Schmitz PG, McCloud LK, Reikes ST, Leonard CL, Gellens ME: Prophylaxis of hemodialysis graft thrombosis with fish oil: Double-blind, randomized prospective trial. J Am Soc Nephrol 2002;13:184–190.

56 Crowther MA, Clase CM, Margetts PJ, et al: Low-intensity warfarin is ineffective for the prevention of PTFE graft failure in patients on hemodialysis: A randomized controlled clinical trial. J Am Soc Nephrol 2002;13:2331–2337.

57 Saran R, Dykstra DM, Wolfe RA, et al: Association between vascular access failure and the use of specific drugs: The dialysis outcomes and practice patterns study (DOPPS). Am J Kidney Dis 2002;40:1255–1263.

58 Gradzki R, Dhingra RK, Port FK, et al: Use of ACE inhibitors is associated with prolonged survival of arteriovenous grafts. Am J Kidney Dis 2001;38:1240–1244.

59 An Expanded Medicare Outpatient End Stage Renal Disease Prospective Payment System. Phase I Report 2002. www.med.umich.edu/kidney/pps/pps.html.

60 Lee H, Manns B, Taub K, et al: Cost analysis of ongoing care of patients with end-stage renal disease: The impact of dialysis modality and dialysis access. Am J Kidney Dis 2002;40:611–622.

Note added in proof:
A recently conducted randomized, placebo-controlled, multicenter trial of clopidogrel plus aspirin versus placebo for the prevention of HD AVG thrombosis was stopped prematurely because of a significantly increased incidence of bleeding events in the treatment arm. There was no significant benefit of active treatment in the prevention of graft thrombosis [Kaufman et al., J Am Soc Nephrol 2003;14:2313–2321].

Rajiv Saran, MD, MS, MRCP, Assistant Professor,
Division of Nephrology, Co-Director, Kidney Epidemiology and Cost Center,
University of Michigan, 315 W. Huron, Suite 240, Ann Arbor, MI 48103–4262 (USA)
Tel. +1 734 998 6611, Fax +1 734 998 6620, E-Mail rsaran@umich.edu

Ronco C, Levin NW (eds): Hemodialysis Vascular Access and Peritoneal Dialysis Access.
Contrib Nephrol. Basel, Karger, 2004, vol 142, pp 29–46

....

Vascular Access: Issues and Management

Anatole Besarab

Division of Nephrology and Hypertension, Henry Ford Hospital, Detroit, Mich., USA

Introduction

Over 300,000 individuals in the United States rely on a vascular access to receive hemodialysis treatment [1]. Expenditures for access care constitute a large fraction of the total cost of caring for hemodialysis patients. In 1997, vascular access accounted for approximately 12% of the USD 10.7 billion that Medicare paid for end-stage renal disease (ESRD) [2]. As the number of diabetics and elderly with ESRD has grown, the establishment and maintenance of functional vascular access sites has grown and is now the second leading cause for hospitalization [3]. Many analyses of the Medicare analysis of spending on hemodialysis found that vascular access is the most requested United States Renal Data System claim, the largest single cause of morbidity, and the major contributor to inadequate hemodialysis [4, 5]. It is not surprising therefore that vascular access continues to be an important area for quality improvement [6–9]. Currently total expenses related to the creation and maintenance of vascular access equal or exceed USD 1 billion dollars [Eggers, pers. commun.].

In 1997, the National Kidney Foundation published the Dialysis Outcomes Quality Initiative (NKF-DOQI) Clinical Practice Guidelines for Vascular Access [10]. These guidelines, now known as the Kidney Disease Outcomes Quality Initiative (K/DOQI), were updated in 2001 [11–13]. The guidelines recommend optimal clinical practices to individuals taking care of dialysis patients in order to improve patient outcomes and survival. Adhering to such guidelines is a critical component in improving vascular access care. To the greatest extent possible, the guidelines are evidence-based using data from the published literature. When this evidence is not available, the opinion of the Vascular Access Working Group is provided and is clearly delineated in the guidelines. Currently the vascular access guidelines are being carefully reviewed and will be updated based on the voluminous literature published in the past 3 years (over 2,000 articles).

Vascular access patency and adequate hemodialysis are essential to the optimal management of ESRD receiving renal replacement therapy with hemodialysis. The first is a necessary prerequisite for the second since achieving adequacy of hemodialysis (whether expressed as Kt/V or as Kt) at low blood flows to the dialyzer prolongs the treatment time, decreasing quality of life for both patient and staff, and increasing labor costs. Thus it is no surprise that two primary goals to improve quality of life and overall outcomes for hemodialysis patients originally put forth in the preamble to the vascular access guidelines were: (1) increase the use of native arteriovenous fistulas (AVFs) and (2) detect access dysfunction prior to the development of thrombosis [12].

In the United States where vascular access has been a 'national embarrassment' until recently, the Center for Medicare/Medicaid Services (CMS; formerly known as HCFA) developed three clinical performance measures for vascular access. Data has been actively collected through its 18 regional networks on the prevalence of autologous AVFs among hemodialysis patients aged 18 and older, on the prevalence of catheters, and on the use of surveillance of accesses to foster the preemptive correction of problems before failure [14]. Recently, CMS has mandated that the networks develop Quality Improvement Projects (QIPs) on vascular access and has set up a National Vascular Access Improvement Initiative (NVAII).

Major Issues

Issues that have evolved in the past few years that need to be addressed include:
(1) Choice of autologous (native) AVF over a bridge graft, or catheter whenever possible
   (a) Revision of targets for autologous AVF construction (CPG 29)
   (b) Need for and effectiveness of preoperative venous imaging studies in achieving the goals (CPG 2)
   (c) Revision of the statements about timing of access placement (CPG 8)
   (d) Impact of the development of the buttonhole technique for cannulating AVF particularly with the increasing use of more than 3×/week dialysis (home, overnight, daily)
(2) Development of other synthetic graft materials (CPG 4)
(3) Preemptive detection of access dysfunction to maintain patency

(a) Efficacy of access surveillance and monitoring (CPG 10) and update on new techniques
(4) Use of thrombolytics (CPG 5H) in catheter-based devices
(5) Redefinition of a dysfunctional access, especially if catheter based on availability of devices able to provide initial flows in excess of 400 ml/min (CPG 5E, CPG 34)
(6) Prevention/treatment of access-related infection

It is beyond the scope of this chapter to cover all the above in depth as some of these topics will be addressed by others. This chapter will address the first five and also discuss the tools that are needed to optimize vascular access care.

Access Dysfunction Leading to Inadequate Hemodialysis

Clinical practice does not consistently achieve the performance levels stipulated by the vascular access guidelines and, as a result, optimal care is denied many hemodialysis patients [14, 15]. Of the estimated 250,000 Americans who received hemodialysis in 2000, approximately 14% did not receive adequate dialysis [16]. This results from low flow rates due to access dysfunction that limit dialysis delivery, extend treatment times, and result in underdialysis. Underdialysis leads to increased morbidity and mortality, decreased quality of life, and increased healthcare costs [17, 18]. Adequate blood flow can be particularly troublesome with tunneled cuffed catheters [19].

Importance of Blood Flow

K/DOQI guidelines 5, 23, and 34 explicitly state that blood pump flow rates of >300 ml/min should be achieved *regardless* of the type of vascular access. By definition a value less than 300 ml/min indicates access dysfunction. Extracorporeal blood flow rates in excess of 300 ml/min are essential for the provision of adequate dialysis within fixed assigned time periods that range from 2.5 to 5 h. Although the USA has been the bastion of 'short efficient' dialysis, the average treatment duration has progressively increased to 3.5 h in the USA over the last decade [14]. In the HEMO study, eKt/V of 1.4 could be achieved in all except the very large patients (110 kg) if a blood flow rate >350 ml/min could be achieved. During the last decade, low blood flows have remained the main obstacle to achieving adequate Kt/V [14].

Most permanent accesses can deliver at least 350 ml/min and most should deliver over 400 ml/min. Flow rates in a mature AVF commonly reach between

600 and 1,200 ml/min [20–24]. Access flow in prosthetic grafts is typically equal to or sometimes greater when constructed at the same arterial site [25, 26]. NKF-K/DOQI guidelines 10 and 11 state that an absolute flow rate of <600 ml/min at any time or a value <1,000 ml/min with a 25% decrease within a 4-month period in fistulas and grafts may indicate an impending problem and warrant further investigation and treatment [12].

Catheter failure is defined in guideline 34 as the inability to achieve flow rates of 300 ml/min or greater. This guideline was established prior to the development of newer catheters that typically can achieve blood flow rates of 400 ml/min or greater reflecting the technologic advancements in catheter design [27–29]. In the future, a value >350 ml/min is likely to be used to define access dysfunction.

Thus monitoring of 'delivered' blood pump flow rates during dialysis is essential, particularly when using catheters, to ensure adequate dialysis and to detect problems while they are still amenable to pharmacological or mechanical intervention. When waiting until access flow rates decrease below 300 ml/min for catheters or 600 ml/min for fistulas and grafts it may be too late for intervention [30]. Early treatment can restore vascular access with minimal discomfort and risk to the patient and prevent unnecessary loss of an access site and the accompanying costs and risk for complications.

The blood pump flow achieved by the prepump pressure is probably the best indicator of access function in catheters and ports [31]. We have found that a ratio of 1.6–2.0 ml/min per mm Hg is routinely achievable (i.e. a blood flow of 400–500 ml/min at pressures of 200–280 mm Hg). A ratio approaching 1.0 indicates dysfunction. The policy in some centers of bypassing the prepump pressure alarm is dangerous and puts the patient at risk of hemolysis [32, 33].

Choosing the Access

The ideal access delivers adequate dialysis flow rates, has a long use life, and has a low rate of complications. The native AVF comes closest to achieving these criteria and it is the preferred method of permanent vascular access in hemodialysis [34, 35]. The autologous wrist AVF has been acknowledged to be the preferred type of *first* hemodialysis access since 1966 [36] and generally the AVF consistently delivers a higher overall performance than either AV grafts or central venous catheters. AVFs have the lowest rates of infection, thrombosis, and stenosis and have the longest use life among different types of access. Investment of time and energy through process improvements require both fiscal and manpower resources. Reduction of catheters and reduction in access events (thrombosis, infection) will automatically result from the processes of increasing native fistulas. Multiple studies show that the number of access events is 3- to 7-fold higher in prosthetic bridge grafts than in native fistulas, contributing to the increased cost of care. The lower event rate translates into lower costs. Several studies have shown lower annual surgical and hospitalization costs associated with the use of native fistulas compared to grafts [37, 38]. The review of Eggers and Milam [38] of Medicare billing revealed that the first-year costs for patients with catheters were USD 86,927 compared to USD 75,611 for grafts and USD 68,002 for fistulas. Although, the second-year costs were lower for all groups, catheters still resulted in the highest costs at USD 57,178 compared to USD 54,555 for grafts and USD 46,689 for fistulas.

Vascular access infectious risks are lowest in patients with AVFs, intermediate in those with grafts, and highest in those with catheters [39]. USRDS data clearly shows that patients receiving catheters and grafts had a higher mortality risk than patients dialyzed with AVFs [40]. Epidemiological evidence indicates that a greater use of AVFs would reduce the rate of infection and occlusion seen in hemodialysis patients [41, 42], be cost-effective [43] and reduce morbidity and mortality [44, 45]. In view of the above facts, it is not surprising that a number of authors have emphasized that the most important policy that should be pursued in the USA is the placement of AVFs [46, 47].

The K/DOQI Goal: Is It Realistic?

While the NKF-K/DOQ guidelines recommend achieving a minimum of >40% placement of AVFs in prevalent patients, the current rate in the USA has slowly crept up from the low 20s (prior to DOQI 9I2 1997) to about 30% as of 2002 [14, 41,48, 49]. Much higher placement rates are found in Europe [46] and in targeted programs in the United States [48–53]. Comparisons of USA, European, and Japanese data coming from Dialysis Outcomes and Practice Patterns Study (DOPPS) indicate that AVF can be created in the majority of patients despite an aging, increasingly diabetic, and 'sicker' (higher comorbidity) population initiating hemodialysis [51]. In fact reports in the USA increasingly indicate that it is possible to achieve over 90% AVF access rate despite increased age, predominance of women, diabetes, and some obesity [48, 53], all factors previously reported to reduce the likelihood of AVF construction [54]. The issue is not whether we can do better, rather what needs to be done. Recent studies using venous evaluations suggest that 70% of patients are candidates for AVFs [55, 56]. Establishing AVF in all of these would bring the USA to the same level as some nations in Europe. Fistula rates are reported to be 84% in Japan, 66% in Australia, and the lowest in Sweden at 55% [51].

Increasing Fistula Use: What Needs to Be Done?

Unfortunately, maturation time for AVFs – 1–4 months – demands adequate planning time [22] Some studies indicate that fistulas can fail to mature in approximately 30–40% of cases [15, 57–59], and this has been cited as a major reason for a decreased use of AVFs versus other types of access in the USA [60].

The critical determinants for creating AVFs are early patient referral, vascular anatomy, and surgical skill. Planning for access must start before the need for dialysis and before the patient is seduced by the painless nature of the catheter. The patients must become their best advocate and be proactive in preserving forearm and elbow veins. This can only occur if they are taught at stage 3–4 CKD and is the nephrologist's responsibility. Permitting an autologous fistula to mature for 1 year does no harm. The nephrologists must remain the central motivator for AVF construction even with untimely referral (after dialysis is initiated) since he can influence the choice of future access.

Intrinsic to a successful program to increase AVF construction is surgical interest, teamwork, long-term vascular access planning, preoperative mapping, and adherence to the philosophy that even those whose initial access is a graft should have an AVF constructed when the graft fails. A common proffered explanation for the lack of AVF is the lateness of the referral for access placement within the USA system [61]. However, a root cause for the disproportionate use of catheters and grafts and the low use of AVF is the failure of the nephrologist/ESRD team to develop a long-term access plan for the patient, initiated promptly with the first dialysis treatment. Process root causes include the lack of a facility vascular access tracking system (database) for monitoring the use of permanent and especially temporary catheters. It is not uncommon for an access to have matured but the catheter continuing in use for the convenience of the patient (painless access) and only being discontinued after a catheter-related infection occurs.

Preoperative venous mapping is essential in deciding where to place the AVF [62–68]. Visual inspection and physical examination have major limitations in the elderly, the obese, and in those with previously failed accesses. A feeding artery with an inner diameter of >2 mm, and a vein >3 mm and contiguous into the thorax are desired. Vascular mapping with appropriate selection of vessels, both arterial and venous, reduces unacceptable early failure rates in these populations to less than 10%. With mapping, diabetics seem to be as good candidates for AVF as patients without diabetes [63] as are those who are obese [67]. If venography must be done, very good alternatives to conventional radiocontrast are CO_2 phlebography and gadoterate meglumine [68]. Magnetic resonance can also be used to evaluate arteries and veins [69].

Patients should be referred to a surgeon months before the need for dialysis [70]. This, although ideal, is not essential for increasing the prevalence of AVFs. Policies to increase the percentage of autologous AVFs result in a greater proportion of AVFs being placed even if they focus on prevalent patients [48, 49, 71]. In most cases, the construction of elbow level fistulas relative to the forearm-wrist fistula increases. It is possible to achieve over 90% AVF access rate despite increased age, predominance of women, diabetes, and some obesity [49], all factors previously reported to reduce the likelihood of AVF construction [54]. In my experience this will require that half of all fistulas be constructed at the elbow, frequently basilic transpositions (unpubl. observations). Intrinsic to a successful program is surgical interest, teamwork, long-term vascular access planning, preoperative mapping, and adherence to the philosophy that even those whose initial access is a graft should have an AVF constructed when the graft fails.

Increasingly in an older increasingly diabetic population, a wrist fistula is not possible. In such patients, options at the elbow (brachiocephalic, transposed brachiobasilic, autogenous vein transfers) can be pursued [72–74]. When the elbow or antecubital veins cannot be used to create an AVF, the end of the cephalic vein can be mobilized and tunneled for an anastomosis with the proximal, above-elbow brachial artery. Sometimes, the use of a short 6-mm-jump graft connecting the above-elbow brachial artery with the cephalic vein when the distance between brachial artery and cephalic vein is too large for direct anastomosis [75] can provide good 1- and 5-year primary patency of 85 and 48%, respectively. These rates are still much better than the corresponding primary 1- and 5-year patency rates of 40 and 10% reported for long jump grafts constructed in the forearm or arm [35]. We must try harder to increase the fraction of patients, currently 29% prevalency [14], who are dialyzed using an AVF.

There had been some concern about the ability of autologous fistulas to tolerate repeated cannulation related to daily dialysis. Several studies document that the AVF not only tolerates such use but is superior to grafts [76, 77].

Prosthetic Grafts

For nearly 2 decades, polytetrafluoroethylene (PTFE) in various formats (extruded, reinforced) has been the material of choice for synthetic bridge grafts. There has been scant progress in this area over the past few years. There is no difference in function or patency between PTFE grafts made by different manufacturers [78, 79]; neither is patency improved by producing an external wrap around the graft [80] or affected by the wall thickness [81]. However, new graft material including polyurethane [82], cryopreserved femoral vein [83, 84], and self-sealing composite material [85] has been tested clinically but to date none of these synthetic materials have had the same biological advantages as native vessels. To prevent anastomosis to an 'unhealthy' vein, some advocate that the venous anastomoses be done to the deep veins of the forearm since these have avoided venipuncture and are larger in diameter [86, 87]. The provision of a cuff or hood at the venous outflow (to decrease shear stress) has produced only a marginal increase in graft patency [88, 89].

In summary, current practice leaves much to be desired [15]. It is essential to reaffirm the superiority of AVFs, and the importance of maintaining adequate dialysis flow and access patency in order to deliver the best possible care to patients receiving hemodialysis. Higher targets for AVFs are needed and grafts only used when native AVF options have been exhausted.

Surveillance and Monitoring

A number of surveillance methods are available to assess access function of permanent accesses; these include intra-access flow (ultrasound dilution, conductance dilution, thermal dilution, or Doppler flow measurement) [90], pressure (static intra-access pressure, dynamic venous dialysis pressure) [91, 92], or recirculation studies [93]. Recently additional flow techniques using glucose dilution [94] and a transcutaneous method that does not require dialysis [95] have been added to our armamentarium. Garland et al. [96] found that reduced access flow (Qa) predicted the presence of stenosis and ultimately thrombosis in both AVFs and grafts. These authors recommended that monthly Qa measurements be taken early in a hemodialysis session, preferably before ultrafiltration begins, as the hemodynamic changes that occur later in a session can affect measurements, an observation noted by Besarab et al. [25] previously. Similarly, the dynamic venous pressure measurement [25, 97] has been reconfigured to be more sensitive for detecting access dysfunction in grafts [92]. The efficacy of such surveillance techniques in detecting access stenosis is proven [92, 98–101].

The main issue for most dialysis clinics is which surveillance test meets their needs. The controversy currently raging is whether pressure or flow better predicts the stenosis and provides sufficient lead time for elective procedures to be performed in grafts, since these are most prone to rapid thrombosis. A detailed discussion is beyond the scope of this section. Absolute flow detects stenosis well but does not predict when thrombosis might occur [102]. Yet several centers and clinics have used flow and particularly a change in flow as a basis for elective referral for angiography and subsequent angioplasty [101, 103, 104]. On the other hand, static venous pressures, although chiefly a function of outlet stenosis, are affected by the adequacy of arterial inflow, as well as surgical technique. A healthy artery in a patient with reasonable cardiac function can produce flows >1,000 ml/min and yet be associated with 'increased' pressures in the access if the venous outflow vein chosen is small. Increasingly, arm grafts with venous outflow diameters of 6–7 mm are anastomosed to veins less than 4 mm in diameter essentially producing a physiological stenosis that may or may not resolve over time depending on the 'health' and ability of the vein to dilate and accommodate the flow. As a result, among patients a single measurement of intra-access pressure correlates imperfectly with a single measurement of flow [105]. Within a given patient, however, changes in flow correlate quite well with changes in venous outlet stenosis and venous pressure [106, 107]. Baseline measurements of the parameter of interest are all important in assessing the initial state of the access when first used (and presumably free of stenosis) and it is the changes over time in the parameter, whether access flow or static pressure, that indicate dysfunction [91, 93, 104]. Any change from baseline must be confirmed to assure that it is a true change and not the result of systemic hemodynamics on flow within the vascular accesses [25]. There is simply no substitute for obtaining many measurements so the true mean is known and changes from the mean discerned (trend analysis). Overall, in grafts there appears to be little advantage of flow measurements over static pressure [99, 105]. Direct access pressure measurements obtained using the venous drip chamber provide a relatively simple, low-cost method of screening vascular accesses for potential complications [106, 107]. Static pressures can also be measured prior to dialysis using a simple device [91]. Vascular accesses that show abnormality and therefore a need for more conclusive testing may then be investigated using the more expensive methods, such as Doppler or angiographic studies [93].

In autologous fistulas, direct measures, such as Doppler studies and access flow measurements (ultrasound dilution technique or others), are more predictive of occlusion in AVFs than indirect measures, such as static and dynamic venous dialysis pressure [101, 108].

Use of Thrombolytics (CPG 21) in Grafts and Fistulas

Occlusion of a permanent vascular access, whether a native fistula or prosthetic graft, remains a major clinical problem. NKF-K/DOQI guideline 21 declined to recommend a preference between surgical thrombectomy and revision and percutaneous mechanical or pharmacomechanical thrombolysis.

These methods were considered equivalent in efficacy. Over the past 3 years the clinical use of percutaneous interventional procedures has grown [109–112]. Pharmacomechanical thrombolysis using urokinase and haparinized saline was initially used [113]. With the removal of urokinase from the market, other thrombolytics were used. Tissue plasminogen activator (tPA) with or without heparin in occluded AV grafts was found to be a safe and effective treatment when used in conjunction with percutaneous transluminal angioplasty (PTA) [110, 114, 115]. Reteplase, another thrombolytic agent, is also efficacious [116]. However, the development of various mechanical devices that break up clot without needing lytics has accelerated [109, 117–119]. There are no comparative trials that assess the relative effectiveness of lytics compared to purely mechanical methods using thrombus homogenizers or thrombus-extracting devices. I am concerned about two issues with the use of these mechanical devices. The first is residual thrombus along the vessel wall that can be seen by intravascular ultrasound but missed by angiography. Such residual may be the reason for earlier failure since it can act as a nidus for new thrombus growth. This may explain the worse outcomes following PTA if a graft first thromboses compared to a simple elective PTA. The second is the potential for embolization without the thrombosis having been injected with lytics. Both aspects are fertile areas for future studies.

Use of Thrombolytics (CPG 5H) in Catheter-Based Devices

With central hemodialysis catheters, it is important to diagnose the source of the 'obstruction' early. Early dysfunction is usually the result of catheter kinking, pinch-off syndrome, vessel or wall impingement from malpositioning [60]. Repositioning of the catheter may eliminate the obstruction. The incidence of thrombosis in central venous catheters ranges considerably among studies because of the variable duration of use, but appears to be approximately 30–40% [120]. Thrombotic occlusion may occur as soon as 24 h after insertion or after continued successful usage.

Replacement of vascular access is time-consuming, inconvenient, costly, and exposes the patient to undue physical risk and psychological stress. In addition, the number of potential vascular access sites is limited. Salvage of an established catheter access is more cost-effective than its replacement. Use of a fibrinolytic involves much less expense that the cost associated with the insertion of a new catheter. The availability of a fibrinolytic for catheter clearance allows treatment of stenosis and thrombotic occlusions at the point of patient care. As the proportion of free-standing hemodialysis centers, as opposed to those located within a hospital, has increased from 56% in 1985 to 82% in 2000 [16], many patients are dialyzed at significant distances from medical centers. Thus thrombolysis of a catheter should be initiated in the dialysis center rather than through referral to hospitals.

Treating thrombotic occlusions at the point of care offers benefits to the patient, caregivers, and the facility. There is limited interruption of therapy, reduced risk of stress for the patient, less staff time expended, and decreased risk of complications. Fibrinolytics are able to successfully restore function in catheter-related thrombosis in approximately 80–96% of cases (see below). During the evidence gathering phase of the first DOQI, there was inadequate data on the use of thrombolytics in catheter clearance. Although more data accumulated by 2000, the FDA threw the whole area into chaos in January 1999 by issuing a warning regarding safety problems associated with the manufacture of Abbokinase urokinase (FDA, Important Drug Warning). Urokinase was subsequently withdrawn from the market and at the time the revised NKF-K/DOQI guidelines were issued in 2000; no FDA-approved agents were available for catheter clearance. Streptokinase could not be used more than once or twice due to immune responses and reteplace and tPA were available only in large-dose vials (for treatment of myocardial infarction or pulmonary embolism), not easily amenable for use in catheters or thrombolysis of grafts. Some centers did aliquot the tPA and stored it at $-20°C$ for catheter clearance use. Such use was off-label and, in general, most free-standing units sent patients to medical centers. With FDA approval of the 2-mg catheter clearance dose of alteplase, this situation has changed.

Current Status of Fibrinolytic Therapy for Occlusion

The choice of a thrombolytic is influenced by efficacy, cost, availability, and in the USA by FDA approval. Alteplase, 2-mg unit dose per port, currently is the only FDA-approved agent for catheter clearance on the market. It has demonstrated efficacy as a thrombolytic in a number of trials [121–124] proving to be as effective as urokinase [123, 124]. It does not need aliquoting and can be reconstituted and administered in the hemodialysis unit. Currently, reptiplase is undergoing trials, and the urokinase that is approved for acute myocardial infarction and pulmonary embolism is being aliquoted (off-label and under sterile conditions) for use in catheters.

Timing of the use of a lytic, affected by efficacy and cost, is also influenced by the need to avoid complications, patient comfort, convenience, and the need to deliver adequate dialysis. The protocol followed is strongly influenced by reimbursement policies by CMMS and other insurers.

Develop/Organize Vascular Access Teams

Improvement in access care requires the integrated cooperation of the *vascular access team* [125–127] and not just one individual. Key members of such a team include nephrologist, radiologist, surgeon, and members of the dialysis staff. The vascular access team allows input from all the members regarding goals, objectives, and changes in processes [128]. A team can define root causes and problems specific to their area, combine skills and resources, and encourage increased performance by the members. However, we need to also develop processes that include healthcare providers not directly involved in dialysis treatments who can address social, insurance, and other issues. We also need a global policy that addresses surgical training, nephrology referral patterns, patient and staff education as well as practices within the dialysis centers that will then optimize AVF placement. In terms of public policy, focus should be directed to all health professionals for education and counseling of pre-ESRD patients. In the inner cities, multiple efforts over time need to be made with the same patients who frequently are apathetic or in denial about the severity of their chronic kidney disease. Because so many of our patients are hospitalized for other comorbidities, hospitals must be included. They need to be mindful of their policies for venipuncture and insertion of central lines in patients with preexisting renal insufficiency. If not established such protocols should be developed along with visual warning displays located prominently within a patient's room.

Develop Databases

Management of access problems requires knowledge about the patient's current as well as past access history. Too often decisions about access are made without an adequate medical record and without planning. Focusing on the immediate problem, the long-term access plan is frequently overlooked or not developed. At a minimum each program should develop a database that defines the procedures that have been performed in given patients, both those detailing the original construction or insertion of vascular accesses as well as interventions upon them.

Such data is crucial to the process of continuous quality improvement. Data should be collected on thrombosis rate, catheter usage, primary (unassisted), and secondary (assisted) patency and then analyzed. Monitoring forms, computer checklists, and means of sharing information among nurse, nephrologist surgeon, and interventionalist need to be developed. The ability to access the data via Internet will improve outcomes.

References

1   US Renal Data System, USRDS 2001 Annual Data Report: Atlas of End-Stage Renal Disease in the United States. Bethesda, National Institutes of Health, National Institute of Diabetes and Digestive and Kidney Diseases, 2001.
2   USRD 1997 Annual Data Report. X. Am J Kidney Dis 1997;30(suppl 2):S160–S177.
3   Rocco MV, Bleyer AJ, Burkart JM: Utilization of inpatient and outpatient resources for the management of hemodialysis access complications. Am J Kidney Dis 1996;28/2:250–256.
4   Feldman HI, Kobrin S, Wasserstein A: Hemodialysis vascular access morbidity. Am Soc Nephrol 1996;7:523–535.
5   Lazarus JM, Huang WH, Lew NL, Lowrie EG: Contribution of vascular access-related disease to morbidity of hemodialysis; in Henry ML, Ferguson RM (eds): Vascular Access for Hemodialysis III. Chicago, Gore & Associates and Precept Press, 1993, pp 23–42.
6   Ascher E, Gade P, Hingorani A, Mazzariol F, Gunduz Y, Fodera M, Yorkovich W: Changes in the practice of angioaccess surgery: Impact of dialysis outcome and quality initiative recommendations. J Vasc Surg 2000;1/1:84–92.
7   Bosch JP, Walters BA: Quality assurance and continuous quality improvement in the management of vascular access. Contrib Nephrol. Basel, Karger, 2002, vol 137, pp 60–99.
8   Collins AJ, Roberts TL, St Peter WL, Chen SC, Ebben J, Constantini E: United States Renal Data System assessment of the impact of the National Kidney Foundation-Dialysis Outcomes Quality Initiative guidelines. Am J Kidney Dis 2002;39:784–795.
9   van Andringa de Kempenaer T, ten Have P, Oskam J: Improving quality of vascular access care for hemodialysis patients. Jt Comm J Qual Saf 2003;29:191–198.
10   NKF-DOQI Clinical Practice Guidelines for Vascular Access. New York, National Kidney Foundation, 1997.
11   Eknoyan G, Levin NW: Impact of the new K/DOQI guidelines. Blood Purif 2002;20:103–108.
12   National Kidney Foundation K/DOQI clinical practice guidelines for vascular access, 2000. Am J Kidney Dis 2001;37(suppl 1):S137–S181.
13   Eknoyan G, Levin NW, Steinberg EP: The dialysis outcomes quality initiative: History, impact, and prospects. Am J Kidney Dis 2000;35/4(suppl 1):S69–S75.
14   Health Care Financing Administration. Annual Report, End Stage Renal Disease Clinical Performance Measures Project. Baltimore, Department of Health and Human Services, Health Care Financing Administration, Office of Clinical Standards and Quality, 2002.
15   Beathard GA: Improving dialysis vascular access. Dialysis Transplant 2002;31:210–217.
16   Tokars JI, Alter MJ, Arduino MJ: National Surveillance of Dialysis-Associated Diseases in the United States, 2000. Atlanta, National Center for Infectious Diseases, Centers for Disease Control and Prevention, Public Health Service, Department of Health and Human Services, 2001.
17   Ifudu O, Macey LJ, Homel P, et al: Determinants of type of initial hemodialysis vascular access. Am J Nephrol 1997;17:425–427.
18   Hakim RA, Breyer J, Ismail N, Schulman G: Effects of dose of dialysis on morbidity and mortality. Am J Kidney Dis 1994;23:661–669.
19   Atherikul K, Schwab SJ, Conlon PJ: Adequacy of haemodialysis with cuffed central-vein catheters. Nephrol Dial Transplant 1998;13:745–749.
20   Konner K: Increasing the proportion of diabetics with AV fistulas. Semin Dial 2001;14:1–4.
21   Wedgewood KR, Wiggins PA, Guillou PJ: A prospective study of end-to-end vs. side-to-side arteriovenous fistulas for haemodialysis. Br J Surg 1984;71:640–642.
22   Begin V, Ethier J, Dumont M, Leblanc M: Prospective evaluation of the intra-access flow of recently created native arteriovenous fistulae. Am J Kidney Dis 2002;40:1277–1282.
23   Johnson CP, Zhu YR, Matt C, Pelz C, Roza AM, Adams MB: Prognostic value of intraoperative blood flow measurements in vascular access surgery. Surgery 1998;124:729–738.
24   Bosman PJ, Boereboom FT, Bakker CJ, Mali WP, Eikelboom BC, Blankestijn PJ, Koomans HA: Access flow measurements in hemodialysis patients: In vivo validation of an ultrasound dilution technique. J Am Soc Nephrol 1996;7:966–969.
25   Besarab A, Lubkowski T, Vu A, Aslam M, Frinak S: Effects of systemic hemodynamics on flow within vascular accesses used for hemodialysis. ASAIO J 2001;47:501–506.

26 Besarab A, Lubkowski T, Ahsan M, Lim T, Frinak S: Access flow (QA) as a predictor of access dysfunction (abstract). J Am Soc Nephrol 1999;11:202A.

27 Beathard GA: Catheter thrombosis. Semin Dial 2001;14:441–445.

28 Work J: Hemodialysis catheters and ports. Semin Nephrol 2002;22:211–220.

29 Canaud B, Leray-Moragues H, Kerkeni N, Bosc JY, Martin K: Effective flow performances and dialysis doses delivered with permanent catheters: A 24-month comparative study of permanent catheters versus arteriovenous vascular accesses. Nephrol Dial Transplant 2002;17:1286–1292.

30 Garland JS, Moist LM, Lindsay RM: Are hemodialysis access flow measurements by ultrasound dilution the standard of care for access surveillance? Adv Ren Replace Ther 2002;9:91–98.

31 Polaschegg HD, Sodemann K, Feldmer B: Enhancing patency, safety and cost effectiveness of catheters. EDTNA ERCA J 2002;28:28–32.

32 Francos GC, Burke JF, Besarab A, Martinez J, Kirkwood RG, Hummel LA: An unsuspected cause of acute hemolysis during hemodialysis. ASAIO Trans 1983;29:140–146.

33 Kameneva MV, Marad PF, Brugger JM, Repko BM, Wang JH, Moran J, Borovetz HS: In vitro evaluation of hemolysis and sublethal blood trauma in a novel subcutaneous vascular access system for hemodialysis. ASAIO J 2002;48/1:34–38.

34 Kinnaert P, Vereerstraeten P, Toussaint C, Van Geertruyden J: Nine years' experience with internal arteriovenous fistulas for hemodialysis: Study of some factors influencing results. Br J Surg 1977;64:242–246.

35 Mehta S: Statistical summary of clinical results of vascular access procedures for hemodialysis; in Sommer BG, Henry ML (eds): Vascular Access for Hemodialysis. Chicago, Gore & Associates and Precept Press, 1991, pp 145–157.

36 Brescio MJ, Cimino JE, Appel K, et al: Chronic hemodialysis using venipuncture and a surgically created arteriovenous fistula. N Engl J Med 1966;275:1089–1092.

37 Feldman HI, Held PJ, Hutchinson JT, Stoiber E, Hartigan MF, Berlin JE: Hemodialysis vascular access morbidity in the United States. Kidney Int 1993;43:1091–1096.

38 Eggers P, Milam R: Trends in vascular access procedures and expenditures in Medicare's ESRD program; in Henry ML (ed): Vascular Access for Hemodialysis. Part VII. Chicago, Gore & Associates, 2001, pp 133–143.

39 Nassar GM, Ayus JC: Infectious complications of the hemodialysis access. Kidney Int 2001;60: 1–13.

40 Dhingra RK, Young EW, Hulbert-Shearon TE, Leavey SF, Port FK: Type of vascular access and mortality in US hemodialysis patients. Kidney Int 2001;60:1443–1451.

41 Sands J, Perry M: Where are all the AV fistulas? Semin Dial 2002;15:146–148.

42 Stevenson KB, Hannah KL, Lowder CA, et al: Epidemiology of hemodialysis vascular access infections from longitudinal infection surveillance data: Predicting the impact of NKF-DOQI Clinical Practice Guidelines for Vascular Access. Am J Kidney Dis 2002;39:549–555.

43 Lee H, Manns B, Taub K, Ghali WA, Dean S, Johnson D, Donaldson C: Cost analysis of ongoing care of patients with end-stage renal disease: The impact of dialysis modality and dialysis access. Am J Kidney Dis 2002;40:611–622.

44 Woods JD, Port FK: The impact of vascular access for haemodialysis on patient morbidity and mortality. Nephrol Dial Transplant 1997;12:657–659.

45 Anel RL, Yevzlin AS, Ivanovich P: Vascular access and patient outcomes in hemodialysis: Questions answered in recent literature. Artif Organs 2003;27:237–241.

46 Besarab A: Vascular access in Europe and the United States: Striking contrasts. Contemp Dial Nephrol 1999;20:22–28.

47 Hakim R, Himmelfarb J: Hemodialysis access failure: A call to action. Kidney Int 1998;54: 1029–1040.

48 Gibson KD, Caps MT, Kohler TR, Hatsukami TS, Gillen DL, Aldassy M, Sherrard DJ, Stehman-Breen C: Assessment of a policy to reduce placement of prosthetic hemodialysis access. Kidney Int 2001;59:2335–2345.

49 Nguyen VD, Griffith C, Robinson KD: Graft free hemodialysis (HD) practice is achievable despite high patient co-morbid factors in a community based dialysis program (abstract). J Am Soc Nephrol 2001;12:299a.

50   Tokars JI, Arduino MJ, Alter MJ: Infection control in hemodialysis units. Infect Dis Clin North Am 2001;15:797–812.

51   Goodkin DA, Mapes DL, Held PJ: The Dialysis Outcomes and Practice Patterns Study (DOPPS): How can we improve the care of hemodialysis patients? Semin Dial 2001;14:157–159.

52   Pisoni RL, Young EW, Dykstra DM, Greenwood RN, Hecking E, Gillespie B, Wolfe RA, Goodkin DA, Held PJ: Vascular access use in Europe and the United States: Results from the DOPPS. Kidney Int 2002;61:305–316.

53   Rayner HC, Pisoni RL, Gillespie BW, Goodkin DA, Akiba T, Akizawa T, Saito A, Young EW, Port FK: Creation, cannulation and survival of arteriovenous fistulae: Data from the Dialysis Outcomes and Practice Patterns Study. Kidney Int 2003;63:323–330.

54   Allon M, Bailey R, Ballard R, Deierhoi MH, Hamrick K, Oser R, Rhynes VK, Robbin ML, Saddekni S, Zeigler ST: A multidisciplinary approach to hemodialysis access: Prospective evaluation. Kidney Int 1998;53:473–479.

55   Huber TS, Seeger JM: Approach to patients with 'complex' hemodialysis access problems. Semin Dial 2003;16:22–29.

56   Mendes RR, Farber MA, Marston WA, Dinwiddie LC, Keagy BA, Burnham SJ: Prediction of wrist arteriovenous fistula maturation with preoperative vein mapping with ultrasonography. J Vasc Surg 2002;36:460–463.

57   Berman SS, Gentile AT: Impact of secondary procedures in autogenous arteriovenous fistula maturation and maintenance. J Vasc Surg 2001;34:866–871.

58   Murphy GJ, Nicholson ML: Autogeneous elbow fistulas: The effect of diabetes mellitus on maturation, patency, and complication rates. Eur J Vasc Endovasc Surg 2002;23:452–457.

59   Allon M, Robbin ML: Increasing arteriovenous fistulas in hemodialysis patients: Problems and solutions. Kidney Int 2002;62:1109–1124.

60   Fan P-Y, Schwab SJ: Vascular access: Concepts for the 1990s. J Am Soc Nephrol 1992;3:1–11.

61   Besarab A, Adams M, Amatucci S, Bowe D, Deane J, Ketchen K, Reynolds K, Tello A: Unraveling the realities of vascular access: The network 11 experience. Adv Ren Replace Ther 2000;4(suppl 1): S65–S70.

62   Lemson MS, Leunissen KML, Tordoir JGM: Does pre-operative duplex examination improve patency rates of Brescia-Climino fistulas? Nephrol Dial Transplant 1998;13:1360–1361.

63   Sedlacek M, Teodorescu V, Falk A, Vassolotti JA, Uribarri J: Hemodialysis access placement with pre-operative noninvasive vascular mapping: Comparison between patients with and without diabetes. Am J Kidney Dis 2001;38:560–564.

64   Ascher E, Hingoran A, Gunduz Y, Yorkovich Y, Ward M, Miranda J, Tsemekhin B, Kleiner M, Greenberg S: The value and limitations of the arm cephalic and basilic vein for arteriovenous access. Ann Vasc Surg 2001;15:89–97.

65   Allon M, Lockhart ME, Lilly RZ, Gallichio MH, Young CJ, Barker J, Deierhoi MH, Robbin ML: Effect of preoperative sonographic mapping on vascular access outcomes in hemodialysis patients. Kidney Int 2001;60:2013–2020.

66   Dalman RL, Harris EJ Jr, Victor BJ, Coogan SM: Transition to all-autogenous hemodialysis access: The role of preoperative vein mapping. Ann Vasc Surg 2002;16:624–630.

67   Vassalotti JA, Falk A, Cohl ED, Uribarri J, Teodorescu V: Obese and non-obese hemodialysis patients have a similar prevalence of functioning arteriovenous fistula using pre-operative vein mapping. Clin Nephrol 2002;58:211–214.

68   Spinosa DJ, Angle JF, Hagspiel KD, Shenk WG 3rd, Matsumoto AH: CO_2 and gadopetetate dimeglumine as alternative contrasts for malfunctioning dialysis grafts and fistulas. Kidney Int 1998;54:945–950.

69   Waldman GJ, Pattynama PM, Chang PC, Verburgh C, Reiber JH, de Roos A: Magnetic resonance angiography of dialysis access shunts: Initial results. Magn Reson Imaging 1996;14:197–200.

70   Astor BC, Eustace MB, Powe NR, Klag MJ, Sadler JJH, Fink NE, Coresh J: Timing of nephrologist referral and arteriovenous use: The CHOICE study. Am J Kidney Dis 2001;38:494–501.

71   Silva MB Jr, Hobson RW, Pappas PJ, Jamil Z, Araki CT, Goldberg MC, Gwertzman G, Padberg FT Jr: A strategy for increasing use of autogenous hemodialysis access procedures: Impact of preoperative noninvasive evaluation. J Vasc Surg 1998;27:302–308.

72   Bender MH, Bruyinckx CM, Gerlag PG: The brachiocephalic elbow fistula: A useful alternative angioaccess for permanent hemodialysis. J Vasc Surg 1994;20:808–813.

73   Gade J, Aabech J, Hansen RI: The upper arm arteriovenous fistula – An alternative for vascular access in haemodialysis. Scand J Urol Nephrol 1995;29:121–124.

74   Lindner J: Transposition of the basilic vein in the arm for vascular access in hemodialysis. Rozhl Chir 1997;76:126–128.

75   Polo JR, Vázquez R, Polo J, Sanabia J, Rueda J, Lopez-Baena JA: Brachiocephalic jump graft fistula. An alternative for dialysis use of elbow crease veins. Am J Kidney Dis 1999;33:904–909.

76   Paterson P: Fistula cannulation: The buttonhole technique. Nephrol Nurs J 2002;29:195.

77   Stansfield G: Cannulation of arteriovenous fistulae. Nurs Times 1987;83:38–39.

78   Hurlbert SN, Mattos MA, Henretta JP, Ramsey DE, Barkmeier LD, Hodgson KJ, Summer DS: Long-term patency rates, complications and cost-effectiveness of polytetrafluoroethylene (PTFE) grafts for hemodialysis access: A prospective study that compares Impra versus Goretex grafts. Cardiovasc Surg 1998;6:652–656.

79   Kaufman JL, Garb JL, Berman JA, Rhee SW, Norris MA, Friedmann P: A prospective comparison of two expanded polytetrafluoroethylene grafts for linear forearm hemodialysis access: Does the manufacturer matter? J Am Coll Surg 1997;185:74–79.

80   Almonacid PJ, Pallares EC, Rodriguez AQ, Valdes JS, Rueda Orgaz JA, Polo JR: Comparative study of use of Diastat versus standard wall PTFE grafts in upper arm hemodialysis access. Ann Vasc Surg 2000;14:659–662.

81   Lenz BJ, Veldenz HC, Dennis JW, Khansarinia S, Atteberry LR: A three-year follow-up on standard versus thin wall ePTFE grafts for hemodialysis. J Vasc Surg 1998;28:464–470.

82   Allen RD, Yuill E, Nankivell BJ, Francis DM: Australian multicentre evaluation of a new polyurethane vascular access graft. Aust NZ J Surg 1996;66:738–742.

83   Bolton WD, Cull DL, Taylor SM, Carsten CG 3rd, Snyder BA, Sullivan TM, Youkey JR, Langan EM 3rd, Gray BH: The use of cryopreserved femoral vein grafts for hemodialysis access in patients at high risk for infection: A word of caution. J Vasc Surg 2002;36:464–468.

84   Matsuura JH, Johansen KH, Rosenthal D, Clark MD, Clarke KA, Kirby LB: Cryopreserved femoral vein grafts for difficult hemodialysis access. Ann Vasc Surg 2000;14:50–55.

85   Nakao A, Miyazaki M, Oka Y, Matsuda H, Oishi M, Kokumai Y, Kunitomo K, Isozaki H, Tanaka N: Creation and use of a composite polyurethane-expanded polytetrafluoroethylene graft for hemodialysis access. Acta Med Okayama 2000;54:91–94.

86   Skandalos I, Chatzibaloglou A, Tsalis K, Tourlis T, Kalpakidis V, Anagnostopoulos T, Dadoukis I, Sombolos K: Prosthetic graft placement using the deep forearm veins in hemodialysis patients: A preliminary report. Nephron 2000;85:346–347.

87   Won T, Min SK, Jang JW, Choi SH, Choi KB, Han JJ, Ahn JH: Early result of arteriovenous graft with deep forearm veins as an outflow in hemodialysis patients. Ann Vasc Surg 2002;16:501–504.

88   Lemson MS, Leunissen KML, Tordoir JGM: Does pre-operative duplex examination improve patency rates of Brescia-Climino fistulas? Nephrol Dial Transplant 1998;13:1360–1361.

89   Sorom AJ, Hughes CB, McCarthy JT, Jenson BM, Prieto M, Panneton JM, Sterioff S, Stegall MD, Nyberg SL: Prospective, randomized evaluation of a cuffed expanded polytetrafluoroethylene graft for hemodialysis vascular access. Surgery 2002;132:135–140.

90   Leypoldt JK: Diagnostic methods for vascular access: Access flow measurements. Contrib Nephrol. Basel, Karger, 2002, vol 137, pp 31–37.

91   Besarab A, Lubkowski T, Frinak S: A simpler method for measuring intra-access pressure (abstract). J Am Soc Nephrol 1999;11:202A.

92   Frinak S, Zasuwa G, Dunfee T, Besarab A, Yee J: Dynamic venous access pressure ratio test for hemodialysis access monitoring. Am J Kidney Dis 2002;40:760–768.

93   Besarab A, Samarapungavan D: Measuring the adequacy of hemodialysis access. Curr Opin Nephrol Hypertens 1996;5:527–531.

94   Magnasco A, Alloatti S, Martinoli C, Solari P: Glucose pump test: A new method for blood flow measurements. Nephrol Dial Transplant 2002;17:2244–2248.

95   Ronco C, Brendolan A, Crepaldi C, D'Intini V, Sergeyeva O, Levin NW: Noninvasive transcutaneous access flow measurement before and after hemodialysis: Impact of hematocrit and blood pressure. Blood Purif 2002;20:376–379.

96   Garland JS, Moist LM, Lindsay RM: Are hemodialysis access flow measurements by ultrasound dilution the standard of care for access surveillance? Adv Ren Replace Ther 2002;9:91–98.

97   Besarab A, Frinak S, Aslam M: Pressure measurements in the surveillance of vascular accesses; in Gray R (ed): A Multidisciplinary Approach for Hemodialysis Access. Philadelphia, Lippincott, Williams, & Wilkins, 2002, chap 21, pp 137–150.

98   Cayco AV, Abu-Alfa AK, Mahnensmith RL, Perazella MA: Reduction in arteriovenous graft impairment: Results of a vascular access surveillance protocol. Am J Kidney Dis 1998;32: 302–308.

99   Bosman PJ, Boereboom FT, Smits HF, Eikelboom BC, Koomans HA, Blankestijn PJ: Pressure or flow recordings for the surveillance of hemodialysis grafts. Kidney Int 1997;52:1084–1088.

100   McCarley P, Wingard RL, Shyr Y, Pettus W, Hakim RM, Ikizler TA: Vascular access blood flow monitoring reduces access morbidity and costs. Kidney Int 2001;60:1164–1172.

101   Besarab A, Sullivan KL, Ross RP, Moritz MJ: Utility of intra-access pressure monitoring in detecting and correcting venous outlet stenoses prior to thrombosis. Kidney Int 1995;47:1364–1373.

102   Paulson WD, Ram SJ, Work J: Access blood flow: Debate continues. Semin Dial 2001;14: 459–460.

103   Krivitski N, Gantela S: Access blood flow: Debate continues. Semin Dial 2001;14:460–461.

104   Besarab A, Lubkowski T, Ahsan M, Lim T, Frinak S: Access flow (QA) as a predictor of access dysfunction (abstract). J Am Soc Nephrol 1999;11:202A.

105   Besarab A, Frinak S: Strategies for prospective detection of graft dysfunction; in Schwab S, Conlon P, Nicholson M. (eds): Hemodialysis Vascular Access. Oxford, Oxford University Press, 2000, pp 157–182.

106   Besarab A, Lubkowski T, Frinak S, Ramanathan S, Escobar F: Detection of strictures and vascular outlet stenoses in vascular accesses: Which test is best? ASAIO J 1997;43:M543–M547.

107   Besarab A, Lubkowski T, Frinak S, Ramanathan S, Escobar F: Detecting vascular access dysfunction. ASAIO J 1997;43:M539–M543.

108   Joseph S, Adler S: Vascular access problems in dialysis patients. Heart Dis 2001;3:242–247.

109   Beathard GA, Marston WA: Endovascular management of thrombosed dialysis access grafts. Am J Kidney Dis 1998;32:172–175.

110   Cooper SG: Original report. Pulse-spray thrombolysis of thrombosed hemodialysis grafts with tissue plasminogen activator. AJR Am J Roentgenol 2003;180:1063–1066.

111   Surlan M, Popovic P: The role of interventional radiology in management of patients with end-stage renal disease. Eur J Radiol 2003;46:96–114.

112   Turmel-Rodrigues L, Pengloan J, Bourquelot P: Interventional radiology in hemodialysis fistulae and grafts: A multidisciplinary approach. Cardiovasc Intervent Radiol 2002;25:3–16.

113   Beathard GA: Mechanical versus pharmacomechanical thrombolysis for the treatment of thrombosed dialysis access grafts: A controlled study. Kidney Int 1994;45:1401–1406.

114   Bookstein JJ, Bookstein FL: Augmented experimental pulse-spray thrombolysis with tissue plasminogen activator, enabling dose reduction by one or more orders of magnitude. J Vasc Interv Radiol 2000;11:299–303.

115   Falk A, Mitty H, Guller J, Teadorescu V, Uribarri J, Vassalotti J: Thrombolysis of clotted hemodialysis grafts with tissue-type plasminogen activator. J Vasc Interv Radiol 2001;12:305–311.

116   Falk A, Guller J, Nowakowski FS, et al: Reteplase in the treatment of thrombosed hemodialysis grafts. J Vasc Interv Radiol 2001;12:1257–1262.

117   Aruny JE, Lewis CA, Cardella JF, Cole PE, Davis A, Drooz AT, Grassi CJ, Gray RJ, Husted JW, Jones MT, McCowan TC, Meranze SG, Van Moore A, Neithamer CD, Oglevie SB, Omary RA, Patel NH, Rholl KS, Roberts AC, Sacks D, Sanchez O, Silverstein MI, Singh H, Swan TL, Towbin RB, et al: Quality improvement guidelines for percutaneous management of the thrombosed or dysfunctional dialysis access. Standards of Practice Committee of the Society of Cardiovascular and Interventional Radiology. J Vasc Interv Radiol 1999;10:491–498.

118   Schmitz-Rode T, Wildberger JE, Hubner D, Wein B, Schurmann K, Gunther RW: Recanalization of thrombosed dialysis access with use of a rotating mini-pigtail catheter: Follow-up study. J Vasc Interv Radiol 2000;11:721–727.

119   Vesely TM: Endovascular intervention for the failing vascular access. Adv Ren Replace Ther 2002;9:99–108.

120 Whitman ED: Complications associated with the use of central venous access devices. Curr Probl Surg 1996;33:319–378.
121 Deitcher SR, Fesen MR, Kiproff PM, et al: Safety and efficacy of alteplase for restoring function in occluded central venous catheters: Results of the cardiovascular thrombolytic to open occluded lines trial. J Clin Oncol 2002;20:317–324.
122 Ponec D, Irwin D, Haire WD, Hill PA, Li X, McCluskey ER; COOL Investigators: Recombinant tissue plasminogen activator (alteplase) for restoration of flow in occluded central venous access devices. J Vasc Interv Radiol 2001;12:951–955.
123 Haire WD, Atkinson JB, Stephens L, Kotulal G: Urokinase versus recombinant tissue plasminogen activator in thrombosed central venous catheters: A double-blinded, randomized trial. Thromb Haemost 1994;72:543–547.
124 Eyrich H, Walton T, Macon EJ, Howe A: Alteplase versus urokinase in restoring blood flow in hemodialysis-catheter thrombosis. Am J Health Syst Pharm 2002;59:1437–1440.
125 Waterhouse D: Vascular access: A role for a renal nurse clinician. EDTNA ERCA J 2002;28/2: 64–69.
126 Wofford S: Care and maintenance of hemodialysis catheters and subcutaneous vascular access devices – A nurse's perspective. Nephrol News Issues 2002;16/9:27–31.
127 Spergel LM: Vascular access: New approaches needed for a more complex ESRD population. Nephrol News Issues 1997;11/2:30–34.
128 Welch KA, Pflederer TA, Knudsen J, Hocking MK: Establishing the vascular access coordinator: Breaking ground for better outcomes. Nephrol News Issues 1998;12/11:43–46.

Anatole Besarab, MD,
Division of Nephrology and Hypertension, Henry Ford Hospital,
CFP 511, 27 99 West Grand Blvd, Detroit, MI 48201 (USA)
Tel. +1 313 916 2713, Fax +1 313 916 2554, E-Mail abesarab@ghsrenal.com

Ronco C, Levin NW (eds): Hemodialysis Vascular Access and Peritoneal Dialysis Access.
Contrib Nephrol. Basel, Karger, 2004, vol 142, pp 47–72

··················

Arteriovenous Fistulas: Different Types and Surgical Techniques

Luisa Berardinelli

UO Chirurgia Vascolare e dei Trapianti di Rene, Ospedale Maggiore
Policlinico – IRCCS e Cattedra di Chirurgia Sostitutiva dei Trapianti d'Organo
e di Organi Artificiali, Università degli Studi di Milano, Milano, Italia

The development of chronic hemodialysis has been strictly connected to the availability of arteries and veins suitable for vascular access formation. In fact, although the treatment of end-stage renal disease with the Kolff artificial kidney has been feasible since 1943, the impossibility of achieving long-term cannulation of the circulatory system restricted hemodialysis to being used as an emergency therapy for acute renal failure until 1960, when Scribner, Dillard and Quinton introduced the first external arteriovenous shunt.

Afterwards other types of external devices came into use, such as the winged-in-line shunt of Ramirez, the subcutaneous shunt of Buselmeier, the femoral shunt of Thomas and the Allen Brown shunt, which all allowed urgent and chronic dialysis. Among these, the Allen Brown shunt that consists of a knitted Dacron-Silastic tube prosthesis with a Dacron-velour sleeve, tightly bound around the silicone tubing distal to the Dacron graft, could easily be adapted to various vessel diameters by an oblique cut and was extensively used by us in adults and children. Our original technique [1] is based on an end-to-side anastomosis between the preclotted Dacron patch to the patient's superficial femoral artery. When acute uremia had to be treated, the venous outflow was obtained by a simple cannulation of the great saphenous vein, using a Ramirez Teflon-Silastic tube. In patients on chronic dialysis, another Allen Brown device can be positioned by an end-to-side or end-to-end suture to the great saphenous vein or, as a second choice, to the common femoral vein. Unfortunately, this interesting device, as well as other external shunts, are now abandoned due to a poor average life span, in favor of percutaneous central vein catheters (CVC).

However, as previous central vein cannulation, particularly if the catheter became infected, represents the main risk factor for central vein stenosis and thrombosis, perhaps a revived type of external shunt could be used as a bridge to permanent vascular access with fewer problems than CVCs. In fact, the frequent need of angioplasty and endovascular stent placement for recurrent stenosis, the costs of these percutaneous procedures, and the subsequent poor quality of life of the patient until a thrombosis of an intrathoracic vein precludes the creation of any vascular access in the upper limb advise that some step backward should be taken with the use of CVCs [2].

The disadvantages of the external shunt as long-term vascular access were overcome by the introduction of the subcutaneous arteriovenous fistula (AVF) of Brescia et al. [3] in 1966. Afterwards the use of synthetic or biological prostheses as arteriovenous grafts (AVG) offered alternative means of continuing the provision of renal replacement therapy.

Recent publications of the Dialysis Outcome Quality Initiatives (DOQI) guidelines [2] have focused attention on reducing reliance on angioaccess grafts or central venous catheters for dialysis access and on promoting an increase of the prevalence of autogenous AVFs among dialysis patients whenever possible. Among the motives of long patency rates, one should not forget the skill of the operating surgeon: Prischl et al. [4] found that the 3-year patency of wrist AVFs varied from 34 to 62% depending on the vascular surgeon.

Planning and Choice of Vascular Access

The first vascular access generally shows patency rates superior to that of all subsequent procedures [5]. As the access-related morbidity in the 1st year of dialysis may constitute up to 50% of all patient care costs [6], the initial assessment and a careful planning appear to be of the utmost importance for long-term access patency and even for patient outcome.

The main guiding principles of access site selection include the patient and staff education about the absolute need to preserve superficial vessels by avoiding venipuncture and peripheral/central intravenous cannulation or invasive monitoring lines, the preemptive fistula construction, the use of upper arms rather than legs, the use of nondominant arm vessels and the construction of the AVF as distally as practical, preserving more proximal sites for subsequent procedures.

The AVF should be created when the creatinine clearance reaches 10 ml/min, in order to allow a sufficient 'maturation' of the vascular access. However, characteristics of the superficial vessels, previous central vein catheterization, body mass index, smoking habit, hypotension, condition of the skin, original end-stage renal disease and patient's life expectancy influence the type and location of vascular access placement.

Simple inspection, palpation of the arterial pulse, the Allen test, the use of a tourniquet applied to the upper arm to produce dilation of the veins, as well as duplex sonography make generally invasive procedures unnecessary. However, ultrasound examination is not reliable to detect occult central venous obstruction.

Venography represents the best modality for detecting peripheral/central vein stenosis with higher sensitivity than duplex sonography [7], whilst the latter provides valuable information about arterial anomalies, wall thickening or calcification and the future risk of steal syndrome. A venogram enlarged to the ipsilateral axillary, subclavian and innominate vein is mandatory in patients with upper arm edema or collateral veins in the chest, who were submitted to intravenous pacemaker, temporary hemoaccess procedures or multiple AVF failures or had prior arm, neck or chest trauma or surgery. CO_2 venography is a particularly useful technique for patients who show venous outflow problems but maintain a remnant renal function. Magnetic resonance imaging that is used for patients who are sensitive to contrast agents and computed tomography are alternative imaging modalities.

Radiocephalic AVF at the wrist remains the procedure of choice; nevertheless, if the patients have no suitable peripheral vessels, more proximal sites of the forearm or the elbow region can be considered as first choice. Vein transposition and angioaccess grafts, involving larger vessels in the upper arm or in the leg, are relegated to third and fourth position, respectively.

Risks of infection and steal syndrome must always be considered whenever larger vessels are adopted for AVF construction. We tend to reserve for selected patients the use of vessels that cannot be ligated in case of complications. The planned strategy of procedural choices based on our current practice is listed in table 1.

Vascular Access Procedures in the Upper Limb

As in uremic patients there is an increased bleeding tendency, regional anesthetic techniques as well as spinal/epidural blocks appear unreliable because of the risk of hematoma with important neurologic sequelae. A brachial plexus block is used by some surgeons. However, local infiltration with 1% lidocaine without epinephrine remains the safest and simplest anesthetic technique, useful for the construction of the most vascular access, also in the lower limb.

However, a well-secured intravenous cannula and careful patient monitoring are indicated, because of the risk of anesthetic toxicity, convulsion and cerebral hypoxia. The patient should be fasting on the day of the operation, even if

Table 1. Strategy for chronic hemodialysis access procedures in the upper limb

First choice
    Autogenous wrist (or snuff-box) radiocephalic direct access
    Autogenous mid-forearm radiocephalic direct access
    Autogenous wrist ulnar-basilic direct access

Second choice (or first choice in children and older or diabetic patients)
    Autogenous direct UAF between brachial artery and an antecubital vein
        Median-cephalic vein
        Median-basilic vein
        'Perforating' vein
        'Comitans' vein
        Basilic vein, mobilized
        Cephalic vein, mobilized

Third choice: AVG access
    Brachial artery-comitans (or forearm basilic/cephalic) vein, loop configuration in
      the forearm
    Radial artery-comitans (or forearm basilic/cephalic) vein, straight configuration in
      the forearm
    Brachial artery-comitans (or basilic) vein, 'O-shaped' configuration in the upper arm
    Brachial artery-comitans (or axillary/basilic) vein, straight configuration in the upper arm
    Brachial artery-comitans (or basilic) vein, straight configuration in the forearm/upper
      arm across the elbow crease
    Brachial artery-comitans (or basilic) vein, loop configuration in the forearm across the
      elbow crease for one or two branches
    Brachial artery-comitans (or axillary or basilic) vein, loop configuration in the upper arm

Third choice in diabetic, septic or hypotensive patients: vein transposition
    Superficial venous transposition in the forearm
    Basilic or cephalic vein transposition in the upper arm

the operation is conducted under local anesthesia. General anesthesia should be reserved for children and uncooperative patients.

The diameter of the vessels used for AVF construction appears to be an important predictor of patency: a vein less than 3 mm in diameter has a greater incidence of failure, as at this size the viscosity of blood becomes a measurable determinant of flow [8]. Although Wong et al. [9] observed that if the diameter of the artery or vein was <1.5 mm, the fistula always failed to mature, no predictive value of vascular diameter could be assessed for fistula outcome by Miller et al. [10].

All vascular access should be performed with optical magnification and using microvascular equipments and techniques. Although upper arm ischemia with arterial tourniquet and general heparinization are employed by some operators, we consider these procedures useless and dangerous.

Native AVFs by Direct Anastomosis

Radiocephalic Wrist AVF

With the patient in a supine position, the whole nondominant arm is cleaned with antiseptic solution, draped and laid on a sterile side table. The forearm is maintained in a neutral position. After local infiltration of lidocaine, a 2.5-cm longitudinal incision is made midway between the radial artery and the cephalic vein. Skin hooks are particularly useful to elevate the skin margins. If the arterial supply shows generally little variation in the upper limbs, the venous drainage evidences considerable variation: however, the cephalic vein is found on the radial border of the wrist and the basilic one on its ulnar border.

The cephalic vein is dissected from the subcutaneous tissue by first placing a vessel loop around the vein for better mobilization with minimal manipulation. Tributary vessels are spared if possible. This single incision is generally enough to expose the radial artery, too. However, separate incisions for the artery and the vein are advocated if these vessels are too distant. We have abandoned curved or transverse incisions due to a poor cosmetic appearance of the scar.

The radial artery is identified between the brachial radialis and the flexor carpi radialis tendons, under the deep fascia of the forearm just above the flexor retinaculum, avoiding to interrupt it and small arterial branches are divided after having been ligated with nonabsorbable 5/0 or 6/0 suture. The two 'venae comitantes' run parallel to the artery on either side and should be carefully dissected. The superficial sensory branch of the radial nerve should not be injured to prevent hypesthesia/paresthesia of the thenar eminence. The radial artery is circumscribed by a vessel loop and the adventitia is denuded only in the selected anastomotic site to prevent damage of the vasa vasorum resulting in intramural degenerative changes, venous aneurysm formation or stenosis. Atraumatic vascular clamps are applied on the radial artery, while a vessel loop is generally enough to stop the bleeding from the vein without trauma. The artery is opened with a 'stab' incision by the scalpel blade No. 15, avoiding an excessive pressure against the vessel which may cause injury to the back wall. The arteriotomy is enlarged using Potts vascular scissors. The vessel lumen is irrigated with heparinized saline. Only local heparinization is advisable.

Four different types of anastomotic connections are used in common practice (fig. 1), each of them having some advantages and disadvantages.

The end-to-end anastomosis (fig. 1a) is our preferred method of wrist AVF construction as it prevents either peripheral ischemia or venous hypertension. This method has the small disadvantage of decreasing the fistula flow by about 15%, in comparison with side-to-side or end vein-to-side artery anastomosis with the subsequent moderate adjunctive risk of thrombosis. On the other hand, the ligation of the distal artery increases collateral blood flow by one half to two thirds [11], the ligation of the vein prevents peripheral venous hypertension and minimal impact on intimal hyperplastic response in the recipient's venous bed can be observed at the anastomotic site, due to flow stability, as turbulence and kinetic energy transfer are in this case equivalent [12]. End-to-end anastomosis of small vessels is traditionally accomplished by the 'triangulation' technique, dividing the vessel circumference into approximate thirds with 8/0 or 9/0 sutures. According to our original techniques, the spaces between the triangulation stitches are filled in with three continuous sutures and interrupted ties. This combination of continuous suture and interrupted ties results in microvascular anastomoses being completed faster with less bleeding than the conventional interrupted method.

Another of our original surgical skills in the end-to-end anastomosis consists of bending the artery so that the anastomosis is performed on the venous side (fig. 1a). The advantage of this model is that less dilatation and aneurysm develop in the proximal vein than if the anastomosis is made in a conventional way, as the smooth muscle wall of the artery is more resistant to shear forces than the vein wall and minimal turbulence can be observed with this configuration. Another advantage of the end-to-end fistula is that an everting suture can easily be performed for the entire circumference with a lower risk of thrombosis whilst the posterior wall of side-to-side or end-to-side AVFs is often anastomosed with an inverting suture.

The end vein-to-side artery [13] anastomosis (fig. 1b) shows a smaller incidence of venous hypertension in the hand but the risk of peripheral ischemia remains the same if compared with the side-to-side AVF. The cephalic vein, beveled in the 'fish-mouthed' configuration according to the length of the arteriotomy, enhances the outflow. The anastomosis begins with two stitches between the 'heel' of the vein and the distal angle of the longitudinal arteriotomy, the third through the apex of the incision and the fourth and the fifth stitches on the side toward the operator. Lateral traction on the free end of the vein enhances exposure of the apex of the arteriotomy. The anastomosis proceeds around the apex leaving loose the suture loops for a more accurate placement of each stitch. Completion of the anastomosis is achieved by joining the suture ends with knots without narrowing the anastomosis.

The standard side-to-side anastomosis (fig. 1c), originally described by Brescia et al. [3], results in the highest fistula flow, due to the retrograde flow in the distal artery, coming from the palmar arches, but presents a risk of peripheral ischemia and distal venous hypertension that can be relieved by distal ligation of the two vessels.

The radial artery and the cephalic vein are mobilized and approximated by one vessel loop. Holding both vessels in a single vascular clamp makes the

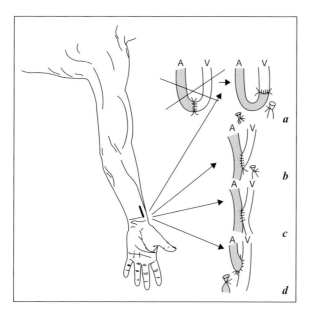

Fig. 1. Radiocephalic wrist AVF configurations. *a* End-to-end with bent artery. *b* End vein-to-side artery. *c* Side-to-side. *d* End artery-to-side vein.

anastomosis easier. A longitudinal incision is also performed on the vein. Two anchoring 7/0 sutures can be useful to retract the lateral walls of the vessels.

The anastomosis is performed using a double-armed monofilament suture of 7/0 (or 8/0) polypropylene. Suturing begins at one corner of the approximated arteriotomy and venotomy, placing the knot on the outside. When the suture of the posterior wall is completed, the needle is passed from the inside to the outside of the vessel; the second double-armed 7/0 suture, previously applied to the opposite corner, is tied. Then, the anastomosis is completed by running the sutures from both ends toward the midline. This technique has the advantage of making the anastomosis easier and of preventing stenosis or dilation of the anastomotic mouth.

The continuous over-and-over suture technique may also be employed, starting the anastomosis in the midline posteriorly with a double-armed 7/0 and proceeding from the outside to the inside. After a last irrigation with heparinized saline, this suture is tied at the midline anteriorly. Frankly, the variation of the side-to-side anastomosis followed by ligature of these vessels distally appears to be intriguing and useless, if compared with end-to-end variation.

End artery-to-side vein (fig. 1d) is a less frequently used technique that prevents the steal syndrome, by which the ulnar artery flow is diverted from the palmar arch into the low-pressure venous system. The distal cephalic vein can be useful for evaluating fistula problems and it can be ligated only when the patient develops venous hypertension. The vascular clamps are released (the one on the venous side by first) and the little bleeding which occurs is controlled by a gentle pressure.

The subcutaneous tissue is closed using interrupted 4/0 or 5/0 fine absorbable monofilament in one or more layers to eliminate the dead space and to give a more accurate approximation. The skin may be closed with interrupted subcuticular sutures of fine absorbable synthetic material and a further application of multiple paper-like adhesive strips. A thrill should be felt over the fistula after wound closure. One-year primary patency rates of wrist AVFs vary from 43% [5] to 93% [14].

Snuff-Box AVF

A more distal variant is the anatomical 'snuff-box' AVF [15] between the tendons of extensor pollicis longus and brevis, which has the unique advantage of preserving the radiocephalic site for a subsequent vascular access in case of failure. Although 5-year cumulative patency of 90% is reported for nondiabetic patients [14], the disadvantages of this AVF are the narrow caliber of the vessels at this site and the poor cosmetic appearance of the bulging veins in the hand.

Ulnar-Basilic AVF

An alternative approach to direct AVF in the wrist is the ulnar-basilic anastomosis [16], which may be considered in case of thrombosis of the cephalic vein and in children, as in these patients it is larger than the radial artery. The ulnar-basilic anastomosis is used less commonly in adults because the vessels are deeper and the intradialytic position is not comfortable. However, the use of the ulnar artery after a failed radiocephalic fistula should be avoided, because of a high risk of hand ischemia.

Mid-Forearm Radiocephalic AVF

After thrombosis of the wrist AVF or if the patients have no suitable peripheral vessels, the radial artery can be utilized in a more proximal site of the forearm, close to the bifurcation of the brachial artery for a side-to-side mid-forearm AVF. A preoperative assessment by Duplex ultrasound should be performed due to a deeper location of the vessels at this site in order to avoid unnecessary surgical exploration. The advantages of this procedure are a lower initial failure rate and fewer complications than with other methods of vascular access.

Upper Arm Fistulas (or Proximal, Elbow or Antecubital Fistulas)

Whenever the forearm vessels are unsuitable for constructing a radiocephalic fistula, a side-to-side upper arm fistula (UAF) using the patient's brachial artery and a native vein (generally the median-basilic vein) should always be preferred to the implantation of a prosthetic graft that presents higher rates of complications and lower long-term patency. First described in 1976 by Someya et al. [17], the UAF represents a good second choice or in some cases an alternative to the forearm fistula.

Our center pursues an aggressive policy of placing autogenous direct upper arm access in 'difficult' patients, whenever an antecubital vein remains patent. In children who have a smaller arterial size or in older or diabetic patients with atherosclerotic or calcified arteries, the UAF can be considered as a first choice procedure with a reported 18-month cumulative patency of 78% versus only 33% for wrist fistula at the same time point in patients with a history of diabetes [18]. In these cases, a UAF between the brachial artery and an antecubital vein allows the blood to flow distally in a reverse fashion, and so enlarging the forearm veins. In contrast, these vessels could be totally destroyed by multiple failed access procedures.

The suitability of the brachial artery at the elbow or in the upper arm can be easily assessed by simple palpation or by a Doppler-sonographic exam, although anatomical malformations can be observed at this site with an incidence of 0.14%. Arteriography should be employed only in highly selected cases because of legal problems or because of a suspicion of anatomical malformations, not well pointed out by Doppler sonography or other noninvasive techniques.

A transverse incision of 2 cm is made in the antecubital fossa above the brachial artery. The antecubital veins lie in the subcutaneous tissue immediately beneath the skin. The brachial artery is mobilized proximally to its bifurcation, dividing the bicipital tendon. Every lymphatic channel should be treated with diathermy to prevent troublesome lymphocele.

A median cephalic or median basilic vein can be used for a side-to-side anastomosis with the brachial artery, using the aforementioned technique. Adventitial bridle resection must be made only in the site near to the anastomosis, to avoid subsequent venous aneurysms.

In case the median-cephalic or median-basilic veins are affected by phlebitic injury or if their diameter is not adequate, the 'perforating' antecubital vein that joins the superficial and deep venous system can be used as an optimal outflow, for an end (vein)-to-side (artery) anastomosis. We and others obtained excellent results with this option [19] with primary patency rates of 80% at 36 months.

Differently from Gracz et al. [20], we prefer not to remove a venous patch from the deep vein, as we believe the deep venous system should remain undamaged to avoid problems of venous drainage in the upper limb. However, our personal opinion is that, in the construction of all UAFs, the perforating vein ought to be always dissected and tied, if its diameter is unsuitable for an end-to-side anastomosis, to maximize the fistula flow in the superficial veins and to prevent discomfort resulting from venous hypertension in the deep region of the elbow joint.

Another technical combination, particularly useful in case the superficial veins at this site are fibrotic or somehow damaged, consists of a side-to-side anastomosis with the 'comitans' vein, which is connected with the superficial venous system [21]. Afterwards, if a scanty maturation of the UAF is observed or if the arterialized vein is too deep for an easy cannulation, a superficialization of the deep vein or a vein transposition can be accomplished. A forearm loop graft may also be inserted in case this AVF is difficult to needle or has a flow too low for efficient dialysis: in this case, the vein enlarged from the arterial-ized flow makes the patient a more suitable candidate for a graft. The cephalic or basilic vein can also be employed for UAF construction after their mobiliza-tion to prevent kinking.

Forearm end vein-to-side artery anastomosis or banding/ligation of the median cubital vein is sometimes advisable to enhance the 'reverse' fistula flow distally in the forearm. Sometimes the competence of distal venous valves ham-pers the development of veins suitable for dialysis cannulation: a valvulotomy can solve this problem [22].

In all upper arm angioaccess, the arteriotomy should never be greater than 75–80% of the proximal arterial diameter, to prevent the steal syndrome and high output heart failure. In any case, once the fistula diameter is equal or greater than 75% of the diameter of the proximal artery, flow is maximized. The patency rates of UAFs are very high, achieving more than 80% at 3 years in our experience and that of others [21, 23].

We usually do not attempt the salvage of an UAF that is failing after a long-term patency: in this case, as well as in the few cases of nonoptimal mat-uration of the venous bed, other technical solutions are advisable, such as mobi-lizing or transposing the basilic/cephalic vein or the placement of a prosthetic graft between the same vessels of the UAF just above.

Secondary Procedures to Enhance 'Maturation' of Autogenous AVFs

Venous branches ligation, balloon angioplasty of AVF inflow or outflow, superficialization of a deep, but otherwise well-functioning AVF, transposition of an arterialized vein to a more proximal, larger artery and interposition of grafts are sometimes required to facilitate the cannulation of an autogenous AVF.

Obesity or a position of wrist, forearm or upper arm native vessels which is too deep is often a reason for vein transposition or graft insertion. Superficialization (or elevation) of a patent and adequate blood flow but failing fistula is a simple and effective method to optimize native AVF utilization in these difficult patients [24].

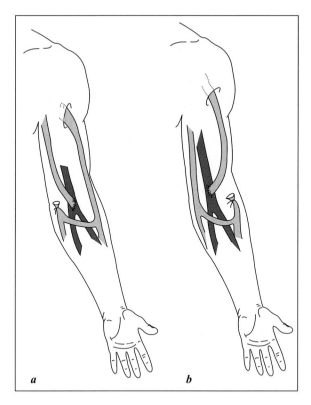

Fig. 2. a. Transposition of the upper arm basilic vein. *b* Transposition of the upper arm cephalic vein.

The most commonly "elevated" arteriovenous communication is the brachiobasilic AVF: the vein is elevated superficial to the surgically reapproximated deep fascia and subcutaneous tissue of the arm [25].

Some forearm veins suitable for AVF formation, such as cephalic or basilic veins, lie in a subcutaneous location too deep, too remote or in a location not readily accessible for a comfortable needle cannulation during hemodialysis. Instead of using a vascular prosthesis, in some patients, such as diabetics or elderly patients, the forearm segment of the selected vein (basilic or cephalic) can be "transposed" into a more superficial position of the forearm to form a J- or U-shaped loop. The beveled free end of the selected vein is anastomosed to the proximal radial or, alternatively, ulnar or brachial artery.

Transposition of the upper arm basilic (fig. 2a) or cephalic vein (fig. 2b) for a brachiobasilic (or brachiocephalic) native AVF construction can be performed by a one-step procedure in obese, diabetic, hypotensive or potentially septic patients, where the use of graft material is not advisable. A two-step procedure can also be adopted: in other words, the arterialized basilic or cephalic vein can be transposed after the construction of an upper arm AVF that, although well functioning, is too deep for easy cannulation. Operative dissection is facilitated with an enlarged, arterialized thick-walled vein, which is mobilized from its subfascial bed in the subcutaneous area, ligating the collaterals. Then, the free end of the vein is anastomosed end-to-side to the brachial artery at the level of the antecubital fossa. Basilic vein dissection can also be performed with a minimal invasive endoscopic technique [26].

As autologous material is employed and only one anastomosis is required, the transposition of the basilic (or cephalic) vein is particularly recommended in the above-mentioned patients, because of more resistance to infection and thrombosis, if compared with the insertion of a prosthetic graft. Furthermore, the insertion of a prosthetic graft is still feasible at a later date, after failed brachiobasilic transposed AVF [27].

Multiple short incisions should always be preferred for dissection of the vein, as this procedure results in better healing and a better cosmetic appearance if compared with a single long incision. Three-year patency rates of transposed brachiobasilic AVFs are reported as ranging from 43 to 64% [28–31]. However, in our experience better results are obtained with basilic transposition than those with cephalic transposition.

AVG Fistulas

The insertion of an AVG remains the method of choice whenever the patient's native vessels have been used up or the vessels are too distant for constructing a native AVF. Although expanded PTFE has become the graft of choice for hemodialysis access, many organic or semiorganic materials are currently available for AVG construction, though not all are well understood, which are more resistant to infection and show the same, if not better, long-term patency. However, the ideal small-diameter prosthesis, which has the same compliance as the native vessels and can be needled immediately for acute uremia treatment, has yet to be developed.

Vascular Substitutes

The autologous saphenous vein was the first type of vascular substitute used for angioaccess grafts, but the increased length of the operation time necessary for its removal, the intention to preserve this vein for potential coronary revascularization or for subsequent use as a bypass graft in peripheral vascular procedures have turned surgeons' attention to other vascular substitutes.

Moreover, discouraging results have been observed with the autologous saphenous vein that present patency rates as low as 20% at 2 years [32] in the upper arm as well as in the groin [33], due to the early occurrence of intimal hyperplasia. Human umbilical vein [34], bovine carotid artery and arterial homograft have also been used in the past and then abandoned due to poor results.

Dacron or polyethylene terephthalate was the first nonbiological material used for angioaccess, but it was soon abandoned because of bleeding and loss of wall integrity. Expanded Teflon or e-polytetrafluoroethylene (e-PTFE), a nontextile material introduced for constructing graft angioaccess in 1977 by Elliott [35], became the preferred material for vascular access, due to its prompt availability and sufficient handleness. Later on, a thin wall configuration became available. Prosthetic rings and coils, applied to the external surface, represent modifications to the basic PTFE, which should make the graft more resistant to kinking and inadvertent compression. However, nonreinforced grafts demonstrated better primary patency versus reinforced grafts [36]. Other modifications of PTFE such as the stretch version, the silicone-coated or carbon-coated grafts and a new multilayered product, the Diastat, that theoretically allowed an early cannulation, did not improve the results. Neither did the venous PTFE cuff at the venous anastomosis, that was recently considered for preventing intimal hyperplasia and improving the patency of PTFE grafts, result in better patency rates [37]. The main problems of all PTFE configurations are the venous outflow tract stenosis, infection and pseudoaneurysm formation [38]. Better results than those with PTFE were obtained, in our hands, with the Hemasite® prosthesis, a totally subcutaneous needleless access device; unfortunately, this interesting vascular access device is no longer sold, because of high rates of thrombosis and infection registered by other investigators.

Plasma-TFE, a Dacron composite graft bonded with a glow discharge polymerization, represents another attempt to lower in vitro thrombogenicity and enhance graft compliance.

Elastic polymers, developed as polyester polyurethane, are more compliant materials, but demonstrated chemical modification and deterioration in vivo, as well as polyether-based polyurethane, susceptible to oxidative degradation. Another vascular access graft made with polyetherurethaneurea allows earlier access, but no difference is found in the patency or complication rates if compared with PTFE vascular access grafts [39].

The patency rates of synthetic materials are not significantly improved by modifications of the luminal surface with pyrolytic carbon coating, heparin binding and electrostatic spinning, adopted to enhance graft compliance and reduce thrombogenicity, platelet deposition and in general the Vroman effect, when compared with those of basic nonorganic grafts.

The current 1-year primary patency rate for PTFE dialysis grafts is 40–50% and there is a 2-year patency rate of about 25% [40, 41].

The reported secondary patency rates of PTFE range from 55 to 75% at 12 months [42] and 1.4 additional procedures per year are required to maintain its patency [43] with a 3- to 6-fold increase if compared with the number of procedures required to maintain the patency of native AVFs [41]. Moreover, the use of AVG is associated with an increased mortality when compared with AVF [44].

The type of graft material used for AVGs may be instrumental in preventing the steal phenomenon: in our experience, biological graft materials appear to be less prone to this complication than PTFE and other synthetic grafts, as they are more easy to be 'capitonated' for matching the vascular substitute to the arteriotomy.

Since the early 1970s [45] more than 1,100 homologous great saphenous veins (HSV) obtained from varicose vein stripping procedures and preserved in a normal refrigerator, according to our original technique, have been used for constructing AVG fistulas. The risk of implanting potentially infected material is minimized by a complete review of the past medical/social history of the 'donor' and by the utilization of the same serological and microbiological laboratory testing procedures adopted for establishing the suitability of solid organs coming from cadaver donors with the exception of histocompatibility testing. In the first period of our experience, the ABO blood group was considered for graft placement. Moreover, recipient T lymphocyte subsets and lymphocytotoxic antibodies were examined after implantation in a small series of our patients with negative signs of immunologic activation. Although in the second period of our experience no effort was made to assign ABO blood-typed or tissue-typed veins to the recipients, no patient showed signs of rejection.

The HSV graft exhibits the best compliance, making it possible to construct a particular access with techniques which are otherwise not feasible with different vascular substitutes. Its patency rate is comparable or even better than that of other grafts, being more resistant to infection. Moreover, venous anastomotic neointimal hyperplasia is averted and the abolition of the prosthesis is not necessary, once the AVG constructed using HSV is closed. However, the great amount of discard, limited availability and tendency for aneurysm formation when used in the lower limb turns our continuous attention to other modern vascular substitutes.

Techniques of cryopreservation potentially allow bank storage of vein allografts for an indefinite period of time, but cause substantial injury to smooth muscle cells, evidenced particularly at reoperations as dangerous tissue cracking. Although some investigators [46] successfully employed a cryopreserved femoral vein for salvaging infected hemodialysis grafts, results reported by us and others [47] recommend that this option should be avoided for the time being.

In the more recent years, besides the HSV graft, other prosthetic materials have been employed and evaluated, such as sheep collagen, bovine mesenteric vein and bovine ureter of a new preparation. These vascular substitutes show less vulnerability to organisms, less compliance mismatch and a smaller incidence of intimal hyperplasia formation, if compared with rigid synthetic graft materials.

The sheep collagen prosthesis is an original biosynthetic material constructed with a polyester mesh, mounted on a flexible silicone mandril and inserted into the subcutaneous trunci muscle of an adult sheep for a period of 12–14 weeks. The collagen tube, formed in straight, J- or U-shaped figures, is harvested and stabilized using glutaraldehyde. As this delicate vascular substitute can easily be damaged by incorrect manipulation, a Fogarty catheter can be useful to drag the ovine collagen graft, greased with sterile Vaseline oil, through the subcutaneous tunnel. The endoskeleton of polyester mesh makes this prosthesis particularly useful for angioaccess graft procedures, constructed using arteries with a large diameter, as the supporting structure provides a barrier to graft dilation and decreases the tendency for aneurysm development. An end-to-end anastomosis of an inverted segment of HSV can enhance the compliance of the whole graft.

Another modern prosthesis is the bovine mesenteric vein that evidences physiologic properties nearly identical to those of the human saphenous vein, due to the high elastin content. The main problem encountered with this prosthesis is an incorrect preparation: the stitch material employed to suture the collateral veins appears to be too thick and positioned without a transfixing suture. Moreover, the ligature is placed too far from the confluence of the collateral veins. A bulging is easily evidenced under pressure: this area of lower resistance becomes a source of vortices with risks of aneurysm formation and thrombosis. A time-consuming procedure of suturing all collateral veins with transfixing 6/0 stitch obviates these inconveniences. We have communicated these problems to the manufacturer who is going to deal with them. Both of these prosthetic materials must be rinsed 3 times and filled with heparin before their use.

The second generation of bovine ureter consists of a collagenous conduit that has been decellularized, so reducing host immune response. The graft compliance is enhanced by no chemical cross-linking using glutaraldehyde fixation; at the same time, the possibility of aldehyde-initiated calcification and the subsequent risk of aneurysmal formation are eliminated. Additional advantages of this graft are the thickness of the graft wall, the absence of valves and tributaries, the virtually unlimited supply, the optimal handling, room temperature preservation and no need of bulky storage equipment or time-consuming rinsing procedures. The only adverse effect evidenced in about 40% of the patients was a reversible edema of the limb where the prosthesis had been positioned and a redness along the graft, which disappeared within 2–4 weeks. A subsequent generation seems to obviate this problem.

Genetic engineering techniques, such as bioresorbable polymers, synthetic protein-based polymers and autologous endothelial cell seeding of prosthetic vascular grafts, are underway to develop new generations of small-caliber vascular substitutes with reduced thrombogenicity, but more extensive studies are required to define their clinical utility.

Most Common Techniques

Low-flow states and hypercoagulable conditions may predispose to graft thrombosis, when not recognized and treated in a timely fashion. Moreover, the artery selected for constructing an AVG fistula must have an adequate inflow, and the vein must show a sufficient outflow.

With regard to the graft configuration, the creation of loop or straight graft fistulas should not depend on a simple technical choice from the vascular surgeon. On the contrary, every effort should be made to save the vascular system of the uremic patient, adopting a critical strategy for a sequential preparation of dialysis access sites.

As the failure of a more distal forearm access still allows the construction of a subsequent access in the same limb, all distal sites should be used before turning to a more proximal location: loop fistulas should be positioned beneath previously failed vascular access, where no other vascular access could be constructed with the patient's native vessels. Sequential graft placement must be considered once reoperation for maintaining patency at a given arteriovenous access has failed.

However, in our experience, although better long-term results are commonly described with straight grafts, the straight forearm graft (fig. 3c) between the radial artery at the wrist and a suitable antecubital vein is a less desirable configuration, as it can expose the patient to the risk of the steal syndrome or early thrombosis, unless a hypertrophied radial artery is present.

The most popular graft configurations are a loop in the forearm and a straight graft in the upper arm, but a number of anatomical variations may be used, depending on the patient's remnant vessels and the level of training of the vascular surgeon.

The loop forearm angioaccess between the brachial artery to its comitans vein, just below the elbow crease, represents the configuration of AVG that we do prefer (fig. 3a). Really, even if there exists only one superficial antecubital vein, as well as the basilic or cephalic vein, it should be reserved for the construction of an elbow fistula with native vessels. The antecubital veins (fig. 3b),

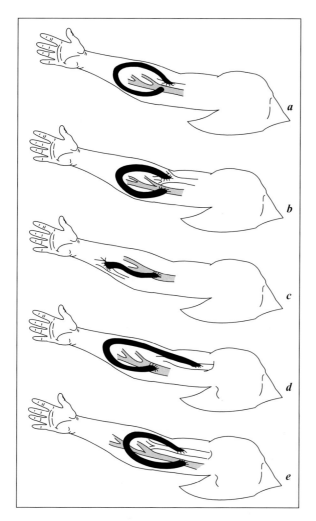

Fig. 3. AVG fistulas. *a* Loop forearm AVG between brachial artery and 'comitans' vein. *b* Loop forearm AVG between brachial artery and cephalic vein. *c* Straight forearm AVG. *d, e* Loop AGV across the elbow crease.

also arterialized by a well-functioning native AVF, should be used only in case they are too deep or unsuitable for dialysis cannulation.

We prefer to use the brachial artery instead of the proximal portion of the radial artery, taking care to perform an arteriotomy not greater than 80% of the arterial diameter, in order to assure a sufficient inflow into the graft access and to prevent the peripheral steal syndrome. A sterile-drape film is placed on the forearm to prevent direct contact between the skin and the graft.

The diameter of the graft used in the upper limb should be 5 or 6 mm in diameter, according to the patient's size. Larger grafts expose the patient to the peripheral steal syndrome.

The brachial artery and the largest brachial vein are identified with the same incision used for the aforementioned upper arm native AVFs. The median nerve lies medial to the artery and must remain untouched. The end-to-side anastomosis between the arterial end of the graft, slightly beveled cut, and the brachial artery is performed first. In this way, the correct shape of the graft can be better determined on the forearm. Moreover, the length of the graft should be proportional to systolic pressure values of the patient, as long grafts are more exposed to thrombosis in hypotensive patients.

After completion of the arterial anastomosis, the free end of the graft is flushed with saline under pressure to check the suture prior to removing the vascular clamps. The distal clamp is removed first from the artery and then the cranial clamp to control bleeding. Then, the graft is filled with heparinized saline and a bulldog clamp is placed at the venous end of the graft.

The subcutaneous tunnel is created by a counterincision near the apex of the loop portion of the graft, according to the course indicated on the volar surface of the forearm by the pulsating graft. It should be deep enough to avoid skin erosion, yet superficial enough to get an easy percutaneous cannulation. A proper placement procedure forecasts the elimination of acute angles at both the arterial and venous anastomoses, in order to prevent graft kinking.

The pulsating graft, greased with Vaseline oil, is passed through the subcutaneous tunnel with a delicate traction simply using a blunted Klemmer to prevent twisting of the graft. However, graft tunnelers can also be used, such as Kelly-Wick or an inflated Fogarty catheter.

The venotomy should be as long as possible to encourage the outflow and the venous end of the graft is tailored obliquely to match. The cranial clamp is removed first from the vein and then the distal clamp for a safe control of bleeding. Lastly, the bulldog clamp placed at the venous end of the graft is removed and a thrill should be at once felt above the efferent vein. The subcutaneous tissue is closed using a 4/0 Vicryl in two layers and the skin with 4/0 nylon. A subcuticular suture should be discouraged due to its closeness to the elbow crease.

A fairly good long-term patency can be achieved by our original 'O-shaped' graft in the distal third of the upper arm (fig. 4e) between the brachial artery and its comitans vein (or basilic vein), which makes it possible to isolate these vessels with only one incision and to preserve the more proximal location for potential future sites in the same extremity [48]. The choice of an adequate graft is crucial, since it must be flexible enough to make a narrow loop. Homologous saphenous veins appear to be the better graft for this procedure.

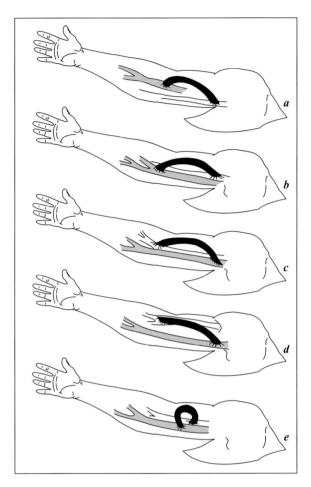

Fig. 4. AVG fistulas. *a* Straight upper arm AVG between brachial artery and axillary vein. *b* Straight upper arm AVG between brachial artery and 'comitans' vein (centripetal flow). *c* Straight upper arm AVG between brachial artery and 'comitans' vein (centrifugal flow). *d* Straight upper arm AVG between brachial artery and cephalic vein. *e* 'O-shaped' AVG.

The bridge graft between the brachial artery and axillary vein (fig. 4a) in a straight configuration is the angioaccess most frequently used in the upper-arm. The skin incisions are longitudinal. The graft, anastomosed end-to-side to the brachial artery which can be isolated just above the antecubital fossa, joins the axillary vein, or basilic vein below the axilla by a subcutaneous tunnel running over the lateral surface of the biceps muscle. The cephalic vein can also be used as outflow.

Other possible variations of bridge grafts can be achieved, isolating the brachial artery below the axilla and a patent vein above the antecubital fossa (fig. 4c, d). This alternative bridge graft is particularly well-suited for elderly or diabetic patients, who are affected by significant peripheral vascular diseases and are more prone to the steal syndrome, as the graft fistula flow is directed in a centrifugal way.

A straight or loop configuration across the joints (fig. 3d, e), which is sometimes used in an attempt to preserve potential future sites in the same limb, should as a rule be avoided, as well as a loop configuration in the upper arm, unless a very compliant graft can be adopted.

Vascular Access Procedures in the Lower Limb

Early experience with vascular access procedures in the groin was discouraging because of high infection rates and the risk of limb amputation. In our experience, groin hemodialysis access is a viable option when superficial vessels in the upper extremity are unavailable and peritoneal dialysis has failed. The excessive widespread use of central venous catheters leading to thrombosis of the chest veins has recently again pointed to the utility of vascular access placed in the groin.

Lower limb autogenous AVF is a rarely performed procedure due to its frequent complications and poor results. Instead, the patient's own autologous saphenous vein, transposed to form a loop and anastomosed end-to-side to the superficial femoral artery, leaving the saphenous vein junction untouched, can be used for a native AVF. The great saphenous vein is freed from the supragenicular level, ligating the confluents by transfixing sutures, and divided distally. The autologous saphenous vein is then transposed to form a J or U loop configuration and anastomosed to a distal superficial femoral artery. However, this technique has almost been abandoned by us, due to a high rate of intimal hyperplasia at the venous anastomosis.

Other lower limb AVFs which employ the autologous saphenous vein [49] are seldom reported in the literature, due to their poor long-term results and the intention to preserve the patient's own saphenous vein for myocardial and peripheral revascularization; moreover, it is often unsuitable for vascular access construction and the incision itself can cause considerable problems in these uremic patients with poor wound healing. An endoscopic vein harvest may reduce morbidity and risk of wound infection.

The transposition of the superficial femoral vein appears to be burdened by too many complications, such as major wound complications, steal syndrome and leg amputation eventually, to be considered as a safe procedure [50].

Table 2. Personal strategy for prosthetic access procedures in the groin in chronic hemodialysis

Femoral (superficial or common) artery-greater saphenous vein (or its junction with common femoral vein) straight access

Femoral (superficial or common) artery-greater saphenous vein (or its junction with common femoral vein) loop access

Femoral (superficial or common) artery-femoral vein loop access

Femoral (superficial or common) artery-external iliac vein loop access

External iliac artery-external iliac vein loop access

The use of a fit vascular prosthesis shortens the operation time and avoids problems of wound healing at the groin incision. In our experience, reinforced sheep collagen or second generation bovine ureter give better results in terms of patency and infection rates, if compared with either autogenous veins or HSV graft and PTFE. As a matter of fact, the HSV graft in the lower limb as well as other nonreinforced biological grafts are more prone to aneurysm formation.

The presence of peripheral arterial disease or venous occlusion is evaluated preoperatively by Doppler sonography. With regard to the strategy for access procedures, our personal guidelines, based on 35 years' experience, suggest a careful policy of native vessel preservation, to maximize the use of potential access sites, also in the lower limb (table 2).

The superficial femoral artery is dissected by a transverse incision 3 cm under the inguinal ligament. The great saphenous vein is identified by a longitudinal incision 3 cm above the knee. If the diameter of the saphenous vein above the knee is over 4 mm, a reinforced biological graft is interposed between

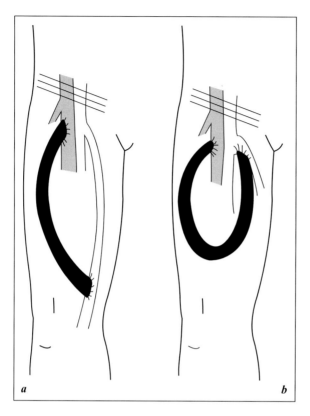

Fig. 5. Prosthetic access procedures in the groin. *a* Superficial femoral artery to greater saphenous vein, straight access. *b* Superficial femoral artery to greater saphenous vein junction with common femoral vein.

these two vessels in a straight configuration (fig. 5a). This should be the preferred procedure in the thigh, as straight graft access through superficial femoral artery-saphenous vein allows the re-use of the same vessels in a more proximal area for a subsequent construction of a new access in a loop configuration (fig. 5b), when the previous one has failed.

The common femoral artery can also be adopted as a second choice inflow, if the superficial femoral artery is obstructed or affected by heavy atherosclerosis, whilst *we* recommend to avoid the use of profunda femoris artery or popliteal artery [51], due to the high risk of critical ischemia of the lower limb and major amputation. Whenever the saphenous vein or its junction with the common femoral vein are unsuitable or failed, the common femoral vein can be directly used for a loop-configured angioaccess graft.

The 1-year primary patency rate ranges from 50 to 71% [52, 53].

Table 3. Personal algorithm of 'extreme' or 'body wall' access procedures

Axillary artery-ipsilateral axillary vein, chest loop access

Axillary artery-ipsilateral jugular (inner/external) vein, chest
(loop or straight) access

Axillary artery-controlateral axillary (or jugular) vein, chest straight access

External iliac artery-external ipsilateral iliac vein, loop access

External iliac artery-external contralateral iliac vein, straight
(or 'cross-over') access

Permanent central venous catheter

Subclavian artery–right atrium bridge

Other alternative vessels, such as distal external iliac artery and vein under the inguinal ligament, can also be employed for 'extreme' angioaccess graft construction in a loop configuration across the groin crease, in patients who are not on the waiting list for kidney transplantation (table 3).

A suitable surgical alternative for patients whose conventional arm sites have been used up is the axillary artery and ipsilateral axillary vein chest loop access. A longitudinal single incision in the axilla makes it possible to identify the two vessels after the resection of the pectoralis minor muscle. The graft joins the artery and the vein by a little counterincision on the anterior wall of the chest in a loop configuration. A patency rate of 60% is described at 3 years [54].

If the ipsilateral axillary vein shows an inadequate outflow, the ipsilateral jugular (inner or external) can be adopted for a straight or looped AVG, as well as the controlateral axillary vein in a straight configuration. The distal segment of the external iliac artery and vein can only be used for an extreme AVG loop construction in the groin, across the inguinal crease, if the patient is not on the waiting list for kidney transplantation. The permanent central venous catheter represents at this stage a valuable alternative to continue the substitution treatment.

In case of superior vena cava occlusion, a subclavian artery-to-right atrium bridge graft was also successfully attempted [55].

Conclusion

Patient-specific factors, such as age, gender, duration of renal replacement therapy and peculiar comorbidities, require a tailored angioaccess for the maintenance of an adequate hemodialysis. The experience of the vascular surgeon plays a substantial role in angioaccess selection.

As significant inferior outcomes of arteriovenous access have been described in patients who had prior temporary access [56], a timely placement of AVF is advocated to avoid as much as possible the long-term use of tunneled central venous catheters. Permanent central venous catheters should be limited to patients with no other potential form of access.

The prompt availability of a well-functioning vascular access for dialysis improves the patient's life expectancy and the quality of his or her life with a substantial reduction of social costs and hospitalization. A vascular access coordinator, an integrated, multidisciplinary approach and a dedicated vascular surgeon are the keys for better success.

References

1   Berardinelli L, Vegeto A: L'accesso vascolare per la dialisi extracorporea. Monografia con video-cassetta (durata 90') UTET. Torino, Periodici Scientifici, 1993.
2   Schwab S, Besarab A, Beathard G: NKF-DOQUI clinical practice guidelines for vascular access. Am J Kidney Dis 1997;30:S150.
3   Brescia M, Cimino JE, Appel K, et al: Chronic haemodialysis using venipuncture and a surgically created arteriovenous fistula. N Engl J Med 1966;275:1089.
4   Prischl FC, Kirchgatterer A, Brandstatter E: Parameters of prognostic relevance to the patency of vascular access in haemodialysis patients. J Am Soc Nephrol 1995;6:1613.
5   Hodges TC, Fillinger MF, Zwolak RM: Longitudinal comparison of dialysis access methods: Risk factors for failure. J Vasc Surg 1997;26:1009.
6   US Renal Data System: US Renal Data System 1997 Annual Report. Washington, 1997, chap 10, p 143.

7   Koksoy C, Kuzu A, Kutlay J, Erden I, Ozcan H, Ergin K: The diagnostic value of color Doppler ultrasound in central venous catheter related thrombosis. Clin Radiol 1995;50:687.
8   Reilly DT, Wood RFM, Bell PRF: Five-year prospective study of dialysis fistulae: Problem patients and their treatment. Br J Surg 1982;69:549.
9   Wong V, Ward R, Taylor J: Factors associated with early failure of arteriovenous fistulae for hemodialysis access. Eur J Vasc Endovasc Surg 1996;12:207.
10 Miller CD, Robbin ML, Allon M: Gender differences in outcome of arteriovenous fistulas in hemodialysis patients. Kidney Int 2003;63:346.
11 Johnson G Jr: Local pathophysiology of an arteriovenous fistula; in Swan KG (ed): Venous Surgery in the Lower Extremity. St Louis, Warren H. Green, 1975, pp 41–50.
12 Fillinger MF, Reinitz ER: Graft geometry and venous intimal-medial hyperplasia in arteriovenous loop grafts. J Vasc Surg 1990;11:556.
13 Tellis VA, Veith FJ, Soberman RJ, et al: Internal arteriovenous fistula for haemodialysis. Surg Gynecol Obstet 1971;132:866.
14 Burkhart HM, Cikrit DF: Arteriovenous fistulae for hemodialysis. Semin Vasc Surg 1997;10/3:162.
15 Mehigan JT, McAlexander RA: Snuffbox arteriovenous fistula for haemodialysis. Am J Surg 1982;143:252.
16 Hanson JS, Carmody M, Keogh B, et al: Access to circulation by permanent arteriovenous fistula in regular dialysis treatment. Br Med J 1967;iv:586.
17 Someya S, Gergan JJ, Khan BD: An upper arm AV fistula for hemodialysis patients with distal access failure. Trans Am Soc Artif Intern Organs 1976;22:398.
18 Hakaim AG, Nalbandian M, Scott T: Superior maturation and patency of primary brachiocephalic and transposed basilic vein arteriovenous fistulae in patients with diabetes. J Vasc Surg 1998;27:154.
19 Sparks SR, Van der Linden JL, Gnanadev DA: Superior patency of perforating antecubital vein arteriovenous fistula for hemodialysis. Ann Vasc Surg 1997;11:165.
20 Gracz KC, Ing TS, Soung LS: Proximal forearm fistula for maintenance dialysis. Kidney Int 1977;11:71.
21 Berardinelli L, Vegeto A: Lessons from 494 permanent accesses in 348 haemodialysis patients older than 65 years of age: 29 years of experience. Nephrol Dial Transplant 1998;13(suppl 7):73.
22 Bell PRF, Wood RFM: Surgical Aspects Dialysis. Edinburgh, Churchill Livingstone, 1983, p 35.
23 Elcheroth J, de Pauw L, Kinnaert P: Elbow arteriovenous fistulas for chronic haemodialysis. Br J Surg 1994;81:982.
24 Weyde W, Krajeweska M, Letachowicz W: Superficialization of the wrist native arteriovenous fistula for effective hemodialysis vascular access construction. Kidney Int 2002;61:1170.
25 Hossny A: Brachiobasilic arteriovenous fistula: Different surgical techniques and their effects on fistula patency and dialysis-related complications. J Vasc Surg 2003;37:821.
26 Tordoir JH, Dammers R, de Brauw M: Video-assisted basilic vein transposition for haemodialysis vascular access. Preliminary experience with a new technique. Nephrol Dial Transplant 2001;16:391.
27 Matsuura JH, Rosenthal D, Clark M: Transposed basilic vein versus PTFE for brachial-axillary arteriovenous fistulas. Am J Surg 1998;176:219.
28 Cantelmo NE, LoGerfo FW, Menzoian JO: Brachiobasilic and brachiocephalic fistulas as secondary angioaccess routes. Surg Gynecol Obstet 1982;155:545.
29 Murphy GJ, White SA, Knight AJ, Doughman TD, Nicholson ML: Long-term results of the transposed autologous brachiobasilic fistula for haemodialysis. Br J Surg 2000;87:819.
30 Coburn MC, Carney WI Jr: Comparison of basilic vein and polytetrafluoroethylene for brachial arteriovenous fistula. J Vasc Surg 1994;20:896.
31 Tsai YT, Lin SH, Lee GC: Arteriovenous fistula using transposed basilic vein in chronic hypotensive hemodialysis patients. Clin Nephrol 2002;57:376.
32 Haimov M, Burrows L, Schanzer H, et al: Experience with arterial substitutes in the construction of vascular access for haemodialysis. J Cardiovasc Surg 1980;21:149.
33 Valenta J, Bilek J, Opatny K: Autogeneous saphenous vein graft as secondary vascular access for haemodialysis. Dial Transplant 1985;14:567.
34 Jorgensen L: Human umbilical vein for vascular access in chronic haemodialysis. Scand J Urol Nephrol 1985;19:49.

35 Elliott MP: Use of e-PTFE grafts for vascular access in haemodialysis: Laboratory and clinical evaluation. Am Surg 1977;43:455.

36 Schuman ES: Reinforced versus nonreinforced PTFE grafts for haemodialysis access surgery. Am J Surg 1997;173:407.

37 Lemson MS, Tordoir JH, van Det RJ, Welten RJ, Burger H, Estourgie RJ, Stroecken HJ, Leunissen KM: Effects of a venous cuff at the venous anastomosis of polytetrafluoroethylene grafts for hemodialysis vascular access. J Vasc Surg 2000;32:1155.

38 Kauffman JL, Garb JL, Berman JA: A prospective comparison of two e-PTFE grafts for linear forearm hemodialysis access: Does the manufacturer matter? J Am Coll Surg 1997;185:74.

39 Glickman MH, Stokes GK, Ross JR, et al: Multicenter evaluation of a polytetrafluoroethylene vascular access graft as compared with the expanded polytetrafluoroethylene vascular access graft in hemodialysis applications. J Vasc Surg 2001;34:465.

40 Hodges TC, Fillinger MF, Zwolak RM: Longitudinal comparison of dialysis access methods: Risk factors for failure. J Vasc Surg 1997;26:1009.

41 Schwab SJ, Harrington JT, Singh A: Vascular access for hemodialysis. Kidney Int 1999;55:2078.

42 Veldenz HC: Selection of graft material for prosthetic arteriovenous access. Int J Artif Organs 2000;23/5:293.

43 Schuman ES, Gross GF, Hayes JF, et al: Long-term patency of polytetrafluoroethylene graft fistulas. Am J Surg 1988;155:644.

44 Dhingra RK, Young EW, Hulbert-Shearon TE: Type of vascular access and mortality in US hemodialysis patients. Kidney Int 2001;60:1443.

45 Vegeto A, Berardinelli L, Malan E: Use of homologous vein grafts for chronic hemodialysis. J Cardiovasc Surg 1977;18:501.

46 Matsuura JH, Rosenthal D, Wellons ED: Hemodialysis graft infections treated with cryopreserved femoral vein. Cardiovasc Surg 2002;10:561.

47 Ruddle AC, George S, Armitage WJ, et al: Venous allografts prepared from stripped long saphenous vein. Is there a need for antibiotic sterilization? Eur J Vasc Endovasc Surg 1998;15:444.

48 Berardinelli L, Beretta C, Pozzoli E: The 'O' shaped graft fistula in the arm: A new procedure for difficult patients on dialysis. 2nd International Congress on Access Surgery, Maastricht, 1990.

49 Cimochowski GE: Use of the spiral vein graft as an arterial substitute for secondary access. Am J Nephrol 1991;11:64.

50 Gradman WS, Cohen W, Haji-Aghaii M: Arteriovenous fistula construction in the thigh with transposed superficial femoral vein: Our initial experience. J Vasc Surg 2001;33:968.

51 Mandel ST, McDougal EG: Popliteal artery to saphenous vein vascular access for hemodialysis. Surg Gynecol Obstet 1985;160:358.

52 Khadra M, Dwyer A, Thompson J: Advantages of PTFE arteriovenous loops in the thigh for hemodialysis access. Excerpta Med 1997;173:280.

53 Tashjian DB, Lipkowitz GS, Madden RL: Safety and efficacy of femoral-based hemodialysis access grafts. J Vasc Surg 2002;35:691.

54 McCann RL: Axillary grafts for difficult hemodialysis access. J Vasc Surg 1996;24:457.

55 Mickley V: Subclavian artery to right atrium haemodialysis bridge graft for superior vena cava occlusion. Nephrol Dial Transplant 1996;11:1361.

56 Rayner HC, Pisoni RL, Gillespie BW: Creation, cannulation and survival of arteriovenous fistulae: Data from the DOPPS. Kidney Int 2003;63:323.

Prof. Luisa Berardinelli
Ospedale Maggiore Policlinico Universitario (IRCCS)
Via Francesco Sforza 35
20122 Milano (Italy)
Tel. +39 0 2 503 20391, Fax +39 02 550 35650, E-Mail luisa.berardinelli@unimi.it

Ronco C, Levin NW (eds): Hemodialysis Vascular Access and Peritoneal Dialysis Access.
Contrib Nephrol. Basel, Karger, 2004, vol 142, pp 73–93

....

Vascular Grafts for Hemodialysis: Types, Sites and Techniques

*David G. Warnock[a], Ashita J. Tolwani[a], Michael Gallichio[b],
Michael Allon[a]*

Departments of [a]Medicine and [b]Surgery, University of Alabama at Birmingham,
Birmingham, Ala., USA

Introduction

This review will summarize the issues surrounding arteriovenous grafts for
hemodialysis from the nephrologic perspective. Rather than focusing on the
details of the surgical techniques, the characteristics of these grafts that impact
on their ultimate success will be considered. The sites, types and other technical considerations of grafts will be discussed in the context of their utilization
for arteriovenous access in the chronic hemodialysis setting. The issues of surveillance and diagnosis of graft dysfunction in established grafts, as well as the
approaches to graft thrombectomy, angioplasty and other forms of endovascular salvage will be addressed in other contributions to the present volume.

Fistulae versus Grafts versus Catheters

The National Kidney Foundation published the Dialysis Outcome Quality
Initiative (DOQI) guidelines in 1997 (updated as K/DOQI in 2000) that specifically addressed the optimal management of vascular access [1, 2]. An important guideline emphasized the desirability of using arteriovenous fistulae over
grafts for chronic dialysis access. As the dialysis population in the US has
become increasingly older, has remained on dialysis for longer periods of time,
and included more patients who were female, diabetic and with extensive atherosclerotic disease, the prevalence of arteriovenous fistulae has not measured
up to the DOQI guidelines [3]. A number of factors may account for this short

fall, but there are important differences between the prevalence of grafts versus fistulae within the US [4, 5], and also when the US experience is compared to other geographic areas [6]. While the prevalence of arteriovenous fistulae was 24% in the US dialysis patient sample, more than 80% of the sampled population in Germany, France, Italy, Britain and Spain were using arteriovenous fistulae for chronic dialysis access [6]. Even more striking is the reported early success of fistula cannulation in the European experience [7], which is not the standard of practice in the US [8]. There are other technical aspects that impact primary surgical success and fistula maturation that do not appear to be optimal in the US experience [3]. Until these factors are better understood, and addressed, the current reliance on arteriovenous grafts in the majority of chronic dialysis patients in the US requires that the possible advantages and clear-cut disadvantages of arteriovenous grafts be fully understood. Despite local preferences, the risk of access failure once established is demonstrably higher with grafts than fistulae [9, 10]. Barriers to optimal access utilization include systematic factors [4, 11] and referral factors [12]. Even if initial arteriovenous fistula formation is not successful, the resultant dilation of the venous outflow system, even on a short-term basis, may facilitate the subsequent conversion to a graft [13].

Once a successful access has been established, it has long been recognized that the long-term patency of fistulae is better than that of grafts. Furthermore, infections, pseudoaneurysms, venous stenosis with elevated pressures, and vascular steal complications are more common with grafts [14]. Consequently, grafts have higher revision rates than fistulae [15, 16]. There is some debate about the patient-specific factors that impact on primary and secondary graft outcome [16, 17], but there is no doubt that a multidisciplinary approach to access management [18], preoperative vascular assessment for optimal access placement, and aggressive monitoring and interventions to ensure access patency will impact positively on overall outcomes, reduce the incidence of accesses that fail before being successfully used, and subsequent interventions for grafts as well as fistulae [3, 19–21]. Continuing progress along these lines has occurred [22], stimulated by the K/DOQI Access guidelines [1, 2].

Various sorts of temporary and semipermanent catheters are described in other contributions to this volume. While the choice between grafts and fistulae is greatly affected by practice patterns and patient demographics, the use of temporary catheters for hemodialysis access is often unavoidable in the setting of late referral, graft dysfunction, and graft removal due to infection. Such catheters offer immediate access, but their use is fraught with short- and longer-term complications that are only too well-known to the practicing nephrologists and dialysis staff.

Sites for Arteriovenous Graft Placement

Upper Extremity

Upper extremity grafts have been a mainstay for chronic hemodialysis access in the US over the last several decades. Loop grafts in the forearm (connecting the brachial artery to an antecubital vein) and upper arm (brachioaxillary) appear to have longer-term patency rates than straight grafts between the radial artery and an antecubital vein in the forearm [23–26], or straight grafts between the brachial artery and internal jugular vein in the upper arm [27]. Straight radial-antecubital polytetrafluoroethylene (PTFE) grafts may have some utility in older patients with concurrent vascular disease since the ulnar circulation and brachial circulation are spared, but suffer from inferior flow velocities and patency rates when compared to other graft locations [28]. Randomized, prospective evaluations of forearm loop grafts have defined optimal flow characteristics, and primary and secondary patency rates that appear to favor 6-mm nontapered loop grafts [29], but also have observed a greater incidence of steal syndromes with 6-mm grafts compared to 4- to 7-mm tapered grafts [30]. Grafts that cross the elbow or utilize antecubital veins can be problematic, especially if only the proximal cephalic vein can be used for dialysis. A brachiocephalic jump graft has been described with a short segment of graft anastomosed to the brachial artery and cephalic vein [31].

Lower Extremity

Thigh grafts have been used when upper arm sites are exhausted or the vessels are too small (e.g., in children), and are definitely more problematic than upper arm grafts. Although not considered a first choice, femoral artery-based hemodialysis access is an option when arteriovenous fistulae in the upper extremity cannot be constructed, or upper extremity accesses have failed, particularly in the setting of central venous stenosis affecting the upper extremities [32]. Thrombosis is a continuing concern that limits graft patency, even more than infection rates [33, 34]. Patency rates are approximately half with lower extremity grafts compared to upper extremity grafts [35], but are still far superior to dialysis catheters. Femoral artery-vein loop grafts can worsen claudication and have even caused vascular insufficiency that has resulted in distal extremity amputation [36, 37]. Similar results have been obtained with arteriovenous fistulae using the superficial femoral vein, which are associated with a high incidence of clinically significant postoperative ischemia requiring reoperation [38]. Chronic dialysis patients have an increased relative risk for occlusive peripheral vascular disease [39], and higher mortality rates following peripheral revascularization procedures [40]. Therefore, chronic dialysis patients who have lower extremity grafts placed because of access failure in their upper extremities due to vascular disease are at significantly greater risk for morbidity and mortality [41, 42].

Other Sites

When the conventional upper and lower extremity access sites have been exhausted, the choices for further access become extremely limited. Alternate dialysis modalities or semichronic venous catheters have to be considered. There is very limited experience with other sites, none of which have proven to be satisfactory. Brachial-jugular grafts [43, 44], axillofemoral grafts [45], and even grafts into the right atrial appendage to bypass central venous obstruction [46] have been described. These approaches can only be considered for the occasional patient in whom all other access sites have failed.

Comparisons between various access sites are summarized in table 1.

Types of Arteriovenous Grafts

PTFE Grafts

PTFE grafts have been used for chronic hemodialysis access for nearly 3 decades. This material has been of considerable utility, and was first used for upper arm grafts in patients who had failed fistulae, or bovine heterologous [47, 48] or saphenous vein grafts [49–52]; even then, complications, including undesirable flow rates, edema, thrombosis, aneurysm formation and associated cardiac failure, were described. This material was also found to be useful for jump grafting of anatomic defects in preexisting grafts and fistulae [53, 54]. While primary patency rates are comparable to fistulae [5], there is a much larger risk of thrombosis with PTFE compared to fistulae, especially at the venous anastomotic site [8]. The original nonreinforced PTFE design appears to be superior to subsequent modifications with external reinforcing [55, 56], but PTFE grafts from the two leading manufacturers (Gore-Tex; W.L. Gore and Associates, Flagstaff, Ariz., USA; Impra; C.R. Bard Inc., Tempe, Ariz., USA) are essentially equivalent [57, 58].

Expanded PTFE (ePTFE; Gore-Tex) has been in use nearly as long as the original nonreinforced PTFE grafts, with the early experience favoring thigh grafts with ePTFE over upper arm grafts [59], and loop grafts over straight grafts [60]. It has been suggested that these grafts could be cannulated relatively early compared to nonreinforced PTFE grafts, thus minimizing the need for using a bridging catheter while the access matures [61]. This theoretical advantage of ePTFE has not been borne out by subsequent studies [55, 56]. Arterial tapers, from 8 to 6 mm, have been used in the upper arm in order to avoid midgraft stenosis observed with other nontapered grafts [25]. A newer

Table 1. Primary and secondary patency rates for hemodialysis vascular access

Reference	Site/material	Interventions (number/access/year)	1-year patency, % primary	1-year patency, % secondary	2-year patency, % primary	2-year patency, % secondary
AV fistulae versus AV grafts						
Gibson et al. [10]	AVF				39.8	64.3
	AVG				24.6*	59.5
Ascher et al. [20]	AVF	0.01	85			
	AVG	0.20	54*			
Astor et al. [17]	AVF	0.39				
	AVG	0.71				
Hodges et al. [15]	AVF		43	46		
	AVG		41	59		
Upper extremity grafts						
Dammers et al. [29]	LALG, PTFE					
	6 mm	0.81	43	91		
	4–7 mm taper	0.74	46	87		
Miller et al. [16]	AVG	1.22	23	65	4	51
Savader et al. [27]	LALG		26	89		30
	UASG		22	52		35
	Branchial-IJ		6*	54		42
Polo et al. [25]	UALG PTFE					
	6–8 mm taper	0.37	73	91		
Bhandari et al. [34]	LALG (saphenous vein)			89.4		89.4
Tordoir et al. [62]	AVG PTFE			74		59
Munda et al. [23]	UALG			60		
	LALG			78		
	LASG			35		
Lower extremity grafts						
Tashjian et al. [32]	LEG		71	83		
Gradman et al. [38]	Fistulae ± PTFE		73	86		
Vogel et al. [35]	LEG			62		
Korzets et al. [36]	LEG			73		
Taylor et al. [37]	LEG (PTFE and bovine)				47	
Bhandari et al. [34]	LEG (PTFE)			84.9		82.3
Slater et al. [33]	LEG (PTFE, 50% patient survival)					80.5

*p < 0.001. Primary failure rates not specified. Primary patency refers to percentage of accesses that are patent at 1 year. Secondary patency refers to percentage of accesses that are usable at 1 year, but required some sort of intervention in the interval. AVF = Arteriovenous fistula; AVG = arteriovenous graft; UALG = upper arm loop graft; UASG = upper arm straight graft; LALG = lower arm loop graft; LASG = lower arm straight graft; LEG = lower extremity graft; IJ = internal jugular.

'stretch' thin wall ePTFE graft appears to have better primary patency rates and less stenoses due to intimal hyperplasia as compared to standard ePTFE grafts [62], and can also be cannulated relatively soon after placement [63]. Mean primary, secondary, and cumulative patency times for the standard wall thickness ePTFE grafts were significantly better than those for the thin wall stretch ePTFE grafts [64]. Another approach was to incorporate a mesh cannulation segment (Diastat graft) to facilitate early cannulation [65], but this material was associated with increased rates of early thrombosis and other complications that offset any advantage of early cannulation [66, 67]. Thrombosis and anastomotic stenosis continue to be problems with ePTFE grafts, and secondary interventions to maintain patency are not uncommon [68]. Cuffed ePTFE grafts were developed to address the problem of recurrent venous stenosis due to intimal hyperplasia at the venous anastomotic site. With this design, the force of the arterial flow is blunted before the venous component of the anastomosis, it appears to have improved primary and overall patency rates compared to standard ePTFE grafts [69, 70]. The reasons for the apparent improvement in patency rates need confirmation and further investigation.

Polyurethane Grafts

The idea of using graft materials that will support immediate cannulation postplacement would have an important practical advantage of eliminating the need for a bridging catheter for dialysis access while the graft is developing. Several materials, including modifications of PTFE mentioned above, have been evaluated for success of early cannulation [71]. A self-sealing PTFE-silicone graft was developed early on [72]. This material appeared to have similar patency rates to PTFE, and fewer pseudoaneurysms, despite relatively greater difficulty with the earlier cannulations [72, 73]. Plasma polymerized woven Dacron tetrafluoroethylene grafts had similar primary patency rates to standard PTFE grafts, but do not perform as well after a thrombotic event [74].

Polyurethane grafts and those coated with gelatin and reinforced with polyester fibers have been used for early cannulation, but have lower primary and overall patency rates compared to standard PTFE [75, 76]. A three-layered cast polyurethane vascular access graft (Thoratec Vectra) has been evaluated, and also had lower primary and secondary patency rates at 1 year than would be expected for PTFE grafts [77]. The marked elasticity of the Vectra graft has posed some placement problems involving suturing of the material, and optimal placement in the subcutaneous tissues. A composite graft with a segment of ePTFE at the anastomosis site has been described that may overcome some of the drawbacks of polyurethane grafts [78].

A multicenter randomized, prospective, controlled study has been carried out to compare the performance of a multilayered, self-sealing polyurethane vascular access graft to ePTFE vascular access grafts for hemodialysis access [79]. Again, there were technical differences at placement, but the polyurethane grafts could be used sooner after placement, and had shorter bleeding times after cannulation, and with comparable long-term patency and complication rates compared to ePTFE [79]. Acceptable long-term patency with these grafts has been confirmed in a subsequent study [80], but this finding was not confirmed by other studies mentioned above [77].

Autologous and Heterologous Vein Grafts

Bovine heterologous [47, 48, 81] or saphenous vein grafts [49–52] were used for hemodialysis access before the advent of PTFE grafts. Saphenous vein grafts are rarely used because of inferior patency rates [82], except perhaps in the thigh [34], and the high prevalence of cardiovascular disease in chronic dialysis patients, and the not infrequent need for coronary bypass surgery utilizing the saphenous veins. PTFE grafts were found to be superior to bovine heterologous grafts with regard to long-term patency, and the latter are rarely used today [83–85]. Cryopreserved autologous femoral vein grafts have been evaluated, and have similar patency rates to PTFE grafts, and may also have some advantage in dealing with infected access sites [86–88]. However, patients at high risk for infection had high rates of graft infection and rupture, particularly when the cryopreserved autologous vein grafts were placed in the thigh position. The replacement of infected PTFE arteriovenous grafts with cryopreserved vein grafts appears to have very limited current utility but may have some benefits in attempts at salvaging infected grafts [89].

Comparisons between various access materials are summarized in table 2.

Techniques

Jump Grafts and Stent Repair

The most common cause of graft failure in patients undergoing hemodialysis is outflow venous stenosis. Jump grafts or bridging grafts have been used to improve venous outflow, alleviate symptoms of venous hypertension, and restore vascular integrity for optimal dialysis. Angiographic studies are used to demonstrate occlusion or stricture of the central venous tract and venous outflow compromise, and to plan optimal intervention [90]. Jump grafts have been described for upper and lower extremity grafts [31, 91, 92]. Jump grafts have also been described as part of the surgical approach to isolating infected segments of existing grafts [93].

Table 2. Comparison of vascular access materials for hemodialysis

Reference	Material	Early use %	6-month patency, %		1-year patency, %		2-year patency, %	
			primary	secondary	primary	secondary	primary	secondary
Wiese et al. [80]	Poly-U	100			67			
Glickman et al. [79]	PTFE	0	47	99	36	80		
	Poly-U	53.9	55	87	44	78		
Cinat et al. [68]	PTFE				43	64		
Ferraresso et al [65]	PTFE (Diastat)	100			56	72		
Kaufman et al. [57]	PTFE (Gortex)				47	69	26	41
	PTFE (Impra)				43	49	30	38
Schuman et al. [55]	PTFE					80		
	Reinforced PTFE					77		
Allen et al. [77]	Poly-U (Thoratec)	100			45	65		
Bartlett et al. [63]	PTFE (Diastat)	58			42			
Tordoir et al. [62]	PTFE PTFE (stretch)							
Nakagawa et al. [76]	PTFE					71		
	PE-PEUG					53		
Helling et al. [74]	PTFE				56	66		
	Plasma-TFE				47	45		
Schanzer et al. [72]	PTFE	0			66	67		
	PTFE-sil	100			63	75		
Rizzuti et al. [60]	PTFE					76		

Primary failure rates not specified. Primary patency refers to percentage of accesses that are patent at 1 year. Secondary patency refers to percentage of accesses that are usable at 1 year, but required some sort of intervention in the interval. Diastat = Expanded PTFE graft with a mesh cannulation segment; Plasma-TFE = plasma polymerized woven Dacron tetrafluoroethylene; Poly-U = polyurethane; PE-PEUG = polyurethane vascular access graft coated with gelatin and reinforced with knitted polyester fibers; PTFE-sil = double wall PTFE graft with a silicone rubber middle layer.

Alternative approaches to dealing with access stenosis have been developed using percutaneous techniques [94]. Flexible, self-expanding metallic endoprostheses were first employed in 1989 for the treatment of venous outflow stenoses [95]; however, the early experience with stents was not favorable [96]. Central venous stenosis of the subclavian or innominate veins is not readily amenable to surgical techniques and has been approached with stenting [97, 98]. Wallstents and Craggstents have been used with better success than the earlier stent models, but recurrent thrombosis is a major obstacle to overall success [99–103]. The long-term utility of these stents, especially when exposed to ongoing needle punctures, is problematic [104]. Stenting is a reasonable approach when surgical access to the site of stenosis is awkward, but does not provide better overall outcome to surgical jump graft repairs of stenotic regions of an access [105]. Wallstents are also useful for pseudoaneurysm revisions and access salvaged and repair [106, 107].

Vascular Steal

The access flow volume is a critical determinant of adequacy of the access for optimal clearance, but excessive arteriovenous flow can compromise arterial perfusion of the more distal aspects of the extremities with resultant ischemic pain ('steal' syndrome). The syndrome is common in diabetics, develops several months after access placement, and can include ischemic pain, tissue loss due to digital ischemia, and trophic changes, and loss of neurologic function. Brachioaxillary grafts have been described as impairing intradialytic coronary perfusion in patients in whom ipsilateral internal thoracic artery grafts were used for myocardial revascularization [108]. Several approaches have been explored to prevent and/or treat distal vascular steal. Tapered grafts have been used, as well as banding of the graft in its mid-portion to limit flow [25, 109]. Partial ligation of the graft combined with distal revascularization has been relatively successful [110]. Monitoring pulse waveforms during the course of banding of the arterial end of a graft can be used to optimize flow through the graft and minimize distal hypoperfusion [111].

Stapled Anastomosis and Vascular Clip Systems

Suturing of artificial vascular access materials at the arterial and venous anastomosis has been well recognized as a potential source of difficulty that can result in immediate graft thrombosis even in the operative setting. This challenge seems to be especially notable with polyurethane grafts [78]. Continued technical developments along these lines may be worthwhile, and include vascular clip systems and reabsorbable cuffs at the anastomosis site [112–114]. The incidence of neointimal hyperplasia may be reduced by nonpenetrating stapling procedures, but no obvious effect on outcome has been appreciated [115]. Venous collars do not improve primary patency rates [116], and may even accelerate stenosis at the venous anastomosis [117].

Infections and Access Salvage

While venous anastomotic hyperplasia and thrombosis are the most commonly encountered problems that limit long-term success of grafts, access infections are equally problematic with even fewer options for graft salvage other than resection [23, 118, 119]. The relative risk of infection with grafts is markedly increased compared to fistulae [120], and graft infections are directly associated with substantial morbidity, prolonged dependence on temporary dialysis catheters, and multiple vascular-access procedures [121].

Graft infections are often associated with sites of damage to the graft wall secondary to trauma associated with cannulation [119, 122]. Careful needle puncture technique, systematic rotation of puncture sites, and the use of rigorous aseptic technique are essential for preserving the long-term structural integrity of PTFE grafts [122]. An improved design of graft materials and cannulation devices would be important developments that could prolong the useful lifetime of grafts [123]. Short-term catheters are often utilized as bridging accesses until more permanent access is available; in this setting there has been understandable interest in self-sealing graft materials that permit immediate cannulation following access construction [72, 124, 125]. Infection rates are clearly higher with grafts than arteriovenous fistulae, but perhaps surprisingly, the infection rate is similar for grafts in the lower extremities compared to upper extremity grafts [32, 36]. It has been possible to isolate infected segments of infected grafts, and bypass these areas with segmental bypass and partial graft excisions [93]. Stenting of an infected access introduces another foreign body at the site of infection [102]. Autologous vein grafts and even heterologous vein grafts may provide some advantages over synthetic materials when salvage of infected grafts is attempted [87, 88, 126–128]. Salvage attempts with infected grafts are uniformly more successful than with infected arteriovenous fistulae [129], but salvage of infected thigh grafts with this approach is only modestly successful [89].

Other Considerations

Predictors of Successful Graft Outcome and Salvage

There is uniform agreement about the desirability of arteriovenous fistulae over grafts [1, 2]. Even if the venous anatomy is such that transposition is required to construct a fistula, the primary and secondary patency rates are better than with grafts [10]. There are a variety of patient demographic and anatomic aspects that require the use of grafts [130, 131]. In a prospective cohort study, diabetes and serum lipoprotein (a) values in the upper tertile (≥ 57 mg/dl) and age were associated with an increased risk of vascular access occlusion in white and Hispanic patients, but not in black patients, while an increased risk of access occlusion in blacks was associated with PTFE grafts compared to fistulae, low systolic blood pressure and diabetes [132]. Miller et al. [16] reported lower primary patency of grafts in patients with hypoalbuminemia. In prospective evaluations, there was an increased risk of vascular access thrombosis associated with decreased access blood flow assessed with ultrasound dilution techniques [80]; the relative short-term risk of PTFE thrombosis decreased directly with access blood flow, with a relative risk of 2.39 for blood flows of 650 ml/min compared to the reference values of 1,134 ml/min [133].

Preoperative vascular mapping by ultrasound before hemodialysis access placement can directly impact surgical management, with an increased number of arteriovenous fistulae, and an improved likelihood of selecting the most appropriate vessels preoperatively to enhance successful outcomes for both fistulae and grafts [21, 134, 135]. Coexistent vascular disease, number of previous access attempts, use of radial artery and brachial veins, and acute arterial angulations are associated with higher risks of primary or early graft failure [15, 136, 137].

Elective correction of abnormalities in PTFE grafts and in arteriovenous fistulae can prolong the useful life of the access when compared to repair after an initial episode of clotting. Elective revision also decreased the subsequent number of clotting episodes per patient year and the total number of interventions (revisions and thrombectomies) per patient year in both grafts and fistulae [138]. While there is debate about the timing of thrombectomy of a clotted access [139], and the relative merits of surgical versus mechanical and enzymatic methods of thrombectomy [140, 141], there is no doubt that preemptive angioplasty of precritical lesions can extend the useful lifetime of a graft [19, 142], even though surgical revision of such grafts is of limited utility [143]. Multiple attempts at salvage with percutaneous rather than surgical approaches are cost-effective [140], and prospective indices for favorable outcomes are being developed [19].

Pharmacologic Approaches to Graft Patency

Failure of arteriovenous accesses used for chronic hemodialysis is most commonly associated with venous stenosis near the anastomosis, and is 3-fold more frequent with grafts (45%) than fistulae (16%) [144]. Failure occurs sooner after graft placement compared to fistulae. Advanced patient age and use of calcium channel blockers may reduce the incidence of intimal hyperplasia, while diabetes and previous time on dialysis seem to predispose to venous stenosis [145]. Angiotensin-converting enzyme inhibitors may also reduce the development of intimal hyperplasia [146]. The possible beneficial effects of aspirin, calcium channel blockers and angiotensin-converting enzyme inhibitors have been supported by a large sample of US hemodialysis patients enrolled in the Dialysis Outcomes and Practice Patterns Study, an international, prospective, observational study [147]. A multicenter, randomized, double-blind, placebo-controlled clinical trial demonstrated that warfarin had no positive benefit on the patency rates of PTFE dialysis grafts, and was associated with an increased frequency of major bleeding episodes [148].

Stenosed venous segments exhibit marked intimal hyperplasia that is almost exclusively smooth muscle cells with extracellular matrix surrounding the smooth muscle cells in the neointima [144]. Uniform intimal gradients of actin, collagen, and proteoglycan suggest that the intimal hyperplasia is a steadily progressive, uniform proliferative response that is very much unlike atherosclerosis. These observations and analyses of hemodynamic stresses have led to the hypothesis that upstream release of platelet-derived growth factor, and shear-induced intimal injury may stimulate the myointimal proliferative response process. Design improvements of the vascular inflow at the site of the venous anastomosis may minimize shear stress-associated vascular remodeling [69, 70].

Intimal hyperplasia is characterized by the presence of smooth muscle cells, accumulation of extracellular matrix components, angiogenesis within the neointima and adventitia, and an active macrophage cell layer lining the PTFE graft material. Platelet-derived growth factor, basic fibroblast growth factor, and vascular endothelial growth factor are expressed by smooth muscle cells within the neointima, by macrophages lining both sides of the PTFE graft, and by vessels within the neointima and adventitia [149]. There appears to be involvement of cell cycle regulators in the intimal hyperplasia process [150]. The nature of the myointimal response at the venous anastomosis, the possible involvement of growth factors, and the similarities to other examples of fibro-muscular hyperplasia has stimulated interest in pharmacologic approaches that would inhibit the proliferative response and thereby prolong the useful lifetime of a graft [151].

A prospective, randomized, double-blind, placebo-controlled, parallel-group study examined the effects of antiplatelet therapy (dipyridamole and/or aspirin) on the rate of thrombosis of PTFE grafts in hemodialysis patients [152]. It appeared that dipyridamole was beneficial in patients with new PTFE grafts while aspirin did not reduce the risk of thrombosis of these grafts. Neither dipyridamole nor aspirin had any beneficial effect in patients with prior thrombosis of PTFE grafts who underwent graft revision [152]. Aspirin and ticlopidine have been shown to reduce in vivo deposition of 111-indium-labeled platelet on PTFE grafts [153]. The direct inhibitory effects of dipyridamole on both platelet-derived growth factor and basic fibroblast growth factor-induced vascular smooth muscle cell proliferation have been demonstrated in vitro [154]. Meta-analyses have suggested that both aspirin and ticlopidine may have beneficial effects on access patency and outcome [155].

A vascular endothelial growth factor D gene in an adenoviral vector that is delivered locally to the adventitial surface of a graft-vein anastomosis by means of a collagen collar device has been suggested for prevention of intimal hyperplasia at the graft-vein anastomosis site [156]. Vascular endothelial growth factor inhibits smooth muscle cell migration and proliferation, associated with increased local production of nitric oxide and prostacyclin; a multicenter prospective trial of the effectiveness of this approach has been proposed [156].

Finally, the NIH has organized a prospective study of access outcomes in a multicenter study by the Dialysis Access Consortium [157]. Two randomized placebo-controlled clinical trials have begun recruitment in January 2003. The first trial is evaluating the effects of the antiplatelet agent, clopidogrel, on prevention of early fistula failure, and the second trial is evaluating the effects of long-acting dipyridamole plus aspirin on hemodialysis graft failure [157].

Conclusions

Grafts are clearly a second choice for hemodialysis access in most patients, with arteriovenous fistulae being much preferred. The major limitation on the patency of grafts is thrombosis, most often due to intimal hyperplasia at the venous anastomosis. Infection rates are higher with grafts than fistulae, and attempts to salvage infected grafts are problematic. Surveillance of access patency has proven to be cost-effective since overall patency is improved for grafts that are prospectively kept patent with angioplasty rather than performing thrombectomy on clotted grafts that invariably have an anatomic defect that is usually at the venous end of the graft. Newer reinforced and multilayer materials have been developed that permit very early cannulation compared to the usual PTFE graft. Although this advantage is very attractive in the section repair of stenoses and/or infected accesses, and would minimize the use of temporary catheters for access, the primary and secondary patency rates for these materials do not yet compare with standard PTFE grafts. Further improvements in the flow characteristics of grafts, and even chronic pharmacologic interventions for high-risk grafts may improve the overall patency rates for grafts.

References

1 NKF-DOQI Clinical Practice Guidelines for Vascular Access: National Kidney Foundation-Dialysis Outcomes Quality Initiative. Am J Kidney Dis 1997;30:S150–S191.
2 III. NKF-K/DOQI Clinical Practice Guidelines for Vascular Access: Update 2000. Am J Kidney Dis 2001;37:S137–S181.
3 Allon M, Robbin ML: Increasing arteriovenous fistulas in hemodialysis patients: Problems and solutions. Kidney Int 2002;62:1109–1124.
4 Hirth RA, Turenne MN, Woods JD, Young EW, Port FK, Pauly MV, Held PJ: Predictors of type of vascular access in hemodialysis patients. JAMA 1996;276:1303–1308.
5 Allon M, Ornt DB, Schwab SJ, Rasmussen C, Delmez JA, Greene T, Kusek JW, Martin AA, Minda S: Factors associated with the prevalence of arteriovenous fistulas in hemodialysis patients in the HEMO study. Hemodialysis (HEMO) Study Group. Kidney Int 2000;58:2178–2185.
6 Pisoni RL, Young EW, Dykstra DM, Greenwood RN, Hecking E, Gillespie B, Wolfe RA, Goodkin DA, Held PJ: Vascular access use in Europe and the United States: Results from the DOPPS. Kidney Int 2002;61:305–316.
7 Rayner HC, Pisoni RL, Gillespie BW, Goodkin DA, Akiba T, Akizawa T, Saito A, Young EW, Port FK: Creation, cannulation and survival of arteriovenous fistulae: Data from the Dialysis Outcomes and Practice Patterns Study. Kidney Int 2003;63:323–330.
8 Culp K, Flanigan M, Taylor L, Rothstein M: Vascular access thrombosis in new hemodialysis patients. Am J Kidney Dis 1995;26:341–346.
9 Young EW, Dykstra DM, Goodkin DA, Mapes DL, Wolfe RA, Held PJ: Hemodialysis vascular access preferences and outcomes in the Dialysis Outcomes and Practice Patterns Study (DOPPS). Kidney Int 2002;61:2266–2271.
10 Gibson KD, Gillen DL, Caps MT, Kohler TR, Sherrard DJ, Stehman-Breen CO: Vascular access survival and incidence of revisions: A comparison of prosthetic grafts, simple autogenous fistulas, and venous transposition fistulas from the United States Renal Data System Dialysis Morbidity and Mortality Study. J Vasc Surg 2001;34:694–700.
11 Sands JJ, Ferrell LM, Perry MA: Systemic barriers to improving vascular access outcomes. Adv Ren Replace Ther 2002;9:109–115.
12 Stehman-Breen CO, Sherrard DJ, Gillen D, Caps M: Determinants of type and timing of initial permanent hemodialysis vascular access. Kidney Int 2000;57:639–645.
13 Keoghane SR, Leow CK, Gray DW: Routine use of arteriovenous fistula construction to dilate the venous outflow prior to insertion of an expanded polytetrafluoroethylene (PTFE) loop graft for dialysis. Nephrol Dial Transplant 1993;8:154–156.
14 Kherlakian GM, Roedersheimer LR, Arbaugh JJ, Newmark KJ, King LR: Comparison of autogenous fistula versus expanded polytetrafluoroethylene graft fistula for angioaccess in hemodialysis. Am J Surg 1986;152:238–243.
15 Hodges TC, Fillinger MF, Zwolak RM, Walsh DB, Bech F, Cronenwett JL: Longitudinal comparison of dialysis access methods: Risk factors for failure. J Vasc Surg 1997;26:1009–1019.
16 Miller PE, Carlton D, Deierhoi MH, Redden DT, Allon M: Natural history of arteriovenous grafts in hemodialysis patients. Am J Kidney Dis 2000;36:68–74.
17 Astor BC, Coresh J, Powe NR, Eustace JA, Klag MJ: Relation between gender and vascular access complications in hemodialysis patients. Am J Kidney Dis 2000;36:1126–1134.
18 Allon M, Bailey R, Ballard R, Deierhoi MH, Hamrick K, Oser R, Rhynes VK, Robbin ML, Saddekni S, Zeigler ST: A multidisciplinary approach to hemodialysis access: Prospective evaluation. Kidney Int 1998;53:473–479.
19 Lilly RZ, Carlton D, Barker J, Saddekni S, Hamrick K, Oser R, Westfall AO, Allon M: Predictors of arteriovenous graft patency after radiologic intervention in hemodialysis patients. Am J Kidney Dis 2001;37:945–953.
20 Ascher E, Gade P, Hingorani A, Mazzariol F, Gunduz Y, Fodera M, Yorkovich W: Changes in the practice of angioaccess surgery: Impact of dialysis outcome and quality initiative recommendations. J Vasc Surg 2000;31:84–92.

21 Allon M, Lockhart ME, Lilly RZ, Gallichio MH, Young CJ, Barker J, Deierhoi MH, Robbin ML: Effect of preoperative sonographic mapping on vascular access outcomes in hemodialysis patients. Kidney Int 2001;60:2013–2020.

22 Fullerton JK, McLafferty RB, Ramsey DE, Solis MS, Gruneiro LA, Hodgson KJ: Pitfalls in achieving the Dialysis Outcome Quality Initiative (DOQI) guidelines for hemodialysis access? Ann Vasc Surg 2002;16:613–617.

23 Munda R, First MR, Alexander JW, Linnemann CC Jr, Fidler JP, Kittur D: Polytetrafluoroethylene graft survival in hemodialysis. JAMA 1983;249:219–222.

24 Hylander B, Fernstrom A, Swedenborg J: Interposition graft fistulas for hemodialysis. Acta Chir Scand 1988;154:107–110.

25 Polo JR, Tejedor A, Polo J, Sanabia J, Calleja J, Gomez F: Long-term follow-up of 6–8 mm brachioaxillary polytetrafluoroethylene grafts for hemodialysis. Artif Organs 1995;19:1181–1184.

26 Lazarides MK, Iatrou CE, Karanikas ID, Kaperonis NM, Petras DI, Zirogiannis PN, Dayantas JN: Factors affecting the lifespan of autologous and synthetic arteriovenous access routes for haemodialysis. Eur J Surg 1996;162:297–301.

27 Savader SJ, Lund GB, Scheel PJ: Forearm loop, upper arm straight, and brachial-internal jugular vein dialysis grafts: A comparison study of graft survival utilizing a combined percutaneous endovascular and surgical maintenance approach. J Vasc Interv Radiol 1999;10:537–545.

28 Pontari MA, McMillen MA: The straight radial-antecubital PTFE angio-access graft in an era of high-flux dialysis. Am J Surg 1991;161:450–453.

29 Dammers R, Planken RN, Pouls KP, Van Det RJ, Burger H, Van der Sande FM, Tordoir JH: Evaluation of 4-mm to 7-mm versus 6-mm prosthetic brachial-antecubital forearm loop access for hemodialysis: Results of a randomized multicenter clinical trial. J Vasc Surg 2003;37:143–148.

30 Dammers R, Planken RN, Pouls KP, van Det RJ, Burger H, van der Sande F, Tordoir JH: Multicenter evaluation of the 4–7 mm versus 6-mm stretch PTFE graft for hemodialysis vascular access: Results of a prospective clinical trial; in Henry M (ed): Vascular Access for Hemodialysis. Arlington Heights, Access Medical Press, 2002, vol 8, pp 75–86.

31 Polo JR, Vazquez R, Polo J, Sanabia J, Rueda JA, Lopez-Baena JA: Brachiocephalic jump graft fistula: An alternative for dialysis use of elbow crease veins. Am J Kidney Dis 1999;33:904–909.

32 Tashjian DB, Lipkowitz GS, Madden RL, Kaufman JL, Rhee SW, Berman J, Norris M, McCall J: Safety and efficacy of femoral-based hemodialysis access grafts. J Vasc Surg 2002;35:691–693.

33 Slater ND, Raftery AT: An evaluation of expanded polytetrafluoroethylene (PTFE) loop grafts in the thigh as vascular access for haemodialysis in patients with access problems. Ann R Coll Surg Engl 1988;70:243–245.

34 Bhandari S, Wilkinson A, Sellars L: Saphenous vein forearm grafts and gortex thigh grafts as alternative forms of vascular access. Clin Nephrol 1995;44:325–328.

35 Vogel KM, Martino MA, O'Brien SP, Kerstein MD: Complications of lower extremity arteriovenous grafts in patients with end-stage renal disease. South Med J 2000;93:593–595.

36 Korzets A, Ori Y, Baytner S, Zevin D, Chagnac A, Weinstein T, Herman M, Agmon M, Gafter U: The femoral artery-femoral vein polytetrafluoroethylene graft: A 14-year retrospective study. Nephrol Dial Transplant 1998;13:1215–1220.

37 Taylor SM, Eaves GL, Weatherford DA, McAlhany JC Jr, Russell HE, Langan EM 3rd: Results and complications of arteriovenous access dialysis grafts in the lower extremity: A five year review. Am Surg 1996;62:188–191.

38 Gradman WS, Cohen W, Haji-Aghaii M: Arteriovenous fistula construction in the thigh with transposed superficial femoral vein: Our initial experience. J Vasc Surg 2001;33:968–975.

39 O'Hare A, Johansen K: Lower-extremity peripheral arterial disease among patients with end-stage renal disease. J Am Soc Nephrol 2001;12:2838–2847.

40 Reddan DN, Marcus RJ, Owen WF Jr, Szczech LA, Landwehr DM: Long-term outcomes of revascularization for peripheral vascular disease in end-stage renal disease patients. Am J Kidney Dis 2001;38:57–63.

41 Ramdev P, Rayan SS, Sheahan M, Hamdan AD, Logerfo FW, Akbari CM, Campbell DR, Pomposelli FB Jr: A decade experience with infrainguinal revascularization in a dialysis-dependent patient population. J Vasc Surg 2002;36:969–974.

42 Biancari F, Kantonen I, Matzke S, Alback A, Roth WD, Edgren J, Lepantalo M: Infrainguinal endovascular and bypass surgery for critical leg ischemia in patients on long-term dialysis. Ann Vasc Surg 2002;16:210–214.

43 Polo JR, Sanabia J, Garcia-Sabrido JL, Luno J, Menarguez C, Echenagusia A: Brachial-jugular polytetrafluoroethylene fistulas for hemodialysis. Am J Kidney Dis 1990;16:465–468.

44 McCann RL: Axillary grafts for difficult hemodialysis access. J Vasc Surg 1996;24:457–461.

45 Rueckmann I, Berry C, Ouriel K, Hoffart N: The synthetic axillofemoral graft for hemodialysis access. ANNA J 1991;18:567–571.

46 El-Sabrout RA, Duncan JM: Right atrial bypass grafting for central venous obstruction associated with dialysis access: Another treatment option. J Vasc Surg 1999;29:472–478.

47 Baker LD Jr, Johnson JM, Goldfarb D: Expanded polytetrafluoroethylene (PTFE) subcutaneous arteriovenous conduit: An improved vascular access for chronic hemodialysis. Trans Am Soc Artif Intern Organs 1976;22:382–387.

48 Elliott MP, Gazzaniga AB, Thomas JM, Haiduc NJ, Rosen SM: Use of expanded polytetrafluoroethylene grafts for vascular access in hemodialysis: Laboratory and clinical evaluation. Am Surg 1977;43:455–459.

49 Lemaitre P, Ackman CF, O'Regan S, Laplante MP, Kaye M: Polytetrafluoroethylene (PTFE) grafts for hemodialysis. 18 months' experience. Clin Nephrol 1978;10:27–31.

50 Haimov M: Clinical experience with the expanded polytetrafluoroethylene vascular prosthesis. Angiology 1978;29:1–6.

51 May J, Harris J, Patrick W: Polytetrafluoroethylene (PTFE) grafts for haemodialysis: Patency and complications compared with those of saphenous vein grafts. Aust NZ J Surg 1979;49:639–642.

52 Haimov H, Giron F, Jacobson JH 2nd: The expanded polytetrafluoroethylene graft. Three years' experience with 362 grafts. Arch Surg 1979;114:673–677.

53 Rapaport A, Noon GP, McCollum CH: Polytetrafluoroethylene (PTFE) grafts for haemodialysis in chronic renal failure: Assessment of durability and function at three years. Aust NZ J Surg 1981; 51:562–566.

54 Raju S: PTFE grafts for hemodialysis access. Techniques for insertion and management of complications. Ann Surg 1987;206:666–673.

55 Schuman ES, Standage BA, Ragsdale JW, Gross GF: Reinforced versus nonreinforced polytetrafluoroethylene grafts for hemodialysis access. Am J Surg 1997;173:407–410.

56 Almonacid PJ, Pallares EC, Rodriguez AQ, Valdes JS, Rueda Orgaz JA, Polo JR: Comparative study of use of Diastat versus standard wall PTFE grafts in upper arm hemodialysis access. Ann Vasc Surg 2000;14:659–662.

57 Kaufman JL, Garb JL, Berman JA, Rhee SW, Norris MA, Friedmann P: A prospective comparison of two expanded polytetrafluoroethylene grafts for linear forearm hemodialysis access: Does the manufacturer matter? J Am Coll Surg 1997;185:74–79.

58 Hurlbert SN, Mattos MA, Henretta JP, Ramsey DE, Barkmeier LD, Hodgson KJ, Summer DS: Long-term patency rates, complications and cost-effectiveness of polytetrafluoroethylene (PTFE) grafts for hemodialysis access: A prospective study that compares Impra versus Gore-Tex grafts. Cardiovasc Surg 1998;6:652–656.

59 Kester RC: Reinforced expanded polytetrafluoroethylene (Gore-Tex) grafts for haemodialysis. Biomater Med Devices Artif Organs 1978;6:331–340.

60 Rizzuti RP, Hale JC, Burkart TE: Extended patency of expanded polytetrafluoroethylene grafts for vascular access using optimal configuration and revisions. Surg Gynecol Obstet 1988;166:23–27.

61 Jaffers G, Angstadt JD, Bowman JS 3rd: Early cannulation of plasma TFE and Gore-Tex grafts for hemodialysis: A prospective randomized study. Am J Nephrol 1991;11:369–373.

62 Tordoir JH, Hofstra L, Leunissen KM, Kitslaar PJ: Early experience with stretch polytetrafluoroethylene grafts for haemodialysis access surgery: Results of a prospective randomised study. Eur J Vasc Endovasc Surg 1995;9:305–309.

63 Bartlett ST, Schweitzer EJ, Roberts JE, Jaekels JL, Sandager GL, Johnson LB, Killewich LA: Early experience with a new ePTFE vascular prosthesis for hemodialysis. Am J Surg 1995;170:118–122.

64 Lenz BJ, Veldenz HC, Dennis JW, Khansarinia S, Atteberry LR: A three-year follow-up on standard versus thin wall ePTFE grafts for hemodialysis. J Vasc Surg 1998;28:464–470.

65 Ferraresso M, Deotto L, Conte F, Sessa A, Mascia G: One-year experience with a new expanded polytetrafluoroethylene vascular graft for hemodialysis. Int J Surg Investig 1999;1:185–190.

66 Coyne DW, Lowell JA, Windus DW, Delmez JA, Shenoy S, Audrain J, Howard TK: Comparison of survival of an expanded polytetrafluoroethylene graft designed for early cannulation to standard wall polytetrafluoroethylene grafts. J Am Coll Surg 1996;183:401–405.

67 Lohr JM, James KV, Hearn AT, Ogden SA: Lessons learned from the DIASTAT vascular access graft. Am J Surg 1996;172:205–209.

68 Cinat ME, Hopkins J, Wilson SE: A prospective evaluation of PTFE graft patency and surveillance techniques in hemodialysis access. Ann Vasc Surg 1999;13:191–198.

69 Nyberg SL, Hughes CB, Valenzuela YM, Jenson BM, Benda MM, McCarthy JT, Sterioff S, Stegall MD: Preliminary experience with a cuffed ePTFE graft for hemodialysis vascular access. ASAIO J 2001;47:333–337.

70 Sorom AJ, Hughes CB, McCarthy JT, Jenson BM, Prieto M, Panneton JM, Sterioff S, Stegall MD, Nyberg SL: Prospective, randomized evaluation of a cuffed expanded polytetrafluoroethylene graft for hemodialysis vascular access. Surgery 2002;132:135–140.

71 Szycher M: End-stage renal disease (ESRD) and vascular access grafting: A critical review. J Biomater Appl 1999;13:297–350.

72 Schanzer H, Martinelli G, Chiang K, Burrows L, Peirce EC 2nd: Clinical trials of a new poly-tetrafluoroethylene-silicone graft. Am J Surg 1989;158:117–120.

73 Schanzer H, Martinelli G, Burrows L, Chiang K, Peirce EC 2nd: Clinical trial of a self-sealing PTFE-silicone dialysis graft. ASAIO Trans 1989;35:211–213.

74 Helling TS, Nelson PW, Shelton L: A prospective evaluation of plasma-TFE and expanded PTFE grafts for routine and early use as vascular access during hemodialysis. Ann Surg 1992;216: 596–599.

75 Ota K, Nakagawa Y, Kitano Y, Oshima T, Teraoka S: Clinical application of modified polyurethane graft to blood access. Artif Organs 1991;15:449–453.

76 Nakagawa Y, Ota K, Sato Y, Teraoka S, Agishi T: Clinical trial of new polyurethane vascular grafts for hemodialysis: Compared with expanded polytetrafluoroethylene grafts. Artif Organs 1995;19: 1227–1232.

77 Allen RD, Yuill E, Nankivell BJ, Francis DM: Australian multicentre evaluation of a new polyurethane vascular access graft. Aust NZ J Surg 1996;66:738–742.

78 Nakao A, Miyazaki M, Oka Y, Matsuda H, Oishi M, Kokumai Y, Kunitomo K, Isozaki H, Tanaka N: Creation and use of a composite polyurethane-expanded polytetrafluoroethylene graft for hemo-dialysis access. Acta Med Okayama 2000;54:91–94.

79 Glickman MH, Stokes GK, Ross JR, Schuman ED, Sternbergh WC 3rd, Lindberg JS, Money SM, Lorber MI: Multicenter evaluation of a polytetrafluoroethylene vascular access graft as compared with the expanded polytetrafluoroethylene vascular access graft in hemodialysis applications. J Vasc Surg 2001;34:465–472.

80 Wiese P, Blume J, Mueller HJ, Renner H, Nonnast-Daniel AB: Clinical and Doppler ultrasonog-raphy data of a polyurethane vascular access graft for haemodialysis: A prospective study. Nephrol Dial Transplant 2003;18:1397–1400.

81 Richie RE, Withers EH, Petracek MR, Conkle DM: Vascular access for chronic hemodialysis: Use of bovine xenografts to create arteriovenous fistulas. South Med J 1978;71:386–388.

82 Haimov M, Burrows L, Schanzer H, Neff M, Baez A, Kwun K, Slifkin R: Experience with arte-rial substitutes in the construction of vascular access for hemodialysis. J Cardiovasc Surg (Torino) 1980;21:149–154.

83 Salmon PA: Vascular access for hemodialysis using bovine heterografts and polytetrafluoroethyl-ene conduits. Can J Surg 1981;24:59–63.

84 Doyle DL, Fry PD: Polytetrafluoroethylene and bovine grafts for vascular access in patients on long-term hemodialysis. Can J Surg 1982;25:379–382.

85 Enzler MA, Rajmon T, Lachat M, Largiader F: Long-term function of vascular access for hemodialysis. Clin Transplant 1996;10:511–515.

86 Bosman PJ, Blankestijn PJ, van der Graaf Y, Heintjes RJ, Koomans HA, Eikelboom BC: A com-parison between PTFE and denatured homologous vein grafts for haemodialysis access:

A prospective randomised multicentre trial. The SMASH Study Group. Study of Graft Materials in Access for Haemodialysis. Eur J Vasc Endovasc Surg 1998;16:126–132.

87   Matsuura JH, Johansen KH, Rosenthal D, Clark MD, Clarke KA, Kirby LB: Cryopreserved femoral vein grafts for difficult hemodialysis access. Ann Vasc Surg 2000;14:50–55.

88   Matsuura JH, Rosenthal D, Wellons ED, Castronovo CS, Fronk D: Hemodialysis graft infections treated with cryopreserved femoral vein. Cardiovasc Surg 2002;10:561–565.

89   Bolton WD, Cull DL, Taylor SM, Carsten CG 3rd, Snyder BA, Sullivan TM, Youkey JR, Langan EM 3rd, Gray BH: The use of cryopreserved femoral vein grafts for hemodialysis access in patients at high risk for infection: A word of caution. J Vasc Surg 2002;36:464–468.

90   Chen CY, Teoh MK: Graft rescue for haemodialysis arterio-venous grafts: Is it worth doing and which factors predict a good outcome? J R Coll Surg Edinb 1998;43:248–250.

91   Ayarragaray JE: Surgical treatment of hemodialysis-related central venous stenosis or occlusion: Another option to maintain vascular access. J Vasc Surg 2003;37:1043–1046.

92   Myers JL, Mukherjee D: Bypass graft to the contralateral internal jugular vein for venous outflow obstruction of a functioning hemodialysis access fistula. J Vasc Surg 2000;32:818–820.

93   Schwab DP, Taylor SM, Cull DL, Langan EM 3rd, Snyder BA, Sullivan TM, Youkey JR: Isolated arteriovenous dialysis access graft segment infection: The results of segmental bypass and partial graft excision. Ann Vasc Surg 2000;14:63–66.

94   Beathard GA: Angioplasty for arteriovenous grafts and fistulae. Semin Nephrol 2002;22: 202–210.

95   Gunther RW, Vorwerk D, Bohndorf K, Klose KC, Kistler D, Mann H, Sieberth HG, el-Din A: Venous stenoses in dialysis shunts: Treatment with self-expanding metallic stents. Radiology 1989;170:401–405.

96   Beathard GA: Gianturco self-expanding stent in the treatment of stenosis in dialysis access grafts. Kidney Int 1993;43:872–877.

97   Shoenfeld R, Hermans H, Novick A, Brener B, Cordero P, Eisenbud D, Mody S, Goldenkranz R, Parsonnet V: Stenting of proximal venous obstructions to maintain hemodialysis access. J Vasc Surg 1994;19:532–539.

98   Vorwerk D, Guenther RW, Mann H, Bohndorf K, Keulers P, Alzen G, Sohn M, Kistler D: Venous stenosis and occlusion in hemodialysis shunts: Follow-up results of stent placement in 65 patients. Radiology 1995;195:140–146.

99   Turmel-Rodrigues LA, Blanchard D, Pengloan J, Sapoval M, Baudin S, Testou D, Mouton A, Abaza M: Wallstents and Craggstents in hemodialysis grafts and fistulas: Results for selective indications. J Vasc Interv Radiol 1997;8:975–982.

100   Funaki B, Szymski GX, Leef JA, Rosenblum JD, Burke R, Hackworth CA: Wallstent deployment to salvage dialysis graft thrombolysis complicated by venous rupture: Early and intermediate results. AJR Am J Roentgenol 1997;169:1435–1437.

101   Vesely TM, Hovsepian DM, Pilgram TK, Coyne DW, Shenoy S: Upper extremity central venous obstruction in hemodialysis patients: Treatment with Wallstents. Radiology 1997;204:343–348.

102   Funaki B, Szymski GX, Leef JA, Funaki AN, Lorenz J, Farrell T, Rosenblum JD, Schmidt J: Treatment of venous outflow stenoses in thigh grafts with Wallstents. AJR Am J Roentgenol 1999; 172:1591–1596.

103   Patel RI, Peck SH, Cooper SG, Epstein DM, Sofocleous CT, Schur I, Falk A: Patency of Wallstents placed across the venous anastomosis of hemodialysis grafts after percutaneous recanalization. Radiology 1998;209:365–370.

104   Zaleski GX, Funaki B, Rosenblum J, Theoharis J, Leef J: Metallic stents deployed in synthetic arteriovenous hemodialysis grafts. AJR Am J Roentgenol 2001;176:1515–1519.

105   Lombardi JV, Dougherty MJ, Veitia N, Somal J, Calligaro KD: A comparison of patch angioplasty and stenting for axillary venous stenoses of thrombosed hemodialysis grafts. Vasc Endovascular Surg 2002;36:223–229.

106   Rajan DK, Clark TW: Patency of Wallstents placed at the venous anastomosis of dialysis grafts for salvage of angioplasty-induced rupture. Cardiovasc Intervent Radiol 2003;26, in press.

107   Lin PH, Johnson CK, Pullium JK, Koffron AJ, Conklin B, Terramani TT, Bush R, Chen C, Lumsden AB: Transluminal stent graft repair with Wallgraft endoprothesis in a porcine arteri-ovenous graft pseudoaneurysm model. J Vasc Surg 2003;37:175–181.

108   Gaudino M, Serricchio M, Luciani N, Giungi S, Salica A, Pola R, Pola P, Luciani G, Possati G: Risks of using internal thoracic artery grafts in patients in chronic hemodialysis via upper extremity arteriovenous fistula. Circulation 2003;107:2653–2655.

109   Rosental JJ, Bell DD, Gaspar MR, Movius HJ, Lemire GG: Prevention of high flow problems of arteriovenous grafts. Development of a new tapered graft. Am J Surg 1980;140:231–233.

110   Knox RC, Berman SS, Hughes JD, Gentile AT, Mills JL: Distal revascularization-interval ligation: A durable and effective treatment for ischemic steal syndrome after hemodialysis access. J Vasc Surg 2002;36:250–256.

111   Mattson WJ: Recognition and treatment of vascular steal secondary to hemodialysis prostheses. Am J Surg 1987;154:198–201.

112   Schild AF, Raines J: Preliminary prospective randomized experience with vascular clips in the creation of arteriovenous fistulae for hemodialysis. Am J Surg 1999;178:33–37.

113   Sumimoto K, Tanaka I, Fukuda Y, Haruta N, Dohi K, Ito H, Tsuchiya T, Ikada Y: Non-suture end-to-end anastomoses between polytetrafluoroethylene graft and vessels for blood access. Panminerva Med 1999;41:72–77.

114   Schild AF, Pruett CS, Newman MI, Raines J, Petersen F, Konkin T, Kim P, Dickson C, Kirsch WM: The utility of the VCS clip for creation of vascular access for hemodialysis: Long-term results and intraoperative benefits. Cardiovasc Surg 2001;9:526–530.

115   Cook JW, Schuman ES, Standage BA, Heinl P: Patency and flow characteristics using stapled vascular anastomoses in dialysis grafts. Am J Surg 2001;181:24–27.

116   Lemson MS, Tordoir JH, van Det RJ, Welten RJ, Burger H, Estourgie RJ, Stroecken HJ, Leunissen KM: Effects of a venous cuff at the venous anastomosis of polytetrafluoroethylene grafts for hemodialysis vascular access. J Vasc Surg 2000;32:1155–1163.

117   Gagne PJ, Martinez J, DeMassi R, Gregory R, Parent FN, Gayle R, Meier GH 3rd, Philput C: The effect of a venous anastomosis Tyrell vein collar on the primary patency of arteriovenous grafts in patients undergoing hemodialysis. J Vasc Surg 2000;32:1149–1154.

118   Etheredge EE, Haid SD, Maeser MN, Sicard GA, Anderson CB: Salvage operations for malfunctioning polytetrafluoroethylene hemodialysis access grafts. Surgery 1983;94:464–470.

119   Tabbara MR, O'Hara PJ, Hertzer NR, Krajewski LP, Beven EG: Surgical management of infected PTFE hemodialysis grafts: Analysis of a 15-year experience. Ann Vasc Surg 1995;9:378–384.

120   Bonomo RA, Rice D, Whalen C, Linn D, Eckstein E, Shlaes DM: Risk factors associated with permanent access-site infections in chronic hemodialysis patients. Infect Control Hosp Epidemiol 1997;18:757–761.

121   Minga TE, Flanagan KH, Allon M: Clinical consequences of infected arteriovenous grafts in hemodialysis patients. Am J Kidney Dis 2001;38:975–978.

122   Delorme JM, Guidoin R, Canizales S, Charara J, How T, Marois Y, Batt M, Hallade P, Ricci M, Picetti C, et al: Vascular access for hemodialysis: Pathologic features of surgically excised ePTFE grafts. Ann Vasc Surg 1992;6:517–524.

123   Ross EA, Verlander JW, Koo LC, Hawkins IF: Minimizing hemodialysis vascular access trauma with an improved needle design. J Am Soc Nephrol 2000;11:1325–1330.

124   Dawidson IJ, Ar'Rajab A, Melone LD, Poole T, Griffin D, Risser R: Early use of the Gore-Tex stretch graft. Blood Purif 1996;14:337–344.

125   Hakaim AG, Scott TE: Durability of early prosthetic dialysis graft cannulation: Results of a prospective, nonrandomized clinical trial. J Vasc Surg 1997;25:1002–1006.

126   Deneuville M: Infection of PTFE grafts used to create arteriovenous fistulas for hemodialysis access. Ann Vasc Surg 2000;14:473–479.

127   Wilson SE: New alternatives in management of the infected vascular prosthesis. Surg Infect (Larchmt) 2001;2:171–177.

128   Lin PH, Brinkman WT, Terramani TT, Lumsden AB: Management of infected hemodialysis access grafts using cryopreserved human vein allografts. Am J Surg 2002;184:31–36.

129   Taylor B, Sigley RD, May KJ: Fate of infected and eroded hemodialysis grafts and autogenous fistulas. Am J Surg 1993;165:632–636.

130   Ifudu O, Macey LJ, Homel P, Hyppolite JC, Hong J, Sumrani N, Distant D, Sommer BG, Friedman EA: Determinants of type of initial hemodialysis vascular access. Am J Nephrol 1997;17:425–427.

131 Rodriguez JA, Armadans L, Ferrer E, Olmos A, Codina S, Bartolome J, Borrellas J, Piera L: The function of permanent vascular access. Nephrol Dial Transplant 2000;15:402–408.

132 Goldwasser P, Avram MM, Collier JT, Michel MA, Gusik SA, Mittman N: Correlates of vascular access occlusion in hemodialysis. Am J Kidney Dis 1994;24:785–794.

133 May RE, Himmelfarb J, Yenicesu M, Knights S, Ikizler TA, Schulman G, Hernanz-Schulman M, Shyr Y, Hakim RM: Predictive measures of vascular access thrombosis: A prospective study. Kidney Int 1997;52:1656–1662.

134 Robbin ML, Gallichio MH, Deierhoi MH, Young CJ, Weber TM, Allon M: US vascular mapping before hemodialysis access placement. Radiology 2000;217:83–88.

135 Wladis AR, Mesh CL, White J, Zenni GC, Fischer DB, Arbaugh JJ: Improving longevity of prosthetic dialysis grafts in patients with disadvantaged venous outflow. J Vasc Surg 2000;32: 997–1005.

136 Khan FA, Vesely TM: Arterial problems associated with dysfunctional hemodialysis grafts: Evaluation of patients at high risk for arterial disease. J Vasc Interv Radiol 2002;13:1109–1114.

137 Rosas SE, Joffe M, Burns JE, Knauss J, Brayman K, Feldman HI: Determinants of successful synthetic hemodialysis vascular access graft placement. J Vasc Surg 2003;37:1036–1042.

138 Sands JJ, Miranda CL: Prolongation of hemodialysis access survival with elective revision. Clin Nephrol 1995;44:329–333.

139 Diskin CJ, Stokes TJ, Panus LW, Thomas J, Lock S: The importance of timing of surgery for hemodialysis vascular access thrombectomy. Nephron 1997;75:233–237.

140 Mansilla AV, Toombs BD, Vaughn WK, Zeledon JI: Patency and life-spans of failing hemodialysis grafts in patients undergoing repeated percutaneous de-clotting. Tex Heart Inst J 2001;28: 249–253.

141 Green LD, Lee DS, Kucey DS: A metaanalysis comparing surgical thrombectomy, mechanical thrombectomy, and pharmacomechanical thrombolysis for thrombosed dialysis grafts. J Vasc Surg 2002;36:939–945.

142 Martin LG, MacDonald MJ, Kikeri D, Cotsonis GA, Harker LA, Lumsden AB: Prophylactic angioplasty reduces thrombosis in virgin ePTFE arteriovenous dialysis grafts with greater than 50% stenosis: Subset analysis of a prospectively randomized study. J Vasc Interv Radiol 1999;10: 389–396.

143 Alexander J, Hood D, Rowe V, Kohl R, Weaver F, Katz S: Does surgical intervention significantly prolong the patency of failed angioaccess grafts previously treated with percutaneous techniques? Ann Vasc Surg 2002;16:197–200.

144 Swedberg SH, Brown BG, Sigley R, Wight TN, Gordon D, Nicholls SC: Intimal fibromuscular hyperplasia at the venous anastomosis of PTFE grafts in hemodialysis patients. Clinical, immunocytochemical, light and electron microscopic assessment. Circulation 1989;80:1726–1736.

145 Taber TE, Maikranz PS, Haag BW, Gaylord GM, Dilley RS, Ehrman KO, Brown PB, Nelson DR, Kay DC, Roberts TL, et al: Maintenance of adequate hemodialysis access. Prevention of neointimal hyperplasia. ASAIO J 1995;41:842–846.

146 Gradzki R, Dhingra RK, Port FK, Roys E, Weitzel WF, Messana JM: Use of ACE inhibitors is associated with prolonged survival of arteriovenous grafts. Am J Kidney Dis 2001;38:1240–1244.

147 Saran R, Dykstra DM, Wolfe RA, Gillespie B, Held PJ, Young EW: Association between vascular access failure and the use of specific drugs: The Dialysis Outcomes and Practice Patterns Study (DOPPS). Am J Kidney Dis 2002;40:1255–1263.

148 Crowther MA, Clase CM, Margetts PJ, Julian J, Lambert K, Sneath D, Nagai R, Wilson S, Ingram AJ: Low-intensity warfarin is ineffective for the prevention of PTFE graft failure in patients on hemodialysis: A randomized controlled trial. J Am Soc Nephrol 2002;13:2331–2337.

149 Roy-Chaudhury P, Kelly BS, Miller MA, Reaves A, Armstrong J, Nanayakkara N, Heffelfinger SC: Venous neointimal hyperplasia in polytetrafluoroethylene dialysis grafts. Kidney Int 2001;59: 2325–2334.

150 De Graaf R, Dammers R, Vainas T, Hoeks AP, Tordoir JH: Detection of cell-cycle regulators in failed arteriovenous fistulas for haemodialysis. Nephrol Dial Transplant 2003;18:814–818.

151 Roy-Chaudhury P, Kelly BS, Zhang J, Narayana A, Desai P, Melham M, Duncan H, Heffelfinger SC: Hemodialysis vascular access dysfunction: From pathophysiology to novel therapies. Blood Purif 2003;21:99–110.

152 Sreedhara R, Himmelfarb J, Lazarus JM, Hakim RM: Anti-platelet therapy in graft thrombosis: Results of a prospective, randomized, double-blind study. Kidney Int 1994;45:1477–1483.

153 Windus DW, Santoro SA, Atkinson R, Royal HD: Effects of antiplatelet drugs on dialysis-associated platelet deposition in polytetrafluoroethylene grafts. Am J Kidney Dis 1997;29:560–564.

154 Himmelfarb J, Couper L: Dipyridamole inhibits PDGF- and bFGF-induced vascular smooth muscle cell proliferation. Kidney Int 1997;52:1671–1677.

155 Da SI, Escofet X, Rutherford PA: Medical adjuvant treatment to increase patency of arteriovenous fistulae and grafts (Cochrane Review). Cochrane Database Syst Rev 2003;CD002786.

156 Fuster V, Charlton P, Boyd A: Clinical protocol. A phase IIb, randomized, multicenter, double-blind study of the efficacy and safety of Trinam (EG004) in stenosis prevention at the graft-vein anastomosis site in dialysis patients. Hum Gene Ther 2001;12:2025–2027.

157 NIDDK/NIH: Dialysis Access Consortium. www.niddk.nih.gov/patient/DAC/DAC.htm 2002: Accessed June 15, 2003.

David G. Warnock, MD,
Room 647 THT, 1530 3rd Avenue South, UAB Station,
Birmingham, AL 35294–0006 (USA)
Tel. +1 205 934 3585, Fax +1 205 934 1879, E-Mail dwarnock@uab.edu

Ronco C, Levin NW (eds): Hemodialysis Vascular Access and Peritoneal Dialysis Access.
Contrib Nephrol. Basel, Karger, 2004, vol 142, pp 94–111

....

Temporary Vascular Access for Hemodialysis Treatment

Current Guidelines and Future Directions

Marcel C. Weijmer[a,b], Piet M. ter Wee[b]

[a] Department of Nephrology, Sint Lucas Andreas Hospital and
[b] Department of Nephrology, Vrije Universiteit Medical Center,
Amsterdam, The Netherlands

In this chapter, temporary vascular access is defined as access to the bloodstream by means of a large-vein catheter for a maximum period of 6 months to make adequate hemodialysis treatment possible. After 6 months patients should have a chronic vascular access such as an arteriovenous fistula, graft or subcutaneous port. This chapter will especially focus on current guidelines and recently published developments. We will discuss future directives that could derive from these developments.

Introduction

In current practice the use of temporary hemodialysis catheters is substantial. From the recent data of the Dialysis Outcomes and Practice Patterns Study (DOPPS), it is recognized that 15–50% of patients in Europe and 60% of patients in the US start hemodialysis treatment with a catheter for vascular access [1]. However, such widespread application of catheters exposes patients to an enhanced risk of catheter-related complications. Because of these complications about 50% of all temporary catheters have to be removed preliminarily and/or replaced, which results in substantial patient morbidity as well as additional consumption of resources, nursing and nephrologists' time [2–4]. Tokars et al. [5] demonstrated in a prospective study performed on 796 hemodialysis patients with a catheter that they had a relative risk of infection of

2.07 compared to patients with an arteriovenous fistula or graft. A third of these patients had to be hospitalized because of their infection.

In order to prevent the most important catheter-related complications, i.e. catheter-related infection and thrombosis, and to optimize the survival of a catheter a number of considerations have to be taken into account; of these an appropriate estimation of the duration for which a catheter will be needed is critically important. Other considerations include decisions on the optimal site and method of cannulation, the type of catheter and whether the catheter should be tunneled or not. In addition, the access team must determine what kind of dressing should be used and whether antimicrobial ointment and/or antimicrobial locking solutions should be applied. A thorough protocol for connecting and disconnecting bloodlines must be available, as well as a protocol on how to treat catheter-related complications. Whether postprocedural checks like chest X-rays, often postponing dialysis treatment, are really needed should be questioned.

Recently the National Kidney Foundation – Dialysis Outcome Quality Initiatives (NKF-DOQI) Clinical Practice Guidelines for Vascular Access have been updated and publicized [6]. These guidelines can be of help when making decisions on hemodialysis catheter-related procedures and on care-giving protocols. However, new strategies that may prevent catheter-related bacteremia and dysfunction, and reduce patient morbidity and mortality have emerged. In this chapter we will discuss current guidelines and recent literature focusing on the decisions a physician and the nursing team have to make when a hemodialysis catheter is needed.

Determination of the Time during Which a Catheter Is Needed

There are numerous clinical situations in dialysis when acute vascular access is required. The specific clinical situation of the patient usually determines how long a dialysis catheter is needed and what the chances for renal recovery are. These two factors determine at large the decisions on the cannulation site and on the type of catheter that is needed.

Acute Renal Failure and Exchange Therapy
In acute renal failure requiring immediate dialysis treatment and for plasma exchange therapy, vascular access by means of a temporary catheter is the best choice. Usually, a femoral catheter will be inserted because treatment can be started without delay, which sometimes is essential in cases of life-threatening hyperkalemia. The cause of renal failure can be analyzed and an approximation of the time period during which dialysis is needed can be made.

Femoral catheters should not be left in place for more than 1 week because, unlike temporary subclavian and jugular catheters, they are associated with an increased risk of infection and dysfunction within 7 days [7, 8]. In case recovery of the renal function is unlikely and the need for chronic dialysis treatment is expected, one should be reluctant to use the subclavian vein because of the high risk of central vein thrombosis [9, 10]. This can compromise arteriovenous access in the future. NKF-DOQI guidelines recommend that when it can be foreseen that a catheter is needed for more than 3 weeks, a tunneled cuffed catheter should be used. However, it has been recognized that this recommendation is largely opinion based. Indeed, recent studies suggest that a tunneled cuffed catheter should be used even earlier. We will discuss this issue in the paragraph on tunneled versus untunneled catheters.

In continuous renal replacement therapy in the intensive care unit (ICU) femoral catheters are frequently used. Although there are no data on double-lumen dialysis catheters in the ICU patient, it has been shown that femoral catheters that are used as infusion catheters have an increased risk of infection [11]. Therefore, subclavian or jugular catheters should be preferred in ICU patients.

Chronic Renal Failure and Failure of Peritoneal Dialysis Treatment
Despite the fact that increasing attention is paid to the timely creation of a functional arteriovenous fistula or graft in the predialysis care, the most common indication for a hemodialysis catheter is the start of dialysis treatment for end-stage renal failure [1]. In most of these patients creation and maturation of a functional arteriovenous access will take at least a few weeks. It is preferable to start with a jugular catheter that can provide adequate dialysis for this period. Whether this should be a tunneled catheter will be discussed in the paragraph on tunneled versus untunneled catheters.

The same accounts for the failure of peritoneal dialysis. Removal of a peritoneal dialysis catheter can be the result of persistent or relapsing peritonitis. Another common cause for interruption of peritoneal dialysis treatment is the failure of ultrafiltration. In both cases vascular access catheters often have to remain in place for months. In a substantial number of these patients, infection or ultrafiltration failure results in a definitive transition to hemodialysis.

Cannulation Sites

Once the duration for which a hemodialysis catheter is needed has been estimated, the next decision that needs to be made is what cannulation site is best. Generally, the femoral, subclavian or internal jugular veins are used.

In patients with exhausted access due to thrombosed veins or infection, exotic routes like translumbar or transhepatic routes may be necessary [12, 13]. Even long-term arterial cannulation has been used for dialysis [14]. Because these routes are rarely necessary, they will not be discussed in detail.

Femoral Vein

The femoral vein is preferred when rapid access is needed because of the underlying condition of the patient or for logistic reasons. Insertion is relatively easy, complications are rare and treatment can be started without delay. In addition, it is the preferred site when patients cannot lie flat because of dyspnea and in case of severe coagulation disturbances. With modern flexible catheters, patients can even be mobilized [15]. According to the NKF-DOQI guidelines, there are data which recommend that untunneled femoral catheters should not be left in place for more than 5–7 days because of the high risk of infections. Oliver et al. [7] demonstrated in a study on 218 patients that the subset of patients with femoral catheters was confronted with a high incidence of bacteremia when the catheter was left in place for more than 1 week (10.7%). However, in this study occlusive dressings were applied and there was no strict protocol for the removal of catheters in case of exit site infection. We found in our prospective study following 83 temporary femoral catheters that 68% had to be removed preliminarily because of complications when left in place for more than 1 week. The bacteremia rate was 7.6 periods/1,000 catheter-days compared to 1.6 periods for tunneled cuffed catheters [8].

Subclavian Vein

The NKF-DOQI guidelines recommend that the subclavian vein should not be used in patients who need permanent vascular access because of a high risk of subclavian vein thrombosis. Schillinger et al. [10] compared in a prospective study the outcome of 50 subclavian with that of 50 jugular hemodialysis catheters and found an incidence of 42% subclavian stenosis compared to 10% jugular stenosis. Subclavian stenosis and occlusion can lead to arm edema and can hamper the development of an adequate arteriovenous fistula or graft in the future. This indicates that in all patients with chronic renal failure, vascular access through the subclavian vein should be avoided. Another disadvantage of subclavian vein cannulation is that it requires more skills of the operator and is associated with more severe insertion complications such as pneumothorax and hemothorax. Notwithstanding these guidelines it was shown in the DOPPS that in the US 46% of all temporary catheters used in patients starting hemodialysis treatment were inserted into the subclavian vein. The reason for this widespread use of subclavian catheters is probably the observation that they have less infectious complications than untunneled jugular catheters [4]. They are more comfortable for the patient and provide reliable blood flow if placed in the right atrial cavity.

In conclusion, the subclavian site should only be used if a catheter is needed in patients with acute renal failure when renal replacement therapy is expected to be temporary and when the jugular site is not available.

Internal Jugular Vein

A hemodialysis catheter in the internal jugular vein is preferred for patients on chronic dialysis treatment. Cannulation is easy, and especially when inserted with the use of ultrasound localization of the vein, the complication rate is extremely low [16]. The right jugular site is preferred because of the straight intravascular route to the right atrial cavity. Left situated jugular catheters can also be used but are associated with more complications and shorter survival compared to right jugular catheters [17, 18].

The most important problem of jugular catheters is that they are uncomfortable for the patient because neck and head movements are limited. This holds especially true for straight, high-inserted, precurved catheters (fig. 1) and jugular catheters with a curved extension (fig. 2). In addition, these catheters have a higher rate of infectious complications compared to subclavian catheters [4, 8]. This is probably because adequate fixation is hampered by continuous movements of these catheters with movements of the head, and by downward pulling of dialysis tubes at the extensions when connected to the hemodialysis machine. In addition, these catheters have an upward directed exit site which in analogy to peritoneal dialysis catheters might be associated with an increased risk of exit site infections as has been demonstrated for peritoneal dialysis catheters [19, 20].

Future guidelines will probably be adapted because of clinical results from recently developed jugular catheters that are more comfortable to the patient and can be immobilized more adequately. Recently, we completed a clinical study with such a novel design, a temporary jugular catheter (11.5-french, polyurethane, Raulerson®, Medcomp, Harleysville, Pa., USA) (fig. 3) [21]. This precurved catheter was inserted into the low jugular site and placed close to the upper border of the clavicle. Thus, the catheter bends over the clavicle and can be immobilized and fixated to the chest wall. Our primary intention was to reduce the discomfort in patients needing a temporary hemodialysis catheter in the jugular vein. We prospectively analyzed infectious complications and catheter removals because of dysfunction. The outcome of 58 precurved jugular catheters was compared with observational data on 104 upward-pointing straight jugular catheters with curved extensions that had been obtained in the period before the introduction of the precurved model. The catheter care protocol was not changed after the introduction of the new catheter. Nine precurved catheters (16%, 5.0/1,000 catheter-days) had to be removed because of

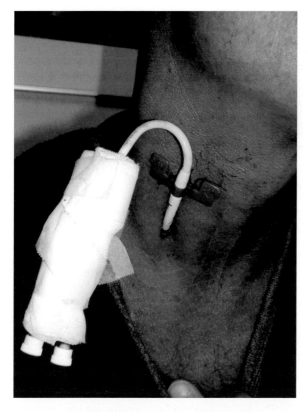

Fig. 1. Uncomfortable position and poor fixation of a straight jugular catheter.

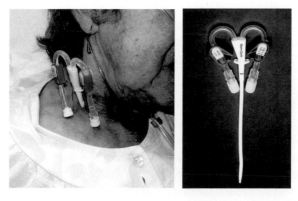

Fig. 2. Uncomfortable position and poor fixation of an untunneled jugular catheter with curved extensions.

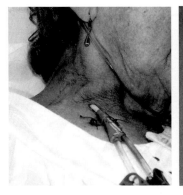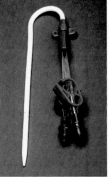

Fig. 3. Comfortable position and better fixation of an untunneled precurved jugular catheter (same patient as in fig. 2).

complications versus 54 straight catheters (56%, 16.9/1,000 catheter-days; $p < 0.01$). There were no periods of bacteremia observed in patients with a precurved catheter and only 1 exit site infection. Seventeen periods of bacteremia (5.3/1,000 catheter-days) and 29 periods of exit site infection (9.0/1,000 catheter-days) occurred in patients with a straight jugular catheter. Infection rates for tunneled catheters were similar during the period when straight jugular catheters were used and the period when precurved jugular catheters were used. This finding makes a time bias as an explanation for the favorable outcome of the precurved model unlikely. The most likely explanation for the low infection rates is the fact that the fixation of these precurved catheters makes it possible to move the head and neck without movement of the catheter. A second advantage could be the downward direction of the exit site.

From this observation, we conclude that a well-positioned, optimally fixated, precurved, untunneled jugular hemodialysis catheter is a safe option when a catheter is needed for access for a period of up to 2–3 months.

Should a Catheter Be Tunneled?

Using the limited data available on complication rates of straight untunneled jugular catheters with curved extensions, the NKF-DOQI guidelines recommend that a tunneled cuffed catheter should be inserted when it can be anticipated that a catheter will be needed for more than 3 weeks [6]. Even when a catheter is needed for less than 3 weeks, inserting a tunneled cuffed catheter is acceptable. The insertion of a tunneled cuffed catheter, however, requires prolonged time for the procedure and special skills of the operator. In addition, its removal is hampered by growth of subcutaneous tissue into the cuff. These drawbacks for the use of tunneled catheters might explain the observation in the DOPPS that untunneled catheters are still widely used beyond the recommended 3-week period. In incident hemodialysis patients, 48% of catheters in the US and 75% of catheters in Europe are untunneled and even in prevalent patients over a third of all catheters are untunneled [1]. As was pointed out recently, there are limited data available in the literature comparing the outcome of untunneled and tunneled cuffed catheters [22].

Reported bacteremia rates vary from 3.8 to 6.5/1,000 catheter-days for untunneled catheters to 1.6–5.5 for tunneled cuffed catheters [2, 4, 7, 23, 24]. In these studies, catheter care protocols and the definitions of complications differ. In addition, because untunneled catheters and tunneled cuffed catheters are used for different clinical situations, the higher incidence of complications in untunneled catheters may be caused by differences in patient characteristics and risk factors for infection. These factors all contribute to the finding that the incidence of catheter-related complications can vary widely between the types of catheters used and between the dialysis centers [5]. Therefore, a comparison of the outcome of untunneled catheters in one center with that of another center is not reliable as was recently clearly pointed out by Lund et al. [25].

Recently, we prospectively studied the outcome of all inserted catheters that had been used consecutively for more than one hemodialysis session in our department [8]. The type of catheter, the duration and place of insertion, and the reason for catheter removal over a 3-year period were analyzed. In addition, all catheter-related infectious complications were evaluated. A total of 272 hemodialysis catheters had been inserted (for a total of 11,612 catheter-days): 37 tunneled cuffed catheters, 83 temporary femoral catheters, 104 untunneled straight temporary jugular catheters with curved extensions (fig. 2) and 48 temporary subclavian catheters. Of the temporary jugular catheters, 55 (53%, 17.1/1,000 catheter-days) had to be removed because of complications. Of the temporary subclavian catheters 24 (50%, 16.1/1,000 catheter-days) and of the tunneled cuffed catheters 11 (30%, 1.8/1,000 catheter-days) had to be removed preliminarily. Infection rates for tunneled cuffed catheters (3.3/1,000 catheter-days) were substantially lower compared to temporary jugular catheters (14.3/1,000 catheter-days). To relate the results to the time recommendations in the NKF-DOQI guidelines, we calculated the patency and infection rates at 14, 21 and 28 days. We observed that for tunneled cuffed catheters actuarial catheter survival was better and infection rates were lower for every time period compared to any of the untunneled catheter groups.

It is not completely clear why tunneled cuffed catheters have a lower risk of infection. One explanation could be that the fixation of tunneled cuffed catheters can be achieved better with the use of a subcutaneous cuff and that bacterial migration from the exit site to the venous entry site is impeded [26]. A recent meta-analysis has clearly demonstrated that cuffing and tunneling of catheters reduces the risk of catheter-related bacteremia by 44–77% [27]. However, this analysis only included nonhemodialysis catheters. Untunneled jugular catheters are more difficult to fixate properly and have an upward-directed exit site.

According to our results, a tunneled cuffed catheter should be used whenever it can be foreseen that a hemodialysis catheter is needed for at least 14 days which is less than currently recommended by the NKF-DOQI. This indicates that almost no untunneled catheters should be used in daily practice.

As discussed in the paragraph on jugular catheters, we recently completed a clinical study with a temporary jugular catheter with a novel design (11.5-french, polyurethane, Raulerson) (fig. 3) [21]. This catheter can be immobilized and fixated better than previous models. In this study we also prospectively compared infectious complications and removals with tunneled cuffed catheters inserted during the same time period. A total of 58 tunneled cuffed catheters, mainly in the right jugular position, could be compared to the group of 58 patients with an untunneled precurved model. Nine precurved catheters (16%, 5.0/1,000 catheter-days) had to be removed because of complications versus 18 tunneled catheters (31%, 2.1/1,000 catheter-days). In tunneled catheters 15 periods of bacteremia (1.8/1,000 catheter-days) and 11 periods of exit site infection (1.3/1,000 catheter-days) were recorded compared to no periods of bacteremia with the novel design catheter and 1 exit site infection. Data were corrected for differences in patient characteristics. The same catheter care protocol was used and not changed at the time of the introduction of the new catheter. This observation was recently confirmed in another catheter trial [28].

In conclusion, recent studies have indicated that straight untunneled jugular catheters should not be used for more than 2 weeks but precurved, well-fixated untunneled jugular catheters can be safely left in place for a period of 2–3 months. Currently developed large-bore untunneled jugular catheters might probably even be used for longer periods but prospectively randomized studies will be needed to estimate whether these catheters can completely replace tunneled cuffed catheters when temporary access is needed.

Tip Design and Catheter Length

Many different catheter types are being offered by manufacturers and most catheters are available in multiple lengths. Both untunneled and tunneled cuffed catheters are available in silicon and different polymer plastics. Despite advertising of different types, limited data are available on what catheter type and material are best. For characterizing catheters, flow curves are often performed in static in vitro models with blood-like substances, not taking into account the possibility of coagulation and pulsatile flow. Furthermore, no model is available for the interdialytic period when the catheter is locked but remains in the blood-stream. So far none of the clinical trials has shown a major difference between different catheters [29, 30].

Geometry and Tip Design

The geometry and tip design of catheters have been determined mainly by methods of trial and error. Multiple side holes were thought to be necessary to secure sufficient inflow in the case of obstruction of some side holes or when a catheter was placed close to the vessel wall. However, side holes can induce thrombosis because they often have an irregular surface [31]. Furthermore, the diameter of the holes is not adapted to actual required flow rates. Despite the various types of catheters available, studies on the influence of tip construction on fluid dynamics are scarce. Recently, De Wachter et al. [32] presented a study on the hemodynamics of a dual-lumen dialysis catheter with 5 arterial side holes and 3 venous ones (Gamcath®, Joka Kathetertechnik, Germany). A computer flow model was used simulating a blood flow of 300 ml/min through the catheter while placed in a 3-cm-wide tube. The sequential placement of the arterial holes was demonstrated to be the reason why mainly the first available hole is employed to draw the blood into a catheter. At the distal holes of the arterial side, a low flow zone was present, suggesting an increased risk of thrombus formation in clinical use (fig. 4). Also, at the venous side the effectiveness of the multiple side hole design was questioned because the first two side holes appeared to be greatly underemployed. At the most proximal venous side hole (closest to the hub), some of the blood is even drawn into the catheter due to the high difference in velocities between catheter and vein. Another disadvantage of multiple side holes is that locking solutions can easily dissolve from the tip. The authors concluded that most currently available temporary catheters can be improved to optimize hemodynamics and reduce dysfunction. We are now using this computer model to analyze different catheter and catheter tip designs to try to determine the optimal tip construction. Preliminary data from this model reveal that double-lumen open shotgun tips are optimal and that a single large side hole is probably sufficient.

The relevance of these findings is supported by the outcomes of two recent clinical trials. Oliver et al. [18] compared a 12-french tapered tip, multiple side hole catheter with a 13.5-french open shotgun tip catheter. They demonstrated that effective blood flow was higher with the shotgun tip catheter and that there was less necessity for reversal of the lumen polarity, a well-known cause of high recirculation rates. We completed a randomized study comparing

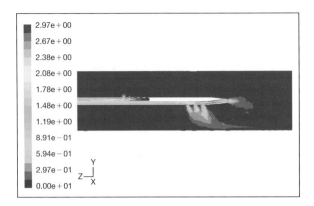

2.97e+00
2.67e+00
2.38e+00
2.08e+00
1.78e+00
1.48e+00
1.19e+00
8.91e−01
5.94e−01
2.97e−01
0.00e+01

Fig. 4. Computer model for estimation of flow distribution through a catheter with multiple side holes. Scale on the left shows flow speed. (By courtesy of D.S. de Wachter; Hydraulics Laboratory, Ibitech, University of Gent, Belgium).

30 consecutively inserted untunneled femoral catheters [33]. Patients were randomized either to a 20- or 24-cm double-lumen catheter with an open shotgun tip (Niagara®, Bard, Salt Lake City, Utah, USA) or to a 20-cm catheter with a tapered tip (Gamcath). Recirculation rates were measured at a blood flow of 200, 250 and 300 ml/min with bloodlines situated normally as well as after the reversal of pools. We could demonstrate a benefit concerning effective blood flow, recirculation rates and early failure rates for the shotgun tip catheter.

For untunneled catheters we conclude that there are good data to support the fact that 11- to 12-french catheters with a multiple side hole design should be replaced by a double-lumen open shotgun tip design with a larger diameter and no more than 1 side hole.

For tunneled cuffed catheters, two prospectively randomized studies of interest have been performed. Trerotola et al. [29] randomized 64 patients to the 14-french Ash-split catheter and 68 to the 14.5-french Opti-flow. Although they concluded that the Ash-split catheter had a better survival, the differences seemed to be caused entirely by insertion problems (kinking) and manufacturing faults (broken hubs). There were no differences in catheter-related bacteremia and late flow problems despite large differences in tip construction. Richard et al. [30] compared 38 Ash-split, 39 Opti-flow, and 36 Tesio catheters. Tesio mean insertion time (42 min) was significantly longer than Ash-split (29 min) or Opti-flow (30 min). There were more insertion complications related to Tesio catheters. Mean flow rates and catheter-related infections were not significantly different among the catheter groups.

We conclude that for tunneled cuffed catheters, one should probably choose a double-lumen catheter for ease of insertion. From currently available models is has not been shown convincingly that one cuffed catheter design is superior over another, provided that they have at least a diameter of 14 french. Therefore, the physicians' experience and cost should play an important role.

The Optimal Length of the Catheter

The current recommendation of the NKF-DOQI is that a femoral catheter should be at least 19 cm long to minimize recirculation [6]. We could show in the aforementioned trial that 24-cm shotgun tip catheters have even lower recirculation rates compared to 20-cm catheters (0 vs. 5%). Also direct dysfunction was lower, probably because longer catheters are better able to reach the inferior vena cava. Thus, for femoral use double-lumen open shotgun tip catheters of at least 24 cm can be recommended [33].

For untunneled and tunneled subclavian and jugular catheters data are less clear. NKF-DOQI guidelines recommend placement of the catheter with the tip adjusted to the level of the caval atrial junction or into the right atrium to ensure optimal blood flow. For untunneled catheters, the catheter length and diameter should be adjusted to the size of the patient. Twardowski and Seger [34] determined the exact distance from an insertion site to the right atrium by magnetic resonance imaging of the dimensions of the venous system of the chest in 31 adult volunteers and correlated them to anthropometrical measurements. The best overall correlations of the lengths and diameters of the large upper body veins were with the body surface area. A table was drawn up to help with the selection of the total catheter length and diameter in relation to the body surface area and insertion site. In general, in patients with a body surface area of 1.5–2.0 m^2 a 12- to 15-cm catheter should be selected for the jugular vein in the low right position and a 15- to 19-cm catheter for the left jugular vein. A 14- to 17-cm catheter should be used for the right subclavian vein and a 17- to 22-cm catheter for the left subclavian vein.

For tunneled cuffed catheters no guidelines for the length are available. In our experience, for the right jugular position (tip to hub) 28 cm are needed for appropriate atrial placement and an adequate tunnel length. For the left jugular vein we use a 32-cm catheter.

Catheter Materials and Coatings

In vitro data on the biocompatibility of polymers used in catheter manufacturing, namely silicon and polyurethane, are conflicting. Likewise, in small randomized trials comparing tunneled cuffed catheters of different materials and construction, no clear benefit of one particular material was found.

For temporary hemodialysis catheters there are no studies available comparing different catheter materials. We compared at our department the patency of temporary polyurethane catheters (Quinton Mahukar®, Quinton, Seattle, Wash., USA and Gamcath 11–11.5 french) and temporary silicone catheters (11.5 french, Medcomp Medical Components, Harleysville, Pa., USA) with a comparable design. There were no significant differences in the sites for insertion (jugular, femoral or subclavian). The same catheter care protocol was applied. A total of 233 temporary polyurethane catheters were compared to 51 temporary silicone catheters. Of polyurethane catheters 49 (21%) had to be removed because of complications (8.2/1,000 catheter-days) and of silicone 22 (43%; 8.9/1,000 catheter-days). Also, there were no differences in infectious complications.

We conclude that to date there is no study that shows an advantage of silicon over polyurethane for the construction of hemodialysis catheters. It might even be the case that silicone catheters are more prone to construction failures because of the difficult manufacturing process necessary [35, 36].

Promising progress is made with the coating of catheters. In ICU patients catheters coated with antibiotics, silver or heparin reduce the number of infections substantially. In a recent review, however, only heparin-coated catheters were considered to be cost-effective [10]. Studies on hemodialysis catheters have been disappointing so far [37]. A problem with bonding of hemodialysis catheters is that they are often needed for a longer period of time and the substance impregnated or bonded on catheters can disappear over time.

Guidelines for Insertion Procedures and Postprocedural Checks

Complications can be minimized when insertion is performed or supervised by an experienced physician. Both untunneled and tunneled cuffed catheters can be safely inserted under local anesthesia by nephrologists or radiologists [25, 38]. The procedure should be strictly aseptic; light sedation can be of help in anxious patients. Ultrasound-guided cannulation has proven to be superior to landmark-guided cannulation and is therefore recommended by the NKF-DOQI [6].

Femoral catheters can be inserted using a blinded percutaneous Seldinger technique, but for femoral catheters it has also been shown in dialysis patients that the procedure time can be significantly shortened with the use of ultrasound guidance [39]. The first attempt success rate increased by 30% and accidental arterial puncture decreased by about 10% [40]. For jugular and subclavian vein cannulation there is also extensive evidence for the use of ultrasound localization of the vein before puncture as well as the use of real time ultrasound-guided cannulation [16, 41]. The risk of complications such as pneumothorax, arterial puncture and fausse route can be decreased to less then 2% and procedure times are shortened. However, long-term patency and the risk of infection were not improved in these trials.

It has been demonstrated that patency rates and recirculation are affected by correct positioning of the tip of the catheter [42, 43]. Preferably, the tip should be at or just below the caval-atrial junction. Fluoroscopy during positioning has been advised by radiologists but is not always available to nephrologists and has not turned out to be better. Using the knowledge from the study of Twardowski and Seger [34] on the correlation between BSA and large vein sizes as discussed in the paragraph on catheter length, correct placement of tunneled catheters is possible without fluoroscopy.

After insertion of tunneled cuffed catheters a chest X-ray is mandatory for evaluating complications and correct positioning of the tip. However, when untunneled jugular catheters are inserted with ultrasound localization, the procedure is uncomplicated and straightforward, the blood flow is good, and there are no postprocedural complaints of the patients; there is convincing evidence that dialysis can be started safely without the use of a chest X-ray and substantial savings can be made [43–45].

Dressings, Antimicrobial Exit Site Applications and Locking Solutions

All hemodialysis catheter manipulations should be performed by carefully instructed dialysis staff. At every dialysis session, the exit site should be cleaned with a chlorhexidine-containing solution as this can reduce infectious complications by 49% compared to the use of povidone iodine [46]. It has been clearly shown that nonocclusive dry gauze dressings should be used for covering the exit site [47]. Recently, antimicrobial ointments have been introduced. Mupirocin ointment and a Polysporin triple antibiotic ointment have been shown to reduce the risk of infectious complications by 70–80% [48–50]. Therefore, mupirocin ointment has been advocated in the latest NKF-DOQI guidelines. However, widespread introduction could lead to the development of mupirocin resistance limiting its application in the future [51, 52].

Catheters have to be locked with a solution for the interdialytic period. Traditionally, heparin is installed but there are no studies to support this practice. Moreover, an increasing number of reports are published showing that leakage of heparin from the tip of the catheter can cause unintentional systemic anticoagulation and clinically relevant bleeding episodes [53, 54]. Antimicrobial locking solutions could be an attractive alternative and will emerge into clinical practice in the near future. It is known from in vitro studies that solutions containing antibiotics can prevent biofilm formation on foreign surfaces [55]. Again, the use of antibiotics in solutions for interdialytic locking of catheters can result in severe side effects caused by leakage from the tip resulting in continuous systemic levels of the antibiotic. Dogra et al. [56] demonstrated in a randomized trial that gentamicin in a lock solution reduced the number of incidents of catheter-related bacteremia but also caused irreversible hearing problems. Trisodium citrate (TSC) has been advocated for locking because it provides local anticoagulation. In vitro it has a broad antimicrobial and antiyeast effect [57]. Ash et al. [58] reported their experience with a hemodialysis patient cohort of 70 patients with 60% tunneled cuffed catheters. After the introduction of TSC 23–47% for catheter locking they observed a decline in the number of patients per month having an episode of bacteremia from 4.5 to 0%. The utilization of urokinase for catheter flow problems also decreased significantly. Additional advantages of TSC are that it prevents unforeseen systemic anticoagulation and is less expensive than heparin. Recently, we finished a double-blind, randomized controlled trial in 291 patients comparing conventional heparin with TSC 30% and could show a 73% reduction of catheter-related bacteremia [28]. We could even show a reduction of bacteremia-related mortality. Furthermore, clinically relevant bleeding episodes were reduced. No clinically relevant side effects occurred during the instillation of TSC into hemodialysis catheters in over 12,000 locking procedures [59]. This is important, as concern has risen over an accident using TSC for catheter locking. However, in this particular case, a large amount (over 10 ml) of TSC was accidentally injected by a physician not aware of the potency of the solution, which stresses the importance of a thorough protocol for these solutions [60].

In conclusion, antimicrobial lock solutions, probably those containing high concentrations of TSC, will replace heparin in the future.

Conclusion

Current guidelines on temporary vascular access by means of a hemodialysis catheter will be influenced by recent developments. It can be expected that the incidence of infectious complications that restrict long-term use of untunneled jugular catheters will decrease with the introduction of antimicrobial ointments, locking solutions and strict protocols. Recent studies on the design and construction of uncuffed jugular catheters have revealed that flow characteristics will improve and better patency rates can be reached. Until now, we can conclude that it is safe to use untunneled precurved jugular catheters for a period of 3 months. As these catheters are easier to insert, it is most likely that further improved novel models will more and more replace tunneled cuffed catheters in the future.

References

1 Pisoni RL, Young EW, Dykstra DM, Greenwood RN, Hecking E, Gillespie B, Wolfe RA, Goodkin DA, Held PJ: Vascular access use in Europe and the United States: Results from the DOPPS. Kidney Int 2002;61:305–316.
2 Little MA, O'Riordan A, Lucey B, Farrell M, Lee M, Conlon PJ, Walshe JJ: A prospective study of complications associated with cuffed, tunnelled haemodialysis catheters. Nephrol Dial Transplant 2001;16:2194–2200.
3 Weijmer MC, ter Wee PM: Temporary vascular access for hemodialysis treatment. Current guidelines and future directions. Contrib Nephrol. Basel, Karger, 2002, vol 137, pp 38–45.
4 Kairaitis LK, Gottlieb T: Outcome and complications of temporary haemodialysis catheters. Nephrol Dial Transplant 1999;14:1710–1714.
5 Tokars JI, Light P, Anderson J, Miller ER, Parrish J, Armistead N, Jarvis WR, Gehr T: A prospective study of vascular access infections at seven outpatient hemodialysis centers. Am J Kidney Dis 2001;37:1232–1240.
6 NKF-K/DOQI Clinical Practice Guidelines for Vascular Access: Update 2000. Am J Kidney Dis 2001;37:S137–S181.
7 Oliver MJ, Callery SM, Thorpe KE, Schwab SJ, Churchill DN: Risk of bacteremia from temporary hemodialysis catheters by site of insertion and duration of use: A prospective study. Kidney Int 2000;58:2543–2545.
8 Weijmer MC, Vervloet MG, ter Wee PM: Tunneled cuffed and temporary jugular catheters for hemodialysis access: Comparison of outcome. J Am Soc Nephrol 2000;11:A1066.
9 Cimochowski GE, Worley E, Rutherford WE, Sartain J, Blondin J, Harter H: Superiority of the internal jugular over the subclavian access for temporary dialysis. Nephron 1990;54:154–161.
10 Schillinger F, Schillinger D, Montagnac R, Milcent T: Postcatheterisation vein stenosis in haemodialysis: Comparative angiographic study of 50 subclavian and 50 internal jugular accesses. Nephrol Dial Transplant 1991;6:722–724.
11 Merrer J, De Jonghe B, Golliot F, Lefrant JY, Raffy B, Barre E, Rigaud JP, Casciani D, Misset B, Bosquet C, Outin H, Brun-Buisson C, Nitenberg G: Complications of femoral and subclavian venous catheterization in critically ill patients: A randomized controlled trial. JAMA 2001;286: 700–707.
12 Po CL, Koolpe HA, Allen S, Alvez LD, Raja RM: Transhepatic PermCath for hemodialysis. Am J Kidney Dis 1994;24:590–591.
13 Gupta A, Karak PK, Saddekni S: Translumbar inferior vena cava catheter for long-term hemodialysis. J Am Soc Nephrol 1995;5:2094–2097.
14 Punzi M, Ferro F, Petrosino F, Masiello P, Villari V, Sica V, Cavaliere G: Use of an intra-aortic Tesio catheter as vascular access for haemodialysis. Nephrol Dial Transplant 2003;18:830–832.
15 Al-Wakeel JS, Milwalli AH, Malik GH, Huraib S, Al-Mohaya S, Abu-Aisha H, Memon N: Dual-lumen femoral vein catheterization as vascular access for hemodialysis – A prospective study. Angiology 1998;49:557–562.
16 Kumwenda MJ: Two different techniques and outcomes for insertion of long-term tunnelled haemodialysis catheters. Nephrol Dial Transplant 1997;12:1013–1016.
17 Wivell W, Bettmann MA, Baxter B, Langdon DR, Remilliard B, Chobanian M: Outcomes and performance of the Tesio twin catheter system placed for hemodialysis access. Radiology 2001; 221:697–703.
18 Oliver MJ, Edwards LJ, Treleaven DJ, Lambert K, Margetts PJ: Randomized study of temporary hemodialysis catheters. Int J Artif Organs 2002;25:40–44.
19 Warady BA, Sullivan EK, Alexander SR: Lessons from the peritoneal dialysis patient database: A report of the North American Pediatric Renal Transplant Cooperative Study. Kidney Int Suppl 1996;53:S68–S71.

20   Golper TA, Brier ME, Bunke M, Schreiber MJ, Bartlett DK, Hamilton RW, Strife F, Hamburger RJ: Risk factors for peritonitis in long-term peritoneal dialysis: The Network 9 peritonitis and catheter survival studies. Academic Subcommittee of the Steering Committee of the Network 9 Peritonitis and Catheter Survival Studies. Am J Kidney Dis 1996;28:428–436.

21   Weijmer MC, Vervloet MG, ter Wee PM: Prospective follow-up of a novel design hemodialysis catheter for the jugular site: Lower infection rates and improved survival. J Am Soc Nephrol 2001; 12:A1575.

22   Mickley V: Central venous catheters: Many questions, few answers. Nephrol Dial Transplant 2002;17:1368–1373.

23   Saad TF: Bacteremia associated with tunneled, cuffed hemodialysis catheters. Am J Kidney Dis 1999;34:1114–1124.

24   Beathard GA: Management of bacteremia associated with tunneled-cuffed hemodialysis catheters. J Am Soc Nephrol 1999;10:1045–1049.

25   Lund GB, Trerotola SO, Scheel PFJ, Savader SJ, Mitchell SE, Venbrux AC, Osterman FA Jr: Outcome of tunneled hemodialysis catheters placed by radiologists. Radiology 1996;198:467–472.

26   Schwab SJ, Buller GL, McCann RL, Bollinger RR, Stickel DL: Prospective evaluation of a Dacron cuffed hemodialysis catheter for prolonged use. Am J Kidney Dis 1988;11:166–169.

27   Randolph AG, Cook DJ, Gonzales CA, Brun-Buisson C: Tunneling short-term central venous catheters to prevent catheter-related infection: A meta-analysis of randomized, controlled trials. Crit Care Med 1998;26:1452–1457.

28   Weijmer MC, van den Dorpel MA, ter Wee PM: Substantial reduction of infectious complications in hemodialysis patients with trisodium citrate 30% as catheter locking solution; a prospective multicenter double-blind randomised controlled trial. CITRATE Study Group. Nephrol Dial Transplant 2003;18:740.

29   Trerotola SO, Kraus MA, Shah H, Namyslowski J, Moresco K: Prospective randomized comparison of step-tip versus split-tip high flow tunneled hemodialysis catheters: Work in progress. J Am Soc Nephrol 1999;10:A1116.

30   Richard HM 3rd, Hastings GS, Boyd-Kranis RL, Murthy R, Radack DM, Santilli JG, Ostergaard C, Coldwell DM: A randomized, prospective evaluation of the Tesio, Ash split, and Opti-flow hemodialysis catheters. J Vasc Interv Radiol 2001;12:431–435.

31   Twardowski ZJ, Moore HL: Side holes at the tip of chronic hemodialysis catheters are harmful. J Vasc Access 2001;1:8–16.

32   De Wachter D, Deserranno D, Verdonck P: Hemodynamic characteristics of a temporary dual lumen catheter for hemodialysis. J Biomech, in press.

33   Weijmer MC, Vervloet MG, ter Wee PM: Long shotgun-tip femoral catheters have better immediate function, better actual blood flow and lower recirculation rates. Nephrol Dial Transplant 2003;18:737.

34   Twardowski ZJ, Seger RM: Dimensions of central venous structures in humans measured in vivo using magnetic resonance imaging: Implications for central-vein catheter dimensions. Int J Artif Organs 2002;25:107–123.

35   Weijmer MC, Kars SM, ter Wee PM: A scanning electron microscopy analysis of a spontaneous hemodialysis catheter fracture. Am J Kidney Dis 2001;38:858–861.

36   Trerotola SO, Kraus M, Shah H, Namyslowski J, Johnson MS, Stecker MS, Ahmad I, McLennan G, Patel NH, O'Brien E, Lane KA, Ambrosius WT: Randomized comparison of split tip versus step tip high-flow hemodialysis catheters. Kidney Int 2002;62:282–289.

37   Trerotola SO, Johnson MS, Shah H, Kraus MA, McKusky MA, Ambrosius WT, Harris VJ, Snidow JJ: Tunneled hemodialysis catheters: Use of a silver-coated catheter for prevention of infection – A randomized study. Radiology 1998;207:491–496.

38   Trerotola SO, Johnson MS, Harris VJ, Shah H, Ambrosius WT, McKusky MA, Kraus MA: Outcome of tunneled hemodialysis catheters placed via the right internal jugular vein by interventional radiologists. Radiology 1997;203:489–495.

39   Kwon TH, Kim YL, Cho DK: Ultrasound-guided cannulation of the femoral vein for acute haemodialysis access. Nephrol Dial Transplant 1997;12:1009–1012.

40   Farrell J, Gellens M: Ultrasound-guided cannulation versus the landmark-guided technique for acute haemodialysis access. Nephrol Dial Transplant 1997;12:1234–1237.

41 Lin BS, Huang TP, Tang GJ, Tarng DC, Kong CW: Ultrasound-guided cannulation of the internal jugular vein for dialysis vascular access in uremic patients. Nephron 1998;78:423–428.
42 Schwab SJ, Beathard G: The hemodialysis catheter conundrum: Hate living with them, but can't live without them. Kidney Int 1999;56:1–17.
43 Work J: Chronic catheter placement. Semin Dial 2001;14:436–440.
44 Guth AA: Routine chest X-rays after insertion of implantable long-term venous catheters: Necessary or not? Am Surg 2001;67:26–29.
45 Farrell J, Walshe J, Gellens M, Martin KJ: Complications associated with insertion of jugular venous catheters for hemodialysis: The value of postprocedural radiograph. Am J Kidney Dis 1997;30:690–692.
46 Chaiyakunapruk N, Veenstra DL, Lipsky BA, Saint S: Chlorhexidine compared with povidone-iodine solution for vascular catheter-site care: A meta-analysis. Ann Intern Med 2002;136:792–801.
47 Conly JM, Grieves K, Peters B: A prospective, randomized study comparing transparent and dry gauze dressings for central venous catheters. J Infect Dis 1989;159:310–319.
48 Sesso R, Barbosa D, Leme IL, Sader H, Canziani ME, Manfredi S, Draibe SA, Pignatari AC: *Staphylococcus aureus* prophylaxis in hemodialysis patients using central venous catheter: Effect of mupirocin ointment. J Am Soc Nephrol 1998;9:1085–1092.
49 Johnson DW, MacGinley R, Kay TD, Hawley CM, Campbell SB, Isbel NM, Hollett P: A random-ized controlled trial of topical exit site mupirocin application in patients with tunnelled, cuffed haemodialysis catheters. Nephrol Dial Transplant 2002;17:1802–1807.
50 Lok CE, Stanley KE, Hux JE, Richardson R, Tobe SW, Conly J: Hemodialysis infection preven-tion with polysporin ointment. J Am Soc Nephrol 2003;14:169–179.
51 Perez-Fontan M, Rosales M, Rodriguez-Carmona A, Falcon TG, Valdes F: Mupirocin resistance after long-term use for *Staphylococcus aureus* colonization in patients undergoing chronic peritoneal dialysis. Am J Kidney Dis 2002;39:337–341.
52 Annigeri R, Conly JM, Vas SI, Dedier H, Prakashan KP, Bargman JM, Jassal V, Oreopoulos DG: Emergence of mupirocin-resistant *Staphylococcus aureus* in chronic peritoneal dialysis patients using mupirocin prophylaxis to prevent exit-site infection. Perit Dial Int 2001;21:554–559.
53 Bayes B, Bonal J, Romero R: Sodium citrate for filling haemodialysis catheters. Nephrol Dial Transplant 1999;14:2532–2533.
54 Moritz ML, Vats A, Ellis D: Systemic anticoagulation and bleeding in children with hemodialysis catheters. Pediatr Nephrol 2003;18:68–70.
55 Costerton JW, Stewart PS, Greenberg EP: Bacterial biofilms: A common cause of persistent infections. Science 1999;284:1318–1322.
56 Dogra GK, Herson H, Hutchison B, Irish AB, Heath CH, Golledge C, Luxton G, Moody H: Prevention of tunneled hemodialysis catheter-related infections using catheter-restricted filling with gentamicin and citrate: A randomized controlled study. J Am Soc Nephrol 2002;13:2133–2139.
57 Weijmer MC, Debets-Ossenkopp YJ, Van de Vondervoort FJ, ter Wee PM: Superior antimicrobial activity of trisodium citrate over heparin for catheter locking. Nephrol Dial Transplant 2002;17: 2189–2195.
58 Ash SR, Mankus RA, Sutton JM, Criswell ER, Crull CC, Velasquez KA, Smeltzer BD, Ing TS: Concentrated sodium citrate (23%) for catheter lock. Hemodial Int 2000;4:22–31.
59 Weijmer MC, van den Dorpel MA, ter Wee PM: Reduction of bleeding complications in hemodialysis patients with high concentration trisodium citrate for hemodialysis catheter locking; a prospective multicenter double-blind randomised controlled trial. CITRATE Study Group. Nephrol Dial Transplant 2003;18:737.
60 FDA Issues Warning on triCitrasol® Dialysis Catheter Anticoagulant. FDA Talk Paper T00-16, April 14, 2000.

Dr. M.C. Weijmer,
Department of Nephrology and Dialysis, Sint Lucas Andreas Hospital,
Postbox 9243, NL–1006 AE Amsterdam (The Netherlands)
Tel. +31 205108911, Fax +31 848339069, E-Mail mc.weijmer@worldonline.nl

Ronco C, Levin NW (eds): Hemodialysis Vascular Access and Peritoneal Dialysis Access.
Contrib Nephrol. Basel, Karger, 2004, vol 142, pp 112–127

....

Hemodialysis Catheters: Materials, Design and Manufacturing

Angela Gloukhoff Wentling

Medcomp, Harleysville, Pa., USA

The utilization of catheters for vascular access to remove and return blood during dialysis increased in the mid-1970s [1]. Legislation in 1972 made it possible for Medicare to pay 80% of treatment costs for dialysis, which increased the number of people eligible for dialysis. Prior to this, dialysis programs were limited in number and size, and not every patient who needed dialysis was accepted. It was the hospital's responsibility to select the patients by way of a 'patient selection' committee [2]. Today, over 3 million hemodialysis catheters are inserted each year in the United States alone [3].

A hemodialysis catheter is a small biocompatible tube made of soft flexible material. It is inserted into a patient's target vein to provide vascular access for hemodialysis. The basic catheter is composed of a lumen (single or bifurcated), hub, extension(s), luer(s), clamp(s), and at times a cuff (fig. 1, 2). Side holes, strain relief, suture wing, and ID ring(s) are other features a hemodialysis catheter may contain. Components are typically made of polymer materials.

Dialysis catheters are available in single, double, and triple lumen configurations. Catheter lumen cross sections can vary in shape such as round, D-shaped, C-shaped, and coaxial (fig. 3). The septum divides the arterial and venous passages to prevent cross flow. The inner lumen is designed with smooth surfaces. Rough surfaces or abrupt edges in the inner lumen may cause hemolysis (destruction of red blood cells) [4].

It is crucial to design the hemodialysis catheter so that the recirculation rate is minimized to promote efficient dialysis. This is done by staggering the tips on the catheter, since the aspirated blood is cycled through the dialysis machine and returned via the venous lumen to the patient's blood [5]. Frequently, the

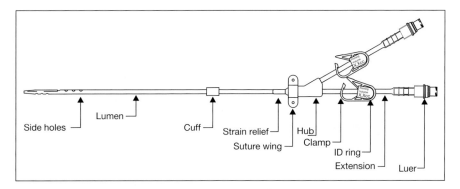

Fig. 1. Hemodialysis catheter components.

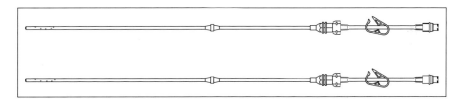

Fig. 2. Two single lumen catheters.

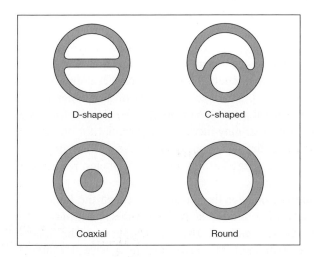

Fig. 3. Lumen configurations.

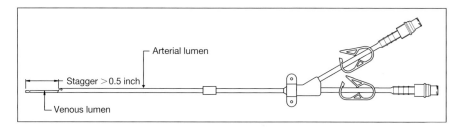

Fig. 4. Hemodialysis catheter with staggered tip.

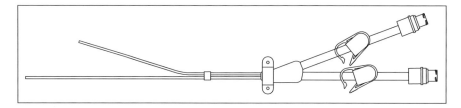

Fig. 5. Hemodialysis catheter with split tip.

venous tip will be longer than the arterial tip with a gap of more than a half inch separating the main arterial and venous orifices (fig. 4). Another design, which incorporates the staggered tips, also goes one step further by having lumens capable of being split at the tip to additionally reduce recirculation (fig. 5). Choosing the right catheter length is vital for both the upper-body (i.e. internal jugular) and lower-body (i.e. femoral) access sites, since recirculation will occur if the catheter length is too short [6].

Tip geometry and side hole diameter configurations are also key design features. Rounding the tip removes any sharp edges, reducing vessel trauma. Some catheter tips are made of a silicone elastomer to further soften the tip, preventing endothelial damage [7]. Strategic placement of side holes on the arterial tip helps to reduce 'arterial sucking' against the vessel wall. Too many side holes or holes that are too large may increase the potential for blood flow through the tip of the catheter after placement between uses. This will permit the catheter lock solutions to be purged at the tip of the catheter, resulting in clotting of the tip [1].

The hub serves as the housing for the transition between the lumen and extensions. The hub can be fixed or removable. A 'fixed hub' is molded onto the lumen and the extension tubes to create an adapting passageway. The internal passageways are not to be obstructed. The main goal is to have the internal passage as uniform as possible throughout the entire catheter. A 'removable hub' is connected to any position on the lumen, making placement easier and requiring fewer measurements. With a removable hub there is potential for disconnection and movement [5]. Some hubs have a strain relief to minimize the potential of lumen kinking at the hub to lumen joint that could result in flow reduction.

Suture wings are provided with some catheters. The suture wings serve as an anchoring device to keep the catheter affixed to the body. This is done by threading sutures through the holes of the suture wings and skin to prevent the catheter from moving back and forth through the exit site. This decreases the chance of dragging bacteria through the tract of the subcutaneous tunnel [1].

Suture wings are available in three configurations: fixed, nonrotating, and rotating. For 'fixed' suture wings, the suture wing is part of the molded hub. This feature eliminates the possibility of the suture wing detaching from the hub. A 'nonrotating' suture is a suture wing made as a separate component that is assembled to the hub or lumen. The only concern with the nonrotating suture wing is the potential movement of the suture wing, since it is not a permanent component of the catheter. Once fixed, it cannot rotate. The 'rotating' suture wing comes attached to the grooves on the hub. It can be rotated so that hub orientation is not a factor.

The luer connectors are found on the catheter extension(s) and allow for a universal connection to bloodlines. The luers on catheters are usually female threaded locking collars with a tapered conical mating surface. The female luers are then engaged to the male luer connectors [8]. Luers are usually color-coded. A red luer signifies a passageway that is reserved for blood removal and is usually referred to as the arterial extension. The blue luer signifies a passageway that is reserved for blood return and is often called the venous extension. Nylon, PVC, ABS, titanium and polycarbonate are a few of the materials frequently used for luers.

Extension tubes are usually clear and round in cross-sectional geometry. Extension tubes provide communication to the dialysis machine bloodline connectors and also provide a clamping area to control blood flow. Some extensions may be opaque to prevent the patient from seeing the blood in the catheter. Depending upon the catheter, there may be one, two, or three extension tubes, which may be curved or straight. Curved extensions are designed so that the luers are positioned away from the patient's face for comfort. The extensions must be able to withstand repeated clamping and are usually made from silicone or polyurethane.

Clamps are installed on each extension tube and are used to control blood flow. Clamps are made of a highly flexible material, such as acetal, that will allow repeated manipulation of the hinged area so that it can bend and return to its original shape without failure. As with the luers, clamps may be color-coded

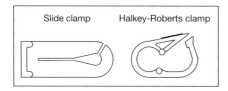

Fig. 6. Clamp styles.

blue and red to distinguish the arterial and venous passageways. A number of clamp styles are available (fig. 6). The most common types are in-line clamps, commonly known as Halkey-Roberts™ clamps, and slide clamps. Slide clamps are usually reserved for extensions with small outer diameters. ID rings with printed information, such as priming volume(s) and catheter contraindications, are now available with the clamp.

The cuff is woven from polyester material. The function of the cuff is to promote tissue ingrowth for catheter stabilization and provide a barrier against microorganisms [1]. It is usually bonded on the lumen about an inch from the hub for long-term catheters. Other cuff designs include the use of a silver-impregnated attachable cuff, such as the VitaCuff® (Bard) [9]. There is no proven advantage of one cuffed catheter design over another. Catheter choice should be based on local experience, goals for use, and cost [10].

Catheters are available with straight or curved lumens. The curved catheter lumen is designed to sit low in the vessel and drape over the collarbone for patient comfort. Curved lumens permit smooth passage of the catheter to the anterior chest wall or the lateral abdominal wall. They provide comfort to the patient and minimize kinking [11].

Three types of curved lumen catheters exist: Raulerson, precurved, and internal jugular (fig. 7). For the 'Raulerson' catheter, the lumen is curved 180° so that it is located directly below the hub and between the extensions. The 'precurved' catheter is designed to be a long-term cuffed lumen catheter. The lumen is curved 180° so that it is located to the outer side of the arterial extension. The arterial tip faces the arterial extension. The total lumen length from the hub is the length designation of the catheter. The 'internal jugular' catheter is used for short-term catheters. The lumen is curved 180° so that the lumen is located to the outer side of the venous extension. The total lumen length from the tip to the suture wing is the length designation of the catheter. The curved section is not considered in the length.

Hemodialysis catheters are divided into two main categories: acute and chronic [12]. Acute catheters are designed for short-term dialysis remaining in the body for less than 30 days. Chronic catheters are designed for long-term dialysis remaining in the body for less than 1 year, although they have been used for longer periods. Typically, hemodialysis catheters are used as a bridging

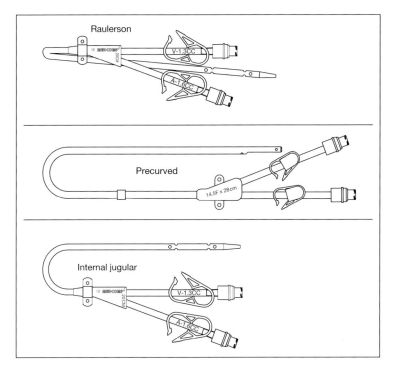

Fig. 7. Curved lumen catheters.

access until a fistula or graft has matured, or as a last resort in the event no alternate venous access site is available [10].

Acute dialysis catheters are typically assembled without a cuff and are designed for short-term use. They are generally designed to have a greater rigidity than chronic catheters with the tip geometry tapered to a point. This allows the catheter to be inserted quickly over the guidewire without the need for a vascular dilator and sheath. The point of the catheter acts as a dilator, expanding the access to the vein upon insertion. Since there is no cuff and the catheter is not tunneled, there is an increased risk of infection if the catheter is left in place in excess of 30 days [13].

Chronic dialysis catheters were introduced when acute silicone catheters emerged with polyester cuffs. Nephrologists noticed that catheters were lasting longer, and began insisting on keeping them in the patient longer [14]. Chronic catheters have also been used for short-term use due to their ability to prevent infection at the access site [15]. Typically, the chronic dialysis catheter has a softer lumen and a blunt tip. Insertion of acute catheters take longer since long-term catheters require a tunnel to be created for the cuff. A tunneler is used to create this passageway. When insertion is completed, the cuff is typically located in the center of the subcutaneous tunnel.

A successfully functioning catheter can be measured by different criteria including catheter design and proper catheter insertion. The primary indication of a good functioning catheter is high blood flow rates with moderate pressure drops. Other indications are the absence of stenosis, thrombosis, or bacterial migration. The lumen should not collapse, crimp, or clot when the catheter is under negative pressure or while being bent during tunneling. Catheters should also be resistant to as many antiseptic agents as possible [1].

Chronic dialysis catheters have their share of advantages and disadvantages. The advantages are they are relatively easy to insert and replace, are universally applicable, and can be inserted in multiple sites with no maturation time. Venipuncture is not required since the catheter now provides venous access over a period of months, improving chances of AV fistula maturation in patients who require immediate hemodialysis. The disadvantages are that they have a high morbidity rate due to thrombosis and infection, although thrombotic complications can be corrected with anticoagulants. In addition the risk of permanent central venous stenosis or occlusion is great [10].

Physicians have the ability to choose the catheter that best fits their application via hospital protocol or experience. In general, the lumen configurations have their advantages and disadvantages. A single lumen catheter, such as the 10-french Tesio® (Medcomp) or the 10-french Tandem-Cath™ Catheter (Tyco), should provide excellent flow rates since the inner lumen cross section is comparatively large. The main disadvantage is that two separate lumens need to be inserted to provide for a two-way flow. This requires increased surgical time and also renders the catheter bulky for the patient. It also increases the chance of catheter infection due to the necessity for two insertion sites. The double lumen catheter is the preferred lumen configuration for most nephrologists. For example, the Split Cath Catheter (Medcomp) double lumen design permits excellent flow rates, while being less bulky, requiring only one insertion site. The triple lumen catheter such as the 12.5-french Mahurkar™ triple lumen catheter (Kendall) provides a third passage. The third passage can be utilized for collecting laboratory specimens, administering blood products, and/or infusing medications. It preserves a patient's peripheral veins by avoiding repeated venipunctures. The addition of a third passage, however, does decrease the inner lumen cross section of the venous and arterial lumens, thereby reducing flow. Additionally, the cost of a triple lumen catheter is usually greater than that of a double lumen catheter.

All components of acute and chronic dialysis catheters are designed to meet specific requirements. It is not sufficient to design the catheter and then have it produced. Engineers are required to follow a proper sequence of steps while designing the catheter from prototype to production, abiding by governmental compliance requirements and maintaining a Design History File (DHF) to document all phases of the design. On average it takes 1–3 years for a new product to reach market.

The design process begins with a conceptual idea for the catheter. Conceptual ideas may be driven by a need in the marketplace or from an improvement to an existing device by the practitioner. The idea is then presented to senior management. If approved, the concept is immediately checked for patentability and processed accordingly. As the design moves forward, a design plan is developed and a DHF is initiated for the project. The DHF keeps track of all phases of the project from design input to market release and is required by all concerned governmental agencies [16].

Catheters are designed and developed in accordance with and under the control of a number of governmental and international standards. A medical device cannot be legally marketed until all governmental clearances are received. For example, in order to market a medical device in the United States, a manufacturer must abide by all FDA Quality Systems Regulations and gain their approval [16]. The catheter manufacturer must submit a premarket notification or 510(k) to prove substantial equivalence to a legally marketed device. This is done to determine if its safety and effectiveness has been compromised [17]. A 510k submission to the FDA is to be reviewed within 90 days of receipt [18]. If the design is such that no substantially equivalent device exists, then a premarket approval is required. In order to market a product to any member of the European Union, the European Medical Device Directives (CE) must be followed and their approval received. A catheter manufacturer must be certified by a notified body to Annex II, V, or VI of the MDD (93/42/EEC) and comply with the requirements of the directive [19]. A technical review is conducted by the certified body, and if all requirements are met a CE clearance letter is issued permitting the sale of the catheter in Europe.

The design process of a hemodialysis catheter requires specific tasks to be documented in the DHF. These tasks in chronological order are design input, design output, design verification, design validation, and design transfer [20]. In design input, the developer is required to document the design requirements for the new hemodialysis catheter by addressing its intended use, which would include the needs of the practitioner and the patient. In design output, procedures for defining and documenting design output are established to allow adequate evaluation for conformance to design input. Design verification confirms that the design output meets the design input requirements by product testing. Design validation confirms the ability of the catheter, as it will be manufactured and packaged, to consistently perform up to the stated specifications. In design transfer the device design is correctly translated into production specifications [16].

After completion of each task, key members of the company made up of managers or directors from different departments examine the DHF. Sales, compliance, engineering, quality control, purchasing, materials, and production are a few examples of departments usually represented. The FDA leaves it up to the manufacturing company to decide when a formal design review is required. The results of the review along with signed and dated approvals are provided for the review [16]. An independent examiner who does not have direct responsibility for the design stage being reviewed is required for each review. Should an audit occur, the auditors will most likely request a review of the product's DHF as it provides detailed compliance information and the product's historical background. The DHF provides proof of compliance of the design and development phases [16].

To manufacture a catheter the manufacturer must follow Good Manufacturing Practices (GMP) and Quality System Regulations (QSR). Standard Operating Procedures (SOPs) must be in place to describe the policies and procedures that the company will use in order to conduct business as a medical device manufacturer. The product must be safe and effective. Emphasis is on cleanliness, training, quality control, design, product reliability, manufacturing repeatability, biocompatibility, in-house procedures, and documented proof of compliance via the DHF [16].

Injection molding, extrusion, tipping, bonding and printing are among the manufacturing processes that are typically used to manufacture a hemodialysis catheter.

Luers, clamps, suture wings, and hubs for dialysis catheters are created by the injection molding process. Injection molding a polymer is a process by which the polymer material, in the form of granules or pellets, is melted and then injected into a mold cavity at a controlled temperature, pressure and rate. When the polymer cools it takes the shape of the cavity. The resulting form usually is a finished part. In this process many details such as bosses, ribs, and screw threads can be formed during the one-step injection molding operation [21].

Extension and lumen tubing are produced utilizing an extrusion process. The extrusion of a polymer requires polymer powder or granules to be melted into a uniform and homogeneous mixture, then forcing it continuously through a die resulting in the desired shape being formed. It is then cooled back to its solid state as it is held in the desired shape so that the end product can be achieved [21].

Tipping, bonding, and printing are additional processes used in catheter manufacture. During the tipping process, holes may be drilled on the sides of the venous and arterial lumen tips. Any square edges on the tips are melted to form a generous radius, which prevents damage to the vessel walls and enhances tip comfort to the patient. Luers are typically joined to the extension by means of solvent bonding or by overmolding. Process selection is material dependent. No matter what joining process is selected it is paramount that all joints are free from leakage in the manufacturing process. Printing is usually the final step. The printing process involves the transfer of a biocompatible ink from a print plate to a specific location on the catheter. Printing typically provides information pertaining to catheter length, french size, priming volume, and company name.

All machines used in the manufacturing process need to be validated [22]. An installation qualification (IQ) is performed to validate the machines. Validation ensures the machines are installed and calibrated to the manufacturer's specifications. All equipment used in the manufacturing process must adhere to a documented schedule of routine maintenance and calibration [22].

An operational qualification (OQ) is performed next. This run establishes, by objective evidence, the process control limits and tasks required to make the finished product meet all predetermined requirements [22]. It is through the OQ that the standard manufacturing parameters are determined.

A performance qualification (PQ) establishes objective evidence that the process, under anticipated conditions, consistently produces a product that meets all predetermined requirements [22]. Typically three separate runs of the product are produced and are identified with a unique lot number. Before each run there is usually a 2- to 3-hour downtime where the machines are powered down. For each run the machines are powered up and the operating parameters are set.

Trained quality assurance personnel ensure the finished product meets established acceptance criteria [16]. Catheters not meeting specifications are rejected and reviewed by appropriate personnel for disposition.

One of the main objectives in designing a catheter is to provide a device capable of producing acceptable flow rates, while maintaining minimal venous pressure. High flow rates maximize the potential for urea reduction in the range of 65% or greater [11]. Emphasis is placed on design tools such as a risk analysis during the development of the catheter to determine and minimize undesirable conditions. In addition, much design input is derived from nephrologists and interventional radiologists. Typical requests are for lumens rigid enough to withstand kinking or collapse during insertion and aspiration. A sturdy lumen facilitates ease of insertion. Wall thickness should be such that it is designed to maximize the lumen inner diameter cross section to allow for maximum urea clearance and blood flow without the need for excessively large outer diameters. The lumen as well as all joints must remain secure when subjected to pull force testing per ISO standards.

The industry standard for unit of measure of the lumen outer diameter is the french size. The catheter french size and lumen length are normally printed on the hub. For a reference, table 1 displays the catheter french size as it relates to the lumen outer diameter in millimeters and inches [23].

Table 1. French size of catheters related to outer diameter of the lumen in millimeters and inches

Catheter french size	Lumen diameter	
	mm	inches
6	2.0	0.079
7	2.3	0.092
8	2.7	0.105
9	3.0	0.118
10	3.3	0.131
11	3.7	0.144
12	4.0	0.158
13	4.3	0.170
14	4.7	0.184
15	5.0	0.197
16	5.3	0.210

Because each anatomy is unique, lumens are designed in various configurations and geometries. Making a lumen large will help if a small clot or fibrous tissue exists. The disadvantage of inserting a large diameter catheter is the increased trauma to the body as opposed to a small catheter [1].

The primary constraints of catheter blood flow are the internal dimensions of the lumen and extension, and tip placement [24]. Blood flow through the catheter is directly proportional to the pressure generated by the blood pump across the catheter and inversely proportional to resistance in the catheter itself where Q_B is the catheter flow, P is the pressure, and R is the resistance as seen in equation 1:

$$QB \sim P/R \tag{1}$$

Laminar flow can be predicted by Poiseuille's equation where k is the proportionality constant, D is the luminal diameter, L is the catheter length, and V is blood viscosity as seen in equation 2:

$$QB = k \times P \times D^4/(L \times V) \tag{2}$$

Jean-Louis Marie Poiseuille, a French physician and physiologist, came up with this formula for the flow rate for laminar (nonturbulent) flow of fluids in circular tubes [25].

A comparison of equations 1 and 2 shows that resistance to flow is directly related to length and inversely proportional to the fourth power of the catheter diameter as seen in equation 3. If resistance within the catheter is the only resistance, doubling the catheter diameter may increase blood flow as much as

16-fold. Flow can be doubled when the diameter is increased by only 19%. Doubling the length will double the resistance to flow [6].

$$R = (L \times V)/(k \times D^4) \tag{3}$$

Material selection is an extremely crucial factor in catheter design. Selected materials should not promote blood coagulation. They must not cause damage to proteins, enzymes, and formed elements of blood, including red blood cells, white blood cells, and platelets. Furthermore, the catheter should not cause hemolysis, red blood cell rupture, or initiation of the platelet release reaction [26].

Materials used in the manufacture of catheters usually fall in the USP Class VI classification. To be classified as an USP Class VI material, the material needs to undergo and pass three distinct tests. The initial test is the acute systemic test, which involves systemically injecting saline, ethanol, polyethylene glycol and cottonseed oil extracts of the test materials into mice. No signs of toxicity should be apparent. The second test is the acute intracutaneous test. This involves injecting saline, ethanol, polyethylene glycol and cottonseed oil extracts of the test material into rabbits. The specimens should show no evidence of erythema (redness of the skin), edema (excessive fluid build-up), scab formation or clinical toxicity [27]. The final test is the implant test. It involves implanting a 1 mm × 1 cm rod of the test material into the paravertebral muscle of a rabbit for 7 days. No signs of hemorrhage, inflammation, necrosis (death of cell tissues), discoloration or encapsulation should be evident [28].

The two most commonly used blood-compatible materials for hemodialysis catheters are silicone and polyurethane [12, 29]. Medical grade silicone rubber has traditionally been considered the standard for long-term access in animals and humans. Silicone is resistant to most chemicals and is also very soft and flexible. However, it is hard to extrude and does not bond easily to other components made of nonsilicone materials. Although it is the softest and least thrombogenic material, its softness requires the use of a sheath or stylet for percutaneous insertion [30]. Polyurethane is the only material on the market that is comparable to silicone rubber with regard to biocompatibility for long-term animal and human vascular access. Its greatest advantage over silicone is its tensile strength. A polyurethane catheter will exhibit better flow rates than a silicone catheter with the same outer lumen diameter (french size), since the polyurethane lumen can be extruded with thinner walls and therefore a larger inner diameter (fig. 8). Polyurethane is more rigid than silicone at room temperature making it easier to insert. Most polyurethanes used for catheter manufacture soften once inserted in the body. It is easily extruded and bonds well with other nonpolyurethane materials. Medications or antimicrobial agents,

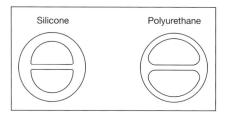

Fig. 8. Inner lumen comparison of silicone versus polyurethane.

such as silver sulfadiazine and chlorhexidine, bond well on polyurethane catheter lumen surfaces [7].

Other materials used to manufacture a catheter are polyethylene and polytetrafluoroethylene. Catheters manufactured with these materials are characteristically rigid at room temperature making it easy to insert the catheters at the bedside. When placed in the body, the material softens, which minimizes the risk of vein puncture during prolonged catheterization. Polyurethane is more flexible and less thrombogenic compared to polyethylene and polytetrafluoroethylene [30].

Site care maintenance must also be examined for catheters. Polyurethane and silicone have different chemical resistance characteristics [12]. Alcohol and chlorhexidine in general are not recommended for cleaning polyurethane catheters. Although a new polyurethane material, Carbothane, has emerged and is capable of being cleaned with alcohol. In general, povidone-iodine is recommended for polyurethane. Alcohol is compatible with silicone. However, not all silicones are compatible with povidone-iodine [31]. Since catheter site care recommendations differ from one manufacturer to another, surgeons or interventional radiologists should check the catheter literature to determine which site cares are acceptable for use.

Catheter lumens can be coated with antiseptics or process treated to reduce blood-borne catheter-related infections, thrombogenicity, and other catheter-related complications without affecting the basic design and function of the catheter [32]. Catheters have been coated with a chlorhexidine and silver sulfadiazine combination, minocycline and rifampin combination, as well as a Heparin™ coat [5, 11]. Ion implantation of silicone rubber has been proven to be a major breakthrough in removing its tacky surface, improving hydrophilicity, and significantly changing the ability of the surface to resist biodeposits in long-term indwelling medical devices [32]. In the ion implantation process, energetic ions are placed onto the catheter surface and penetrate into the surface region, creating significant changes in the structure of the surface region of the catheter [32]. Silver is a known bacteriostatic/bactericidal agent having been used for many medical applications, including the therapeutic use of silver-based compounds for severe burns. Spire Corporation developed a silver-based film that is applied to finished catheters known as Spi-Argent™. It has a low coefficient of friction, is uniform, and has good adhesion. The Institute for Blood Purification in Germany claims thrombus formation or bacterial attachment is decreased with Spi-Argent-treated silicone rubber catheters. Spi-Argent-coated catheter samples were stored in high-humidity chambers at a temperature of 75°C for 2 weeks and showed no sign of degradation. The Spi-Argent™ showed a very low rate of leaching [32].

Ethylene oxide sterilization is the most common sterilization method for catheters. It is the least aggressive form of sterilization for many plastics. Other sterilization methods include steam autoclave, irradiation (gamma, electron beam, or beta), dry heat, cold sterilization, and disinfectants [33]. The catheter package will state the recommended method of sterilization.

Drawing blood from a central vein at 200–400 ml/min is more complex than one would think. Vein walls are thin and the pressure in central veins is much lower than in arteries. Negative pressure is created when blood is removed through the lumen which can cause the vein wall to collapse around the lumen. This in turn blocks the lumen. If a fibrous tissue sheath or a clot forms around the catheter tip, the entry section of the catheter will become smaller and the velocity of the blood flow will increase. This increased blood velocity creates a greater negative pressure around the catheter tip and increases the chance that the vein wall will be pulled over the tip [1].

Pressure in the central vein is close to atmospheric (760 mm Hg); therefore, the maximum negative pressure that can be generated on the inflow side (central vein to pump inflow) is −760 mm Hg at sea level. This pressure range, however, will not be exceeded since most blood pumps are only capable of generating up to −500 mm Hg. Typical pressures for hemodialysis catheters are −250 mm Hg for the arterial lumen and +250 mm Hg for the venous lumen [6].

In summary, dialysis catheters are available as acute and chronic catheters. The acute catheter is usually used for less than 30 days and normally does not have a cuff. The chronic catheter has a cuff and is used for less than 12 months. Hemodialysis catheters are primarily made of silicone or polyurethane. They are available as single, double, and triple lumen catheters. Physicians can choose the catheter that best fits their needs based on experience and potential requirements. A successful functioning catheter is dependent on catheter design and insertion. The catheters are developed in accordance with governmental standards where the device will be sold. A DHF is maintained during the catheter development. Documentation must include design input, design output, design verification, design validation, and design transfer with appropriate reviews. To manufacture a dialysis catheter, the manufacturer must follow Good Manufacturing Practices (GMP) and Quality System Regulations (QSR). Injection molding, extrusion, tipping, bonding, and printing are among the manufacturing processes that are utilized to make the dialysis catheters. All machines used in the manufacturing process must be validated. IQ, OQ, and PQ are all included in the validation procedure. Catheter length, tips, side holes, hub, suture wing, ID ring(s), strain relief, luer(s), extension(s), clamp(s), cuff(s), lumen, and material are all vital components and features of a dialysis catheter. Each component and catheter has been designed with specific functions in mind, tested to government standards, and is integral to the dialysis system.

References

1   Ash SR: The evolution and function of central venous catheters for dialysis. Semin Dial 2001;14: 416–424.
2   National Kidney Foundation of East Tennessee: History of Dialysis. Available from URL: http://www.kidneyetn.org/nkfethistdial.html.
3   Ahmad I, Ray C: Complications of central venous access devices; in Central Venous Access. Philadelphia, Lippincott Williams & Wilkins, 2001, pp 151–162.
4   Dictionary.com. Lexico Publishing Group, LLC, 2003. Available from URL: http://www. dictionary.com.
5   Venous Access. Available from URL: http://www.venousaccess.com.
6   Depner TA: Catheter performance. Semin Dial 2001;14:425–431.
7   Namyslowski J, Charles R: Short and intermediate term central venous catheters; in Ray C (ed): Central Venous Access. Philadelphia, Lippincott Williams & Wilkins, 2001, pp 57–59.
8   Life-Assist Inc: Luer-Slip vs. Luer-Lock. Available from URL: http://www.life-assist.com/lockslip.html.
9   Maki DG, Cobb L, Garman JK, Shapiro JM, Ringer M, Helgerson RB: An attachable silver-impregnated cuff for prevention of infection with central venous catheters: A prospective randomized multicenter trial. Am J Med 1988;85:307–314.
10 Schwab S, Besarab A, Beathard G, Levine M, Brouwer D, McCann R, et al: NKF-DOQI Clinical Practice Guidelines for Vascular Access. New York, National Kidney Foundation, 1997, pp 26–28.
11 Besarab A, Raja R: Vascular access for hemodialysis; in Daugirdas J, Blake P, Ing T, et al (eds): Handbook of Dialysis, ed 3. Baltimore, Lippincott Williams & Wilkins, 2001, pp 67–70.
12 Medcomp Training Manual. Harleysville, Medcomp, 1999.
13 Wilson S: Vascular Access Principles and Practice, ed 3. St Louis, Mosby, 1996.
14 McDowell DE, Moss AH, Vasilakis C, Bell R, Pillai L: Percutaneously placed dual-lumen silicone catheters for long-term hemodialysis. Am Surg 1993;59:569–573.
15 Moss AH, McLaughlin MM, Lempert KD, Holley JL: Use of a silicone catheter with a Dacron cuff for dialysis short-term vascular access. Am J Kidney Dis 1988;12:492–498.
16 Code of Federal Regulations 21 Part 820. RAPS, 2000, pp 138–150.
17 Practical Engineering Data & Tools for Medical Device Professionals. 510K Regulations. Available from URL: http://www.engineeringreference.com/Regulations/510K.htm.
18 Practical Engineering Data & Tools for Medical Device Professionals. Foreign Regulations. Available from URL: http://www.engineeringreference.com/Regulations/foreignregs.htm
19 Practical Engineering Data & Tools for Medical Device Professionals. CE Marking. Available from URL: http://www.engineeringreference.com/Regulations/cemarking.htm.
20 Medcomp, DC-300 Design Plan. Harleysville, Medcomp, 2002.
21 Plastics Handbook. Modern Plastics Magazine Staff (ed.), McGraw-Hill, 1994, pp 152–170.
22 MDI Consultants Inc. Department of Health, Education, and Welfare Food and Drug Administration: Guidelines on General Principles of Process Validation. Great Neck, NY, 1987, pp 1–10.
23 Martech-MDI. French Scale. Harleysville, Pa, 1996.

24   Schwab S, Beathard G: The hemodialysis catheter conundrum: Hate living with them, but can't live without them. Kidney Int 1999;56:1–17.
25   American Cancer Society. Available from URL: http://www.todayinsci.com/12/12_26.htm.
26   Park J, Lakes R: Biomaterials: An Introduction, ed 2. New York, Plenum Press, 1992.
27   Geneva Laboratories Inc. Available from URL: http://www.genevalabs.com/biocompa.htm.
28   Catalog. Woburn, Thermedics Inc. Polymer Products, Biocompatibility/Biostability, 2000.
29   Access Technologies. Available from URL: http://www.norfolkaccess.com/Catheters.html.
30   Berkoben M, Schwab S: Hemodialysis vascular access; in Henrich W (ed): Principles and Practice of Dialysis, ed 2. Baltimore, Lippincott Williams & Wilkins, 1999, pp 41–47.
31   Dinwiddie L: Cleansing agents used for hemodialsyis catheter care. Nephrol Nurs J 2002;29: 599–613.
32   Sioshansi P: New processes for surface treatment of catheters. Artif Organs 1994;18/4:266–271.
33   The Effect of Sterilization Methods on Plastics and Elastomers. New York, Plastics Design Library, 1994.

Angela Gloukhoff Wentling,
Medcomp,
1499 Delp Drive, Harleysville, PA 19438 (USA)
Tel. +1 215 256 4201, Fax +1 215 256 0839, E-Mail Agloukhoff@hotmail.com

Ronco C, Levin NW (eds): Hemodialysis Vascular Access and Peritoneal Dialysis Access.
Contrib Nephrol. Basel, Karger, 2004, vol 142, pp 128–152

....

Chronic Central Venous Catheters for Dialysis and the Ash Split Cath® Catheter: Rationale and Clinical Experience

Stephen R. Ash

Dialysis Center for Greater Lafayette, Nephrology Department of
Arnett Clinic and R&D, Ash Access Technology and HemoCleanse, Inc.,
Lafayette, Ind., and Purdue University, West Lafayette, Ind., USA

History and Challenges of Chronic Central Venous Catheters for Hemodialysis

The use of central venous catheters (CVC) for removing and returning blood during dialysis is commonplace now but in the late 1970s this concept revolutionized dialysis [1]. Before the development of CVC dialysis was possible only with a catheter within an artery, either through the internal/external arteriovenous (AV) silicone shunt or through separate catheters placed into an artery and a vein and removed after each treatment. The development of CVC for dialysis was not simple. Drawing blood from a central vein at 200–400 ml/min is a delicate and somewhat unpredictable process. The pressure in central veins is much lower than in arteries and vein walls are thinner and more distensible, even though the flow of blood though central veins is the same as through central arteries. Removal of blood through the ports of a CVC in a vein creates a negative pressure around these ports due to direct suction or due to the Bernoulli effect. This negative pressure can cause the vein wall to collapse around the ports and obstruct flow into the ports, even if the flow through the vein is much higher than the flow of blood through the catheter. If a fibrous tissue sheath forms around the catheter and reaches the tip or if clots form around the tip, the entry port to the catheter becomes smaller and the velocity of blood flow is increased. The increased blood velocity creates a greater negative pressure around the ports, and increases the tendency to pull the vein wall over the tip.

There are four solutions to the problem of providing sufficient blood outflow through dual-lumen CVC for dialysis. (1) Place the removal and return lumens within the right atrium, where the tips cannot rest against a venous wall and only one lumen usually rests against the atrial wall. (2) Position the catheter with the removal lumen on the inside of the catheter curve, positioning this lumen away from the vein wall. (3) Use a large catheter so that the removal lumen cannot be blocked by a small clot or a small amount of fibrous tissue. (4) Provide multiple blood entry ports in all directions around the circumference of each catheter tip, so that some of the ports are always facing away from the vein wall.

There are problems and limitations of each of these approaches. Positioning the tips of the removal and return lumens at the middle of the atrium is somewhat difficult, especially since the relative positions of the catheter and the heart change when the patient stands up after lying on the procedure table. Positioning the catheter so that the removal lumen is on the inside of the catheter curve is not always easy, as the catheter course through the subcutaneous tissue and central veins is rather complex and tortuous. Placing a larger catheter is always more difficult and somewhat more traumatic than placing a smaller catheter, especially if the larger catheter is not round in shape. Providing multiple side holes in all directions around the catheter tips requires that two catheters be placed, or that one catheter must separate into two separate tips. Side holes in a catheter also have disadvantages. If they are too large or too many, blood will quickly flow through the tip of the catheter after placement and between uses, removing catheter lock solutions and promoting clotting at the tip. If they are too small or too few then blood will flow in and out only through the tip of the catheter, thus diminishing any advantage of the side holes.

CVC for dialysis are classified into either 'acute' or 'chronic' catheters, depending on whether the catheters are expected to be used for only several days or months to years. Acute CVC are designed to be placed with a minimum amount of effort. Generally, acute CVC for dialysis are relatively rigid, pointed catheters with a conically shaped tip and central lumen so that the catheter can be advanced into the vein directly over a guidewire. The guidewire is inserted through a needle placed into a vein, and the point of the catheter follows the guidewire while the catheter body dilates the entry site and the catheter is advanced into the vein. Acute CVC for dialysis have no subcutaneous cuff or locking device.

Chronic CVC for dialysis are soft, blunt-tipped catheters and have a subcutaneous 'cuff' for tissue ingrowth or a plastic 'grommet' to immobilize the catheters below the skin surface. Chronic CVC are generally placed through internal jugular (IJ) veins into the superior vena cava (SVC) with the goal of placing the tips of the catheter at the junction of the SVC and the right atrium. Alternative venous access points are external jugular veins, subclavian veins and femoral veins. Due to their blunt shape chronic CVC have traditionally been placed through a 'split sheath,' which is a cylindrical thin-walled plastic device advanced into the vein over a dilator. The dilator has a central lumen that follows the guidewire. The guidewire and dilator are then removed and the split sheath opening is closed with a finger to prevent excessive bleeding. The catheter is then inserted through the split sheath into the central vein. The split sheath is split along two preformed grooves, and the halves are retracted around the catheter, leaving it in position within the central vein. More recently, techniques have been developed to allow placement of chronic CVC to be performed over a guidewire placed through a previously dilated tract, in a manner similar to acute CVC for dialysis (see below).

Chronic CVC for dialysis have a subcutaneous tunnel leading from the vein insertion site to a distant exit site. A Dacron® cuff (or sometimes a solid plastic grommet) attached to the catheter fixes the catheter in position and prevents bacteria at the exit site from migrating around the catheter. The cuff also serves as the outer limit for the fibrous tunnel that develops around the catheter from the central vein. The tunnel is similar to a vein wall and is contiguous with the IJ vein (or other vein of insertion). The tunnel stops at the Dacron cuff where it melds into the fibrous tissue surrounding the cuff. Without the cuff, this tunnel continues all of the way to the skin exit site over time, creating potential for back-and-forth movement of the catheter and potential for bacterial migration around the catheter. Canaud et al. [2, 3] devised a catheter system comprised of two 10-French catheters, each placed into the vena cava and with tips lending to the right atrium. Flow rate was excellent over many months of use. Tesio added subcutaneous cuffs and the catheter became more popular. More recent versions of the Canaud catheters have included a subcutaneous plastic grommet to fix the catheter limbs.

Placing a chronic CVC for dialysis requires additional skill and takes 10–20 min more time than placing an acute CVC, but with proper equipment the placement and care can done in the ICU setting. For catheters placed into previously uncannulated right IJ veins fluoroscopy is not required for most chronic CVC; tip position can be adequately positioned in the right atrium by using external landmarks (tip of catheter 2 inches above the bottom of the sternum). Placing one chronic catheter can often provide access throughout the entire course of the acute renal failure episode and avoid the need for several acute catheter placements. Using a chronic CVC for acute dialysis provides higher blood flow rates, longer duration of use, diminished risk of infection, and less trauma to veins over the course of treatments (due to use of only one catheter vs. many acute catheters). The placement of a chronic CVC in patients with acute renal failure can minimize physician work, maximize dialysis efficiency and minimize catheter complications. One exception in which an acute CVC should be placed is in patients with suspected septicemia. In these patients placing an acute CVC for dialysis until the septicemia is cleared is a logical choice.

Features for Successful Function of Chronic CVC for Dialysis

The requirements for successful function of chronic CVC for dialysis include numerous elements: provision of high blood flow rates at moderate pressure drops consistently throughout each dialysis without outflow failure regardless of patient fluid status (even when volume depletion decreases the size and stiffness of the SVC), minimal trauma to the vein, to avoid intimal trauma and resultant vein stenosis or thrombosis, resistance to occlusion by fibrous sheathing, prevention of bacterial migration around the catheter or contamination of the catheter lumen, avoidance of clotting at the tip or within the catheter, limited removal or activation of white cells or platelets, avoidance of lumen collapse under negative pressure or crimping of catheter segments at points of bending, physical strength and integrity to avoid breaks or disconnections of any component (ability to replace broken connectors is desirable), resistance to deterioration of the catheter material by antiseptic agents that might be applied at the skin surface, placement procedures with minimum trauma, difficulty and risk, and radiopaque appearance on X-ray, for evaluation of placement and long-term location.

The evolution of chronic CVC for dialysis is a history of new ideas being applied to solve these requirements for CVC, while simultaneously creating designs that are relatively easy to insert [4].

Designs of Chronic CVC for Dialysis

Figure 1 includes schematic diagrams of chronic CVC used for dialysis from the 1960s to the present. The design and function of these catheters are described below, in the order of increasing complexity of the devices.

(a) Canaud designed two 10-French catheters for hemodialysis to be placed side by side through the jugular vein and SVC into the right atrium [2, 3]. Each catheter has side holes arranged in a spiral around the tip of the catheter. The catheters initially had no cuffs, but more recently are secured by a subcutaneous grommet (a plastic component connecting the two catheters). Tesio added subcutaneous Dacron cuffs to each of these catheters, to fix the catheters in position in the subcutaneous tract [5, 6]. Canaud and Tesio catheters have been used for dialysis access for months to years, though usually with the use of radiologic procedures to restore patency. The largest resistance to the use of the Canaud or Tesio catheters is from surgeons and radiologists who do not wish to perform two separate IJ punctures for guidewire placement, two catheter insertions through split sheaths, and two separate tunneling procedures.

(b) Mahurkar designed a chronic CVC of soft materials and blunt tips and double-d blood flow lumens [1]. Each D-shaped lumen ended in a single port. The arterial lumen entry port was proximal to the venous port. The double-d design allowed a relatively low hydraulic resistance, as with acute catheters. A subcutaneous cuff fixed the catheter in position within the subcutaneous space. The catheter was placed through a single split sheath into position with tips within the right atrium. There have been several recent variations on this catheter design. One is the Opti-Flow catheter, which has a return lumen that is somewhat round in shape, and a removal lumen that is more C-shaped. This same general design is included in the LifeJet, Circle C, More-Flow and HemoGlide catheters. Another variation is the Dura-Flow catheter. In this catheter (constructed of Carbothane®) the arterial lumen is back-cut, creating a shape which may be less likely to be blocked by fibrosis or clot. The venous lumen also enlarges from D-shape to circular, resulting in a larger end port also making it somewhat more resistant to blockage.

(c) Quinton designed the PermCath dual lumen chronic catheter, an oval-shaped chronic catheter of about 20-French circumference and including two cylindrical 8-French lumens [7, 8]. The tip was cut to create two entry ports the shorter being the arterial and the longer being the return lumen. The catheter was the first chronic catheter for dialysis, and the first hemodialysis catheter to employ a subcutaneous cuff, yet it is still being placed and used. The catheter is placed through an oval-shaped split sheath that is advanced over a guidewire and an oval-shaped, pointed dilator. It is one of a few chronic CVC for dialysis made of silicone. An adaptation of this shape is used in the Niagara acute catheter, having a preformed 180° bend to conform over the clavicle and point downward.

(d) Uldall created a chronic catheter with roughly the same body shape as the Quinton PermCath, but with a two separate tips and a thin wall and collapsible return lumen. The collapsible return lumen allows the distal portion of the device to be inserted through a cylindrical split sheath, like most chronic catheters, instead of an oval-shaped split sheath. The mid-body of the catheter is oval shaped, and advances into the vein after the split sheath is removed.

(e) The Ash Split Cath chronic catheter (fig. 1, 2) has a double-d configuration in the mid-body, but separates into two separate distal tips, each with side holes in all directions. One goal of having two tips was to combine the

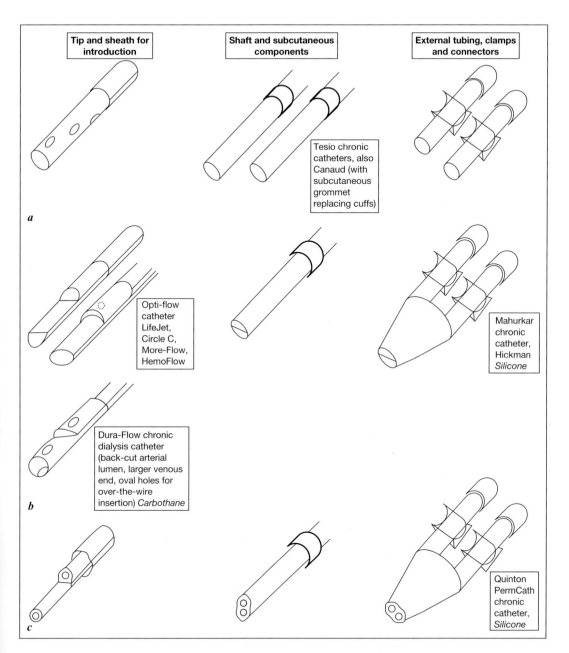

Tip and sheath for introduction	Shaft and subcutaneous components	External tubing, clamps and connectors

a — Tesio chronic catheters, also Canaud (with subcutaneous grommet replacing cuffs)

b — Opti-flow catheter LifeJet, Circle C, More-Flow, HemoFlow — Mahurkar chronic catheter, Hickman *Silicone*

Dura-Flow chronic dialysis catheter (back-cut arterial lumen, larger venous end, oval holes for over-the-wire insertion) *Carbothane*

c — Quinton PermCath chronic catheter, *Silicone*

Fig. 1. Physical components and designs of chronic CVC for dialysis. Thin lines represent the catheter bodies and a sheath for insertion. Heavy lines are subcutaneous cuffs or grommets (labeled G). Material of body construction is polyurethane unless otherwise indicated (silicone or Carbothane®). See text for discussion.

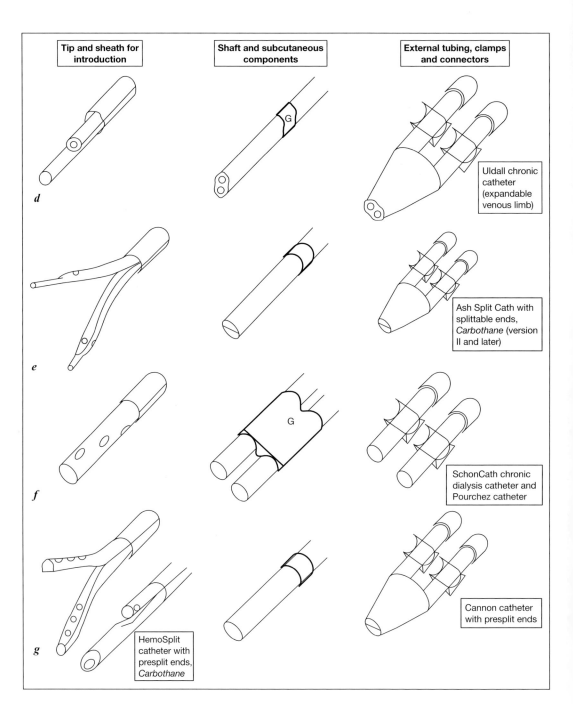

Tip and sheath for introduction	Shaft and subcutaneous components	External tubing, clamps and connectors

d — Uldall chronic catheter (expandable venous limb)

e — Ash Split Cath with splittable ends, *Carbothane* (version II and later)

f — SchonCath chronic dialysis catheter and Pourchez catheter

g — HemoSplit catheter with presplit ends, *Carbothane* / Cannon catheter with presplit ends

Fig. 1. (continued).

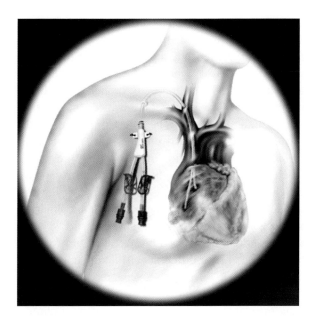

Fig. 2. Ash Split Cath in position with tips in the right atrium.

simplicity of placement of a single-body cylindrical catheter with the low hydraulic resistance of double-d lumens and the excellent hydraulic properties of blood flow through holes on all sides of each distal limb (similar to the Tesio catheters). Another goal was to purposefully separate the limbs of the catheter, making them softer and more flexible and thus diminishing and distributing contact pressure of the catheter limbs against the wall of the vena cava (also similar to Tesio catheters). A unique feature is the step-down in diameter at the tip of the removal and return limbs. This step-down slightly increases the pressure drop at the tip, assuring that blood will enter or exit through all of the side holes, at almost any blood flow rate (in comparison to the Tesio catheter which passes blood through the side holes only when flow is over 300 ml/min). The catheter is tunneled from the exit site through the primary incision with the tips together. The tips are split to the length desired, the cylindrical split sheath is advanced into the SVC and the dilator removed. The tips are grasped together and advanced through the split sheath, and the split sheath removed. The catheter may also be placed over a guidewire (see below). Overall hydraulic function of the catheter is similar to the Tesio and Canaud catheters, with higher flow and less recirculation that other single-body catheters [1, 9]. The Split Cath II and later versions are constructed of Carbothane.

(f) The SchonCath includes two catheters with intravenous and subcutaneous portions identical to the Canaud catheters and Tesio catheters (but without the subcutaneous cuffs). Instead of cuffs, there is a plastic grommet that fixes the two catheters together. Initially this grommet was placed in the subcutaneous space below the primary incision but more recently the grommet has been modified to enter the jugular vein as an oval shape linking the two catheters. The internal catheter portions are placed into the central vein through an oval split sheath placed over guidewire and dilator. The grommet is advanced into the hole in the IJ vein to block bleeding through the hole. The external portions of the catheter are tunneled independently to exit sites from the primary incisions. Hydraulic function and long-term results of function of this catheter are similar to the Canaud and Tesio catheters. The Pourchez catheter also has two separate Tesio-like tips and like the Schon catheter has a cylindrical shape of the part entering the vein. However, like the Uldall or Quinton catheter the cylindrical shape continues through the subcutaneous course through the exit site.

(g) The Cannon catheter has a double-d-shaped body ending in two separate tips, similar to the Split Cath. One major difference is that the tips are preformed to separate at an angle of about 30°. This preset separation requires that the catheter tips be placed within the right atrium rather than 'at the junction of the SVC and the right atrium' (as stated in product literature of most chronic CVC). Another difference is that while there is a slight step-down in size and a circular shape of the tip of the return lumen, the arterial lumen is D-shaped. Finally, the side hole position is designed so that during 'over-the-wire' insertion (described below) the guidewire enters the venous (return) lumen, passes out through the first side hole and then crosses over the arterial (outflow) tip to enter a side hole on the outside of the arterial tip. This wire passage may help to make the catheter advance over a guidewire more easily in spite of the relatively large size of the venous tip. Finally, the catheter is tunneled from inside-out, interfacing with a hub having two D-shaped stainless connectors. The HemoSplit catheter also has preformed split cylindrical ends leading from a double-d body, but the degree of separation of the tips is much lower, about 10°. The venous end is larger than the arterial end but smaller than the body of the catheter.

Material/Design Requirements for Successful Chronic CVC for Dialysis

The materials used for chronic CVC for dialysis have evolved over the years as more options have existed, but the requirements have stayed the same or become more stringent. In some ways, requirements are intrinsically contradictory:

Thickness: To provide maximal blood flow, the inner lumens of CVC for dialysis must be as large as possible, while the overall size as small as possible. Therefore, the catheter walls should necessarily be as thin as possible.

Strength: The body of the catheter, hub joints, and connectors and tubing clamp segments must be strong enough to avoid cracks or breaks on the body of the catheter, at the hub joints, or in the connectors or tubing clamp segments. This requirement has become more stringent as chronic catheters are used for longer periods of time (up to several years for some chronic CVC).

Flexibility: Chronic CVC have a relatively straight course within the vein, but bend fairly sharply in the subcutaneous tunnel. Also they remain within the SVC or femoral vein for a long time, with some continued pressure on the vein wall. Therefore the body of the catheter must have flexibility. The tips and material of the catheter should be as soft as possible.

Rigidity: During placement, while the catheter is relatively straight, it must be rigid enough to slide over a guidewire (for acute CVC or over-the-wire placement of chronic CVC) or through a split sheath (for chronic CVC). Therefore there is a limit to the intrinsic softness of a catheter. Some catheter materials such as polyurethanes have thermoplastic qualities, so that they have some rigidity during placement and are softer when they reach body temperature. Catheters must also be rigid enough to avoid collapse of the removal lumen under negative pressures up to 350 mm Hg.

Resistance to crimping: When chronic CVC are bent, they must resist the tendency to have a lumen collapse or 'crimp' or 'kink' at the apex of the bend in the subcutaneous tunnel. The solution is partly solved by materials; generally softer materials have less tendency to crimp. Design is also important; oval-shaped catheters bend naturally without kinking in the direction perpendicular to the flat surface, double-d catheter configurations bend easily in the direction perpendicular to the flat internal wall, and relatively thick walls in cylindrical catheter limbs help prevent bending.

Moldability: With the increasing complexity of CVC designs, it has become necessary to change diameters and shapes of the body components after the body of the CVC is extruded. This requires that the material is moldable under heat or stress, to obtain the desired shape.

Bondability: The various components of a CVC must all be glued or welded together to create a catheter with overall integrity. Materials that dissolve into solvents allow solvent glues to make the strongest bonds. Materials that can be heat welded can also create solid bonds. Bondability requires that connectors be made of plastic materials rather than metal, in general.

Conformance to the body shape: At the skin surface, the catheter usually penetrates the skin at some upward angle to the skin surface. The external portions of the catheter are sutured or taped to the skin surface, meaning that there is some degree of bend at the exit site. Further, the external connections and extension tubings must be bandaged next to the skin. Some catheter designs include increased material at the skin exit site (such as the Split Cath XL).

Some acute catheters have a 180° bend preformed in the body of the catheter to bend over the clavicle, or a 150° bend preformed into the clamping segment. The materials chosen must have the capability to be formed into these relatively permanent shapes.

Effective clamping and expansion of extension tubings: The extension tubings of chronic CVC for dialysis must remain clamped between dialysis procedures, to serve as a second-line defense against bleeding or air passage in case the cap comes off of the connectors. The tubings must also be clamped whenever the cap is removed for connection to dialysis lines or injection with a syringe. During dialysis however the tubings must expand to allow passage of blood and avoid collapse (especially on the arterial limb). Rotating the position of the clamp on the tubing is helpful, but most extension tubings still develop a 'set' over time and require some squeezing and coaxing to open properly. Some materials like silicone function better in this regard than polyurethane.

Resistance to dissolution by chemicals: For almost every material there is a nemesis, a chemical that will dissolve the material. Stringent chemicals are often used as antiseptics at the exit site and on catheter hubs. Catheters should be created of materials that resist dissolution by commonly used antiseptics such as alcohols, iodine, or peroxide.

Radiopacity: In order for plastic materials to be visualized on x-ray they need to contain some elements with high atomic density to be seen on x-ray. Barium is the most commonly added component, which is mixed in with the plastic before extrusion. It is the barium which makes the catheter materials white (rather than nearly clear, as natural silicone and polyurethane). If too little barium is added, the catheter is barely visible. If too much is added then the structural integrity and surface properties of the materials are affected.

The materials used for acute and chronic CVC for dialysis have included: polyethylene, Teflon, silicone, polyurethane, and Carbothane (polyurethane/ polycarbonate copolymer).

Polyethylene is intrinsically somewhat rigid. Therefore, it was well suited for acute CVC that require relative rigidity and a pointed tip to follow over a guidewire, such as Shaldon catheters. However, in more complex forms it becomes too rigid, it is difficult to glue to dissimilar materials (though it can be heat welded), kinks when bent and is difficult to extrude with thin walls. Its stiffness is too great for safe use in any chronic CVC.

Teflon is also quite rigid, and has been used for over-the-guidewire acute CVC. However, it cannot be molded after extrusion and is difficult to glue to any material, including Teflon. It is not used in any CVC for dialysis at this time, though it is used in peripheral intravenous catheters.

Silicone is intrinsically a soft and flexible material, an advantage for chronic CVC. However, to have sufficient strength it must be somewhat thick.

Silicone catheters generally require a thicker wall than catheters of other materials to avoid lumen collapse, provide some rigidity and avoid kinking. Silicone is easily and strongly glued to other silicone components by solvent glues, but difficult to glue to other materials. It is used in several chronic CVC, but less than other materials. Silicone is greatly weakened by iodine, but is only slightly degraded by povidone-iodine solutions or peroxide. It is compatible with most alcohols and ointments.

Polyurethane can be created in forms that are fairly rigid or soft and flexible. It has a high material strength, so that catheter walls can be made quite thin with preservation of some rigidity in the longitudinal axis and avoidance of lumen collapse at high negative pressures. Polyurethane has thermoplastic properties, becoming softer at body temperature, especially Tecothane®, a mixture of polyurethanes of differing molecular weight. Polyurethane can be easily bonded to several types of plastic materials, and has excellent moldability. Most CVC today are made from polyurethanes. Polyurethane's nemesis is alcohol. Ointments containing polyethylene glycol (such as Mupirocin® ointment or crème or povidone-iodine ointment) can weaken the catheter considerably. One antibiotic ointment that can safely be used at the exit site of polyurethane catheters is Neosporin®, which has a petroleum base.

Polyurethane/polycarbonate copolymers (such as Carbothane) have all of the advantages of polyurethane, but with a greater strength. Catheters created from copolymers can have thinner walls and the same physical properties as catheters made from polyurethane. The copolymer materials are resistant to iodine, peroxide, and alcohols. Copolymer materials will be used for construction of most chronic CVC in the future, and possibly also acute CVC.

Merely inspecting a catheter, it is difficult to determine the material from which it is made. It is important to have a list of chronic CVC used in a dialysis unit, their material and what chemicals must be avoided. For current CVC used for dialysis table 1 elucidates the materials of construction and incompatible chemicals.

Clinical Effectiveness and Survival of the Split Cath: Results in One Dialysis Center

The Split Cath has been on the market for 5 years, so considerable clinical experience has been gained with this catheter. At the Dialysis Center for Greater Lafayette we have performed a prospective, observational study on the success of the Split Cath catheter since 1998, with early data reported in 2002 [10]. Including satellite units the Dialysis Center provides hemodialysis for about 150 ESRD patients. Due to positive early experience with the Split Cath,

Table 1. Materials of construction and incompatible chemicals

Material	Incompatible chemicals
Polyurethane	Alcohols including isopropyl alcohol and ointments containing polyethylene glycol (PEG) such as Mupirocin ointment and crème and povidone-iodine ointment; povidone-iodine solution is ok; possible deterioration with chlorhexidine
Silicone	Tincture of iodine; potential degradation by povidone-iodine solution over long times
Carbothane	None known

this catheter quickly became the standard access for initiating dialysis in patients requiring chronic vascular access for dialysis. The Split Cath was placed in the right or left IJ vein of 265 unselected and consecutive adult ESRD patients beginning dialysis or continuing dialysis after failure of another access. The IJ catheters of this study were intended as a permanent access or as a 'bridge' access until creation and development of a fistula or graft. Placement of 80% of the catheters was by nephrologists, the rest being placed by radiologists. Approximately 80% of the catheters were placed in the right IJ vein, and 20% were placed in the left IJ vein. For right jugular placement, the 28-cm catheter was used. For left jugular placement, the 32-cm catheter was used. All catheters were placed percutaneously, using ultrasound guidance for needle insertion into the vein. Catheters in the jugular veins were tunneled in a gently arcuate direction to an exit site under the lateral clavicle, and the cuff placed generally at least 2 cm below the exit site. For right IJ catheters, the catheter tips were positioned in the center of the atrium using external landmarks (positioning the tip 2 inches above the bottom of the sternum), or by fluoroscopy. Fluoroscopy was used to confirm guidewire and catheter tip position when placing catheters in the left IJ or in external jugular veins. Exit site care of the catheters was by strict protocol which included: patient and nurse wearing masks, nurse wearing nonsterile gloves, sterile drape placed under the catheter, 5 min povidone-iodine soak of connectors before removing caps, dressing change at the start of dialysis rather than the end, swabbing the exit site with povidone-iodine solution after each dialysis and bandaging with gauze and nonocclusive dressing. Patients were advised to not remove the dressing before the next dialysis and to avoid water contact of the dressing. Heparin lock was on average 5,000 units per catheter lumen, filling the exact catheter volume (in some patients, 10,000 units per lumen). Nurses were trained to carefully inspect the catheter with each use and report any apparent problems with the catheter, exit site or tunnel.

Removal of Split Cath catheters was performed when the catheters were no longer needed, or when catheter failures occurred making the catheter unusable or risky to use (such as outflow failure, break or disconnection, exit site infection, or presumed catheter-related bloodstream infection, CRBSI). The nephrologists merely followed the standard definitions of catheter failure when determining that a catheter should be removed: blood flow rate less than 250 ml/min, evidence of CRBSI, or persistent exit site infection. Failure of flow was defined as inability of the catheter to reproducibly deliver blood flow rates of 250 ml/min or greater. Fibrinolytic therapy (urokinase initially and tPA later) was used to improve flow in catheters when flow diminished. Catheter injection with radiopaque dye and brushing of the catheters was performed in radiology if fibrinolytic therapy did not provide sufficient improvement in flow, and in some cases 4-hour infusions of tPA were used if brushing did not restore catheter flow. Catheter sheath stripping was not performed on any of the catheters (our practice has been that if the radiologic procedure indicates a catheter sheath, the catheter is removed and replaced in another site or through the same internal tract with a separate exit site).

For the 265 patients receiving the IJ Split Caths, the average follow-up was 28 months. During this time there were 57 failures of the catheter necessitating catheter removal or replacement. Breakdown of cause of catheter failures was as follows: 55% of catheter failures were due to infection (most in the presence of signs of bacteremia, some with exit infection), 28% were due to lack of flow (exclusively outflow failure), and 18% were due to breaks or leaks in the catheter. Figure 3 indicates the life table analysis of the percentage of Split Cath catheters remaining without failure over 24 months. The percentage of catheters remaining failure-free at 12 months was 81%. By Kaplan-Maier analysis, the projected failure-free half-life of the Split Cath catheter is 30 months.

A comparison was also made of the flow rate and venous and arterial pressures of the Split Cath, from venous and arterial pressures and blood flow data automatically collected each half hour during dialysis (Centry Net) and stored in a clinical computer system (Velos). The average hydraulic resistance of the arterial limb is 0.66 ± 0.17 mm Hg/ml/min and the venous limb hydraulic resistance is 0.57 ± 0.11 mm Hg/ml/min. By comparison, the hydraulic resistance of the arterial limb of grafts and fistulas in the same unit is 0.51 ± 0.23 mm Hg/ml/min and of the venous limb 0.52 ± 0.13 mm Hg/ml/min (without correction for graft/fistula pressure, which augments flow on the arterial side and diminishes flow on the venous side). The hydraulic resistance of blood flow is not significantly different between the Split Cath and the grafts and fistulas in our unit ($p > 0.10$). Further, the average flow rates during

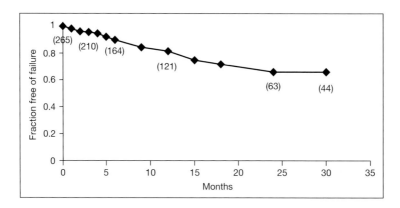

Fig. 3. Life table analysis of percentage of Split Cath catheters functioning without failure (1998–2003). The number of catheters placed or in use is given in parentheses. The percentage of catheters remaining failure-free at 12 months is 80%. By Kaplan-Maier analysis, the projected half-life of the Split Cath catheter is 30 months.

hemodialysis with the Split Cath (266 ± 59 ml/min) were not different from blood flow rates during dialysis with grafts or fistulas (295 ± 46 ml/min, p > 0.10) [11].

This prospective, observational study of Split Cath catheters in adult patients was not randomized and therefore did not directly compare longevity without complication of the Split Cath to grafts, fistulas, or any other type of chronic CVC for dialysis. However, the conclusion of the study is rather simple. The average 30-month failure-free survival of Split Caths in our unit is better than the results using AV grafts in most studies (with interventions). In the past and in DOQI documents, chronic CVC for dialysis have been maligned as having higher complication rates, resulting in lower blood flow rates, and being less desirable than fistulas or grafts. In our study, the Split Cath provided the same blood flow rate and the same hydraulic resistance (statistically) as when dialysis is performed by needles in grafts and fistulas.

There are several reasons for the success of the Split Cath in our study, most of which would apply to successful use of any chronic CVC for dialysis:

Catheters are placed by small incisions and ultrasonic technique, rather than by dissection, resulting in less trauma and dissection in the area of the IJ vein

Most catheters were placed by three nephrologists with considerable skill in placement; some were placed by a few radiologists also with considerable skill

Catheter insertion point is in the IJ veins; results when catheters must be placed in other veins are less positive

Catheter care and access in the dialysis units is by strict protocol; especially important is the training of each nurse and technician to inspect each catheter at the start of each dialysis procedure and report any problems promptly

The incidence of CRBSI is low in the dialysis units, averaging 1/1,000 patient-days as opposed to the 3–4/1,000 patient-days demonstrated in most studies of CRBSI [1]

Patients are instructed to avoid changing the exit site bandage or getting the bandage wet

Catheters are usually removed if there is evidence or suspicion of CRBSI and if signs of infection fail to clear rapidly with antibiotics

If catheters are replaced over a guidewire for reasons of loss of flow or exit infection; the catheter is first tunneled from a separate exit site and then inserted into the central vein over a guidewire

The success of the use of Split Cath catheters in our units should be replicable in any other dialysis unit following the same general approach to catheter placement, use, care and replacement. Other chronic CVC for dialysis may also be proven to have the same overall success, following the same general techniques.

Studies of Split Cath and Other Chronic CVC for Dialysis

There have been a number of studies of the Split Cath as a chronic CVC for dialysis. Some like our study above were observational studies and some were randomized, prospectively controlled comparing the effectiveness of the catheter to other catheters (table 2).

Trerotola et al. [9] performed a randomized study of 12 ESRD patients receiving 14-French Split Cath catheters placed versus 12 patients receiving 13.5-French Hickman catheters. Weekly for 6 weeks the blood flow rate was measured using Transonic flow monitors, while the blood pump was set at speeds of 200, 300, 350, 400 ml/min and as high as possible with sustained flow. The measured blood flow rate at the highest pump (QbEff) setting was 422 ± 12 ml/min for the Split Cath and 359 ± 13 ml/min for the Hickman ($p < 0.005$). Recirculation was significantly less at all pump settings for the Split Cath patients ($p = 0.01$–0.06), though for both catheters it remained below 6%. One Split Cath failed at day 7 with poor flow and was removed and a fibrous sheath was noted (it was not stated whether the patient had previously had an IJ catheter for dialysis). Of patients with Hickman catheters 38% required urokinase infusion during the study. Three insertion complications occurred with the Split Cath group, two catheters with kinking (improved with manipulation) and two with bleeding from the catheter exit site (resolving with compression, occurring after heparin loading of the catheter).

Richard et al. [12] performed a randomized study comparing the Split Cath, Opti-Flow and Tesio catheters in 113 placements in ESRD patients. Maximum (effective) blood flow rates were compared between the catheters immediately after placement, and 30 and 90 days after placement. Blood flow rate tended to be higher with the Split Cath but results were not significantly

Table 2. Randomized, prospectively controlled studies of the Split Cath versus other chronic CVC

Year	First author	Ref. No.	Duration of study	Catheter types, number	Function of catheters, ml/min	Survival of catheters
1999	Trerotola	9	6 weeks	Split Cath, 12	QbEff = 422 Recirc = 1.3%	92% at 6 weeks
				Hickman, 12	QbEff = 359 Recirc = 5.6%	62% at 6 weeks not needing urokinase
2001	Richard	12	120 days, mean	Split Cath, 38	QbEff = 338 at 90 days	Mean catheter survival 302 days Cath inf'n/100 days = 0.12
				Opti-Flow, 39	QbEff = 327 at 90 days	Mean catheter survival 176 days Cath inf'n/100 days = 0.35
				Tesio, 36	QbEff = 297 at 90 days	Mean catheter survival 264 days Cath inf'n/100 days = 0.14
2002	Trerotola	13	100 days, mean	Split Cath, 64	QbEff = 363 at 6 months Recirc = 1.7 at 3 months	78% at 120 days Late cx/100 days = 0.22
				Opti-Flow, 68	QbEff = 366 at 6 months Recirc = 9.5 at 3 months	64% at 120 days Late cx/100 days = 0.43

QbEff = Measured blood flow at highest pump setting with sustained flow; Cath inf'n = catheter infection complitations; cx = complications.

different. Failure-free survival of the catheters was analyzed with an average follow-up of 120 days. Though statistically not significant, the predicted lifespan appeared higher for the Split Cath and Tesio catheters than the Opti-Flow. Placement complications occurred only with Tesio and Opti-Flow catheters.

Trerotola et al. [13] also performed a randomized study comparing the Split Cath and Opti-Flow catheters in 132 placements in ESRD patients.

Table 3. Observational studies on the success of the Split Cath

Year	First author	Ref. No.	Duration of study	Catheter types, number	Function of catheters, ml/min	Survival of catheters
1998	Mankus	11	2 months	Split Cath, 10 Hickman, 22 Tesio, 17	Ave Qb = 295 Ave Qb = 279 Ave Qb = 300	– – –
2000	Conz	14	4–8 months	Split Cath, 7	Ave Qb = 250	100%
2001	Conz	15	3 months	Split Cath, 5 geriatric patients	Ave Qb = 250 Recirc <2%	100%
2002	Ewing	16	183 days	Split Cath, 118 Radiologic placement	URR near prescribed 66%	54% at 90 days
2002	Gallieni	17	260 days	Split Cath, 28	Ave Qb = 308 at 12 months	96% survival and primary patency
2003	Cetinkaya	18	360 days	Split Cath, 92	Thrombosis in 16%	Mean survival 289 days Cath infection = 0.82/1,000 patient-days

Ave Qb = Average blood flow rate during a dialysis procedure; URR = urea reduction ratio.

Complications during placement were no different for the two catheters and ranged 15–17% (mostly kinking). Opti-Flow delivered significantly higher flow rates when tested at 1 month, but there was no significant difference in flow at 6 months. Recirculation was always less with the Split Cath catheter but not always significantly lower. The Split Cath had a significantly longer half-life, partly due to a lower infection rate but also due to some mechanical failures of the Opti-Flow. Postulating on reasons that the Split Cath might have lower infection rates, the authors suggested that the 'self-cleaning' function of the Split Cath, with continuous flow through all side holes, may diminish fibrin sheath and therefore decrease the opportunity for bacterial colonization.

In addition to these randomized studies there have been a number of observational studies on the success of the Split Cath, as shown in table 3.

Mankus et al. [11] published the first paper on the Split Cath and confirmed hydraulic function similar to both the Mahurkar (Hickman) and Tesio Twin catheters. Conz et al. [14, 15] demonstrated in a small number of patients with failure of fistula development and other geriatric patients that the Split Cath provides the prescribed blood flow (a relatively low 250 ml/min) over 3–8 months without failure or complication. Ewing et al. [16] placed 118 Split Caths in ESRD patients who were awaiting fistula creation or had no other access possible. Flow rate was satisfactory according to unit prescriptions. The 3-month infection rate was 18.6% (2.4/1,000 patient-days), but only one third of these catheters required removal. Gallieni et al. [17] placed 28 Split Cath catheters in patients who were not candidates for surgical AV fistula or graft placement. Only one catheter failed during mean a follow-up of 260 days, and there was a 96% primary patency rate. Cetinkaya et al. [18] placed 92 Split Caths in ESRD patients for whom it was planned as the permanent vascular access. The catheter-related infection rate was 0.82 espisodes/1,000 patient-days, and the mean duration of catheter survival was 289 days. All of these prospective observational studies were performed in centers in which the Split Cath was a relatively new access device. Given this background, the results of use of the catheter for long-term dialysis were satisfactory to very positive.

Comparison of Complications of AV Fistulas, AV Grafts, and Chronic CVC for Dialysis

Regarding the incidence of complications with various types of access devices, there is no doubt that the AV fistula is the safest and most effective access for chronic dialysis. However, there is reason to question whether grafts have fewer or more complications than CVC. There have actually been few studies comparing the overall complications of these three types of dialysis access over time. A prospective, multicenter study of vascular access was performed and recently reported by the Research Board of the European Dialysis and Transplant Nurses Association/European Renal Care Association. The study followed the incidence of complications of AV fistulas, AV grafts and chronic CVC for dialysis in 1,380 ESRD patients in Europe for a 1-year period [19]. At the start of the study 77% of patients had an AV fistula, 10% had an AV graft and 13% had a chronic CVC for dialysis. As expected, AV fistulas had the lowest incidence of complications, 15.5% in 1 year. The overall complications for AV grafts was 37.3% over the year and chronic CVC for dialysis had a complication rate of 27.5%. Of types of complications, infection was higher for CVC and thrombosis was higher for AV grafts as shown in table 4. The conclusion of the study was that AV fistulas are the preferred access for chronic dialysis. However, judging by the incidence of complications chronic CVC for dialysis are at least as successful as AV grafts.

Table 4. Incidence of complications in 1 year in 1,380 patients with AV fistula, AV graft, and catheter, and distribution of main complications per type of vascular access [from Research Board of the EDTN/ERCA, 9]

Access type	Patients with complications %	Distribution of complications (total 100%), %				
		thrombosis	stenosis	infection	bleeding	flow problem
AV fistula	15.5	36	28	15	15	7
AV graft	37.3	45	26	6	21	2
Chronic CVC	27.5	18	8	47	8	18

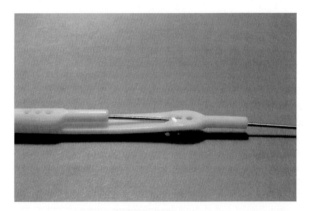

Fig. 4. Ash Split Cath with guidewire threaded through both the venous and arterial limbs, for placement over a guidewire through the IJ vein to the SVC and right atrium.

Advancements in Catheter Placement; the 'Over-the-Wire' Technique

Placement of split-tipped chronic catheters such as the Split Cath has been greatly simplified by the use of the 'over-the-wire' technique [20]. In this technique a guidewire is placed as usual and the tract dilated as usual. The outside end of the guidewire is threaded through the venous end of the catheter and then made to exit from an inside side hole. The wire is then directed through the arterial end of the catheter and advanced through the outside connector (fig. 4). A hemostat is placed on the outside end of the wire and the catheter is advanced over the wire until the tip is at the skin surface. For catheters like the Cannon catheter which are advanced into the vein and then tunneled outward to the skin, the placement is directly along the line of the guidewire and the guidewire can be held relatively constant in position. For catheters like the Split Cath the catheter is first tunneled from a skin exit site to primary incision, the guidewire placed through the catheter and the catheter advanced in an arcuate manner along the guidewire and into the vein while the guidewire is intermittently retracted. When the catheter forms an acute arc over the primary incision (over the IJ vein) pushing the arc downward completes the insertion. Using the 'over-the-guidewire' technique for chronic and acute split catheters has several advantages versus using the split sheath:

The procedure is simpler and avoids need to learn how to grasp the ends of the catheter to insert them into the sheath, and how to split and remove the sheath from around the catheter

There is less blood loss and a lower risk of air entry to the vein versus the split sheath (even when the sheath is 'pinched' after the dilator is removed)

There is less bleeding around the catheter after placement, since the vein entry hole is the size of the catheter, not the size of the larger split sheath

The technique is suitable for any vein, including femoral veins where the pressure of the blood and the bend of the inguinal vein can make use of the split sheath problematic

For chronic CVC for dialysis there are some problems of placement which are specific to the over-the-wire technique:

If the catheter is advanced slowly, then excessive bleeding can still occur as blood exits the arterial lumen around the guidewire (this can be minimized by closing the arterial clamp over the guidewire, as suggested by Patel et al. [20])

As blood exits slowly through the arterial lumen it can clot, causing flow problems during the first dialysis treatment

If the central venous pressure is very low , then air can still enter the venous system during placement through the arterial lumen and around the guidewire

The guidewire cannot be held in constant position while the catheter is advanced; rather the catheter is usually advanced and then the guidewire retracted. If the guidewire is clamped within the arterial extension set then the entire catheter must be advanced with the guidewire

When placing catheters that have already been tunneled under the skin from exit site to primary incision, the catheter becomes sharply arcuate just above the skin as it follows the guidewire out of the primary incision and then back into the vein. This last portion of the catheter must be compressed under the skin through the primary incision. At this time it is impossible to retract the guidewire or prevent it from advancing further into the vena cava or into the right atrium

The guidewire is always bent at the point of arcuate bend of the previously tunneled catheter. This bend in the guidewire and the passage of the guidewire through several holes at the end of the catheter means that there is resistance to movement of the guidewire when removed from the catheter. The guidewire requires more force for removal from the catheter, and there is more stress on the guidewire. In fact during guidewire removal in this procedure, some guidewires have fractured, with the outer spiral winding separating from the inner wire. Careful traction of both the spiral winding and internal wire usually allow the guidewire to be removed intact

The placement procedure is made easier by a Teflon-coated wire such as the Glidewire® (Boston Scientific) as suggested by Patel et al. [20]. This guidewire costs about USD 80.

The long (150 cm) length of the guidewire makes the control of the end of the wire during catheter placement of the catheter more difficult, and the outer coating of this Glidewire can still occasionally fracture from the internal wire if significant force is needed in removal of the guidewire

Chronic CVC which can be placed over a guidewire must have relatively small tips for both arterial and venous lumens, and must have side holes properly placed to allow exit of the wire from the medial side of the venous lumen to enter into the arterial lumen. The Split Cath has small enough tips to make the procedure relatively easy. The Dura-Flow catheter has a guidewire on the outside of the arterial lumen to receive the guidewire, assuring that the catheter follows on one side of the guidewire and making placement easier in spite of the large lumen sizes

These problems and risks of 'over-the-wire' placement can be minimized by some logical steps. First, using an ultrasound machine the patient can be positioned so that the jugular vein is moderately distended but not overly distended, before placing the first needle into the vein. This assures only a modest central venous pressure, which minimizes blood loss through the catheter during advancement of the catheter over the guidewire, and also minimizes the risk of air entering the vena cava. Using fluoroscopy or cardiac monitoring it is possible to advance the tip of the guidewire past the heart and into the inferior vena cava (in most cases). This means that advancing the wire during catheter placement has less risk. Creating a wider than usual primary incision over the jugular vein means that there is a less sharply arcuate bend in this part of the catheter as it is compressed under the skin. Using a Teflon-coated wire such as the Glidewire, which has greater flexibility and resiliency, means that there is less tendency for the wire to bend or kink at the primary incision during placement.

In spite of some potential problems, the over-the-guidewire technique has moderate safety advantages over split sheath placement techniques for chronic CVC for dialysis. Training is easier for the procedure, though there is still a need to learn as regards the proper force and direction for and 'feel' of advancing the catheter into the IJ vein. Further, anyone placing catheters using the over-the-wire technique must also be skilled in the use of the split sheath since in some patients advancement of the catheter over the guidewire is not possible. This is especially likely in patients who have had previous chronic or acute catheters in the IJ, and have scarring of the vein wall [20]. The over-the-wire technique is also more suited to performance in the ICU than the split sheath technique. This means that soft dual-tipped chronic CVC can be placed for treatment of patients with acute renal failure with less risk and difficulty. The use of a chronic tunneled and cuffed CVC for patients with acute renal failure provides advantages of increased blood flow, more stable blood flow, less venous irritation and much greater duration of use versus acute catheters. Patients with soft chronic catheters in the femoral location may walk or sit when desired, and all patients with IJ catheters can walk or sit as desired. Most importantly, the fact that only one catheter is needed for the course of acute renal failure means that there is significantly less vein trauma as opposed to the usual course of changing the acute catheter every 5 days or so. If the patient recovers in other ways but still has renal failure, the chronic CVC is already in place for beginning chronic dialysis therapy.

Future Trends

The advent of successful chronic CVC for dialysis has been a great advance for patients with ESRD, those beginning hemodialysis and for many who remain on dialysis for many years. It has been only 15 years since the PermCath was introduced. Only a few years ago, many authors routinely repeated statements that chronic CVC for dialysis were usable for at most 3 months. Now, longevity and adequate function of chronic CVC for dialysis are maintained for a year or more on average. Though alternative access by AV fistula should always be investigated and attempted when likely to work, the chronic CVC for dialysis serves as a workable alternative to AV grafts.

In spite of the advances, chronic CVC still have significant problems and limitations. For each of these problems, there will exist a solution which will advance the technology and benefits of chronic CVC for dialysis.

Catheter-related infections: Catheter materials, chemical impregnation methods or catheter locks must be found to kill bacteria in the biofilm layers both on the outside and inside of chronic CVC for dialysis, in order to decrease this most common complication of the catheters. The antibacterial effect must remain for many months rather than a week or so (as acute catheter treatments).

Catheter fibrous sheathing: Catheter material, chemical impregnations, shapes or blood flow patterns must be found to prevent the growth of fibrous sheaths around the catheter bodies, which leads eventually to loss of flow. Some degree of sheath probably forms on every chronic catheter placed in the vena cava, and limits eventual flow of many.

Central venous stenosis: Methods to distribute or diminish 'wear' on the vena cava must be evolved to avoid this serious and still frequent complication. Avoiding use of acute dialysis catheters diminishes the frequency of central venous stenosis.

External component bulk: Patients bandage and keep dry the hubs, extension tubings, clamps and connectors, but many also complain about the general bulk of the catheters components on their bodies. Also, the preclusion of showering is a real bother to many patients. Subcutaneous ports were proposed as one solution (LifeSite, BioLink) but clearly are not the answer for most long-term patients. Eventually more radical skin level 'connectology' will be applied.

External component breakage: More durable yet still light-weight components are possible. Simplifying the entire catheter design to limit the size and number of glued connections is a partial solution.

With a few more improvements, chronic CVC for dialysis could become a painless, effective and safe long-term access for the majority of dialysis patients and perfectly acceptable as an alternative to AV grafts.

References

1   Schwab SJ, Beathard G: The hemodialysis conundrum: Hate living with them, but can't live without them. Kidney Int 1999;56:1–17.
2   Canaud B, Leray-Moragues H, Garrigues V, Mion C: Permanent twin catheter: A vascular access option of choice for haemodialysis in elderly patients. Nephrol Dial Transplant 1998;7:82–88.
3   Canaud B, Leray-Moragues H, Kamoun K, Garrigue V: Temporary vascular access for extracorporeal therapies. Ther Apher 2000;4:249–255.
4   Ash SR: The evolution and function of central venous catheters for dialysis. Semin Dial 2001;14:416–424.
5   Tesio F, De Bax H, Panarello G, Calianno G, Quaia P, Raimondi A, Schinella D: Double catheterization of the internal jugular vein for hemodialysis: Indications, techniques, and clinical results. Artif Organs 1994;18:301–304.
6   Prabhu PN, Kerns SR, Sabatelli FW, Hawkins IF, Ross EA: Long-term performance and complications of the Tesio twin catheter system for hemodialysis access. Am J Kidney Dis 1997;30: 213–218.
7   Blake PG, Huraib S, Wu G, Uldall PR: The use of dual lumen jugular venous catheters as definitive long term access for haemodialysis. Int J Artif Organs 1990;13:26–31.
8   Schwab SJ, Buller GL, McCann RL, Bollinger RR, Stickel DL: Prospective evaluation of a Dacron cuffed hemodialysis catheter for prolonged use. Am J Kidney Dis 1988;1:166–169.
9   Trerotola SO, Shah H, Johnson M, Namyslowski J, Moresco K, Patel N, Kraus M, Gassensmith C, Ambrosius WT: Randomized comparison of high-flow versus conventional hemodialysis catheters. J Vasc Interv Radiol 1999;10:1032–1038.
10   Ash SR, Mankus RA, Sutton JM, Spray M: The Ash Split Cath as long-term IJ access: Hydraulic performance and longevity. J Vasc Access 2002;3:3–9.
11   Mankus RA, Ash SR, Sutton JM: Comparison of blood flow rates and hydraulic resistance between the Mahurkar catheter, the Tesio twin catheter, and the Ash Split Cath. ASAIO J 1998;44: M532–M534.
12   Richard HM, Hastings GS, Boyd-Kranis RL, Murthy R, Radack DM, Santilli JG, Ostergaard C, Coldwell DM: A randomized, prospective evaluation of the Tesio, Ash Split, and Opti-flow hemodialysis catheters. J Vasc Interv Radiol 2001;12:431–435.
13   Trerotola SO, Kraus M, Shah H, Namyslowski J, Johnson MS, Stecker MS, Ahmad I, McLennan G, Patel NH, O'Brien E, Lane KA, Ambrosius WT: Randomized comparison of split tip versus step tip high flow hemodialysis catheters. Kidney Int 2002;62:282–289.
14   Conz PA, Crepaldi C, La Greca G: Slow maturation of arterio-venous fistula in seven uremic patients: Use of Ash Split Cath as temporary, prolonged vascular access. J Vasc Access 2000;1: 51–53.
15   Conz PA, Catalon C, Rissioli E, Normanno M, Fabbian F, Preciso G: Ash Split Cath in geriatric dialyzed patients. Int J Artif Organs 2001;24:663–665.
16   Ewing F, Patel D, Petherick A, Winney R, McBride K: Radiologic placement of the Ash Split haemodialysis catheter: A prospective analysis of outcome and complications. Nephrol Dial Transplant 2002;17:614–619.

17   Gallieni M, Conz PA, Rissioli E, Butti A, Brancaccio D: Placement, performance and complica-
      tions of the Ash Split Cath hemodialysis catheter. Int J Artif Organs 2002;25:1137–1143.
18   Cetinkaya R, Odabas AR, Unlu Y, Selcuk Y, Ates A, Ceviz M: Using cuffed and tunnelled central
      venous catheters as permanent vascular access for hemodialysis: A prospective study. Ren Fail
      2003;25:431–438.
19   Elseviers MM, Van Waeleghem J-P: Identifying vascular access complications among ESRD
      patients in Europe. Nephrol News Issues 2003;17/8:61–99.
20   Patel A, Hofkin S, Ball D, Cohen G, Smith DC: Sheathless technique of Ash Split-Cath insertion.
      J Vasc Interv Radiol 2001;12:376–378.

Stephen R. Ash, MD, FACP,
3601 Sagamore Parkway North,
Lafayette, IN 47904 (USA)
Tel. +1 765 742 4813 #208, Fax +1 765 742 4823, E-Mail sash@hemocleanse.com

Ronco C, Levin NW (eds): Hemodialysis Vascular Access and Peritoneal Dialysis Access.
Contrib Nephrol. Basel, Karger, 2004, vol 142, pp 153–158

....

Long-Term Vascular Access:
The Tesio Catheter

F. Tesio, G. Panarello

Department of Nephrology and Dialysis, S. Maria degli Angeli Hospital,
Pordenone, Italy

Introduction

Extracorporeal blood purification treatments are universally increasing, mainly due to the increasing number of patients being treated and the increasing medical conditions for which such a therapy is indicated. For over 40 years, the Cimino-Brescia fistula has remained the gold standard for hemodialytic vascular access. The introduction of artificial vascular grafts, used when superficial veins have been exhausted, has been efficacious but is still plagued with the frequent problems of thrombosis, stenosis and infection, which limits its use [1]. On the other hand, because of the advanced age of dialyzed patients with multiple comorbidities, proximally placed fistulas can compromise cardiac function [2]. Thus, the role for central venous catheters has increased even though complications such as thrombosis, infections, catheter dysfunction and stenosis exist [3]. Of particular importance is the increased incidence of serious catheter-related infections such as septicemia, osteomyelitis and endocarditis [4].

We studied a catheter designed to decrease such complications.

Materials and Methods

Central Venous Catheterization

Femoral catheterization is complicated by a higher incidence of infection due to its position and thromboembolic events due to irregular flow and the presence of a positive venous pressure [5]. Subclavian catheterization is complicated by potential stenosis due to

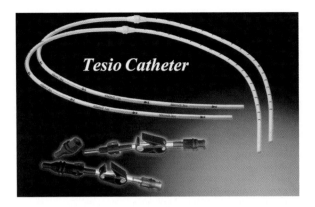

Fig. 1. Spi-Silicone catheter.

vascular dynamics related to flow, inflammation and duration in situ [6]. Such a stenosis can create potential problems for future arteriovenous vascular access. Cimochowski et al. [7] retrospectively studied 52 hemodialysis patients and found a suclavian stenosis in 58% compared to no stenosis found in patients with right internal jugular catheterization. According to the author, the stenosis was found at the point of decubitus of the catheter where its impact on the vein wall was exacerbated by the vessel anatomy, cardiac and blood pump dynamics and movement of the arm.

Our catheter was designed specifically for use in the internal jugular vein.

Materials

In a previous study, 12 of 28 patients with a polyurethane central venous catheter were found to have an asymptomatic thrombosis 15 days after insertion compared with 3 of 28 using a silicone catheter [8]. We chose Spi-Silicone material (fig. 1) for our catheter based on the work of Sioshansi [9] and Bambauer et al. [10]. This material has a free electric charge which modifies the superficial property of the silicon increasing the hydrophilic component and the tension to a critical surface tension of $26\,dyn/cm^2$, which is the ideal value to resist biodeposits when exposed to body fluids thus ideal for long-term usage. With this material, Suzuki et al. [11] demonstrated less thrombosis and infections.

For short- to medium-term catheter usage, among the polyurethane catheters, Bio-Flex® (fig. 2) seems to be the most functional and biocompatible.

The Double Catheter

While we were studying the properties of the material used for long-term catheterization, Canaud et al. [12] published optimal results using two catheters in different positions for long-term access. This technique has the disadvantage of two insertion points but multiple benefits such as: (1) two individual puncture sites of 2.2 mm rarely create a stenosis, compared to a double lumen catheter which has a puncture diameter of 6 mm, (2) the two catheters can be used, removed or replaced separately if infected or dysfunctional, and (3) positioning can be optimized to minimize recirculation [13].

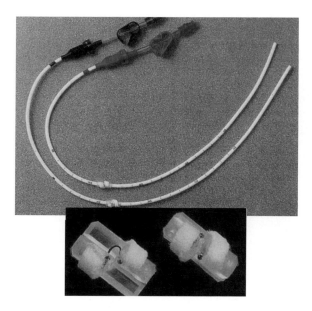

Fig. 2. Bio-Flex catheter with mobile clips.

Catheter Positioning

Once we chose the internal jugular vein as the preferred site, we designed a catheter that had a subcutaneous tunnel of 6–8 cm in the anterior thoracic region before the connection to the extracorporeal circuit. The catheter must be correctly inserted into the vein with the distal lumen in the right atrium (fig. 3), before proceeding to the tunnelization. The distal exit site and the internal point of adherence decrease the risk of infection [9]. The anchor point of the catheter is a swelling made of the same material situated in the center of the tunnel.

In the end, we designed a vascular access requiring ultrasound-guided insertion as described by Cavatorta et al. [14] with the following kit (fig. 4): (1) two individual catheters made of Spi-Silicone or polyurethane Bio-Flex® of 40 cm length and 2–3 mm internal diameter (10–12 gauge), which permits a blood flow of 400 ml/min and low resistance; the anchor point is located at 20–30 cm from the tip covered by a Dacron wrap, (2) two needles for vessel insertion and guidewires, (3) two needles (Redon®) for subcutaneous tunnelization, (4) two external connections to close or access the catheters, and (5) two caps and suture material.

Discussion

Central venous catheters are essential for the treatment of multiple conditions (renal, hematological, oncological and surgical) despite the associated

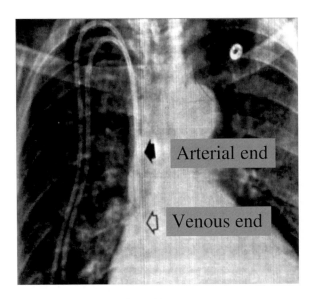

Fig. 3. Catheters in position.

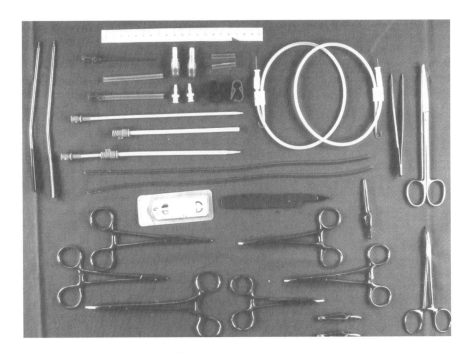

Fig. 4. Tesio Cath implant kit.

complications. Problems such as malfunction, bleeding, thrombosis, infection and stenosis may occur with long-term catheterization.

This catheter was designed to reduce the complications using: (1) the internal jugular vein for access because of its linear anatomy, (2) tunnelization to reduce infection, (3) Spi-Silicone and Bioflex material characterized by flexibility, softness and optimal biocompatibility reducing vascular damage and diminishing the 'fibrin sleeve', (4) a retroclavicular insertion prevents kinking but must be performed using ultrasound guidance, and (5) the design optimizes blood flow and resistance and two separate catheters minimize recirculation and can be exchanged separately in case of malfunction or infection.

Conclusion

The Tesio catheter, using two separate catheters, is ideal for medium- or long-term use. In our experience, excellent biocompatibility, flexibility and a long subcutaneous component with an anchor system reduce the common complications associated with catheters.

The native arteriovenous fistula is the gold standard; however, such a catheter can be an alternative solution in the elderly with cardiovascular instability or poor peripheral venous access. In these patients, it is advised to avoid a proximal arteriovenous fistula which can worsen cardiac failure.

References

1   Pisoni RL, Young EW, Dykstra DM, et al: Vascular access use in Europe and the United States: Results from the DOPPS. Kidney Int 2002;61:305–316.
2   Pastan S, Soucie JM, McClellan M: Vascular access and increased risk of death among hemodialysis patients. Kidney Int 2002;62:620–626.
3   NKF-DOQI Clinical Practice Guidelines for Vascular Access. New York, National Kidney Foundation, 1997, pp 22–23.
4   Nassar GM, Ayus JC: Infectious complications of the hemodialysis access. Kidney Int 2001; 60:1–13.
5   Trottier SJ, Veremakis C, O'Brien RN, Auer AI: Femoral deep vein thrombosis associated with central venous catheterization: Result from a prospective randomized trial. Crit Care Med 1995; 23/1:52–58.
6   Schwab SJ, Beathard G: The hemodialysis catheter conundrum. Hate living with them, but can't live without them. Kidney Int 1999;56:1–17.
7   Cimochowski GE, Worley E, Rutherford WE, et al: Superiority of the internal jugular over the subclavian access for temporary hemodialysis. Nephron 1990;54:154–161.
8   de Cicco M, Panarello G, Chiaradia V, Tesio F, et al: Source and route of microbial colonization of parenteral nutrition catheters. Lancet 1989;ii:1258–1261.
9   Sioshansi P: New processes for surface treatment of catheters. Artif Organs 1994;18/4:266–271.
10 Bambauer R, Mestres P, Pirrung KJ, Sioshansi P: Scanning microscopic investigation of catheters for blood access. Artif Organs 1994;18/4:272–275.

11   Suzuki Y, Kusakabe M, Akiha H, et al: In vivo evaluation of antithrombogenicity for ion implanted silicone rubber using indium-tropolone platelets. Jpn J Artif Organs 1990;19:1902–1905.
12   Canaud B, Berard JJ, Joyeux H, Mion C: Internal jugular vein cannulation using 2 silastic catheters. Nephron 1986;43:133–138.
13   Prabhu N, Kerns SR, Sabatelli FW, Hawkins IF, Ross EA: Long-term performance and complications of the Tesio Twin Catheter System for Hemodialysis Access. Am J Kidney Dis 1997; 30/2:213–218.
14   Cavatorta F, Zollo A, Fiorini F: Il catetere venoso centrale in dialisi; in Andreucci VE (ed): Aspetti Tecnici in Nefrologia. Genova, Accademia Nazionale di Medicina, 2000, vol 11.

Dr. Franco Tesio
Department of Nephrology and Dialysis
S. Maria degli Angeli Hospital
via Montereale 24
1–33170 Pordenone (Italy)
Tel. +39 04 34 39 9478, E-Mail segreteria.dialisi@aopn.fvg.it

Ronco C, Levin NW (eds): Hemodialysis Vascular Access and Peritoneal Dialysis Access.
Contrib Nephrol. Basel, Karger, 2004, vol 142, pp 159–177

....

Vascular Access for Acute Extracorporeal Renal Replacement Therapies

Antonio Granata[a]*, Vincenzo D'Intini*[b]*, Rinaldo Bellomo*[c]*,*
Claudio Ronco[b]

[a] Divisione di Nefrologia, A.O. Vittorio Emanuele, Catania, and
[b] Department of Nephrology, San Bortolo Hospital, Vicenza, Italy;
[c] Department of Intensive Care, Austin Repatriation Medical Centre,
Melbourne, Australia

Introduction

Since its introduction, the use of central double-lumen venous catheters (CVC or better abbreviated as DLHDC) has facilitated the implementation of extracorporeal renal replacement therapy (RRT). The use of DLHDCs has grown exponentially and now is fundamental and a basic prerequisite in the management of a broad range of both renal and nonrenal clinical scenarios. Such catheters have revolutionized clinical practice permitting the application of new therapeutic technologies aiding the management of the patient with acute and chronic problems.

The use of DLHDCs, when RRT is indicated in the acute situation, is fundamental for immediate vascular access and the clinician has at his disposal a wide range of DLHDCs with different characteristics to optimize therapy. In the chronic setting, some 60% of new patients commencing chronic dialysis with an overall prevalence of 30% are now using a catheter for dialysis access [1].

The ideal temporary DLHDC must be easy and quick to insert, be simple and safe to use for nursing staff, avoid major risks both at the time of insertion and during continuing use, avoid long-term damage to central vessels, be made of biocompatible material to prevent thrombosis, and be capable of providing adequate blood flows (100–400 ml/min) with low recirculation at low hydrostatic pressures.

Despite advances in design and material, DLHDCs are associated with significant acute and long-term morbidity. Life-threatening complications

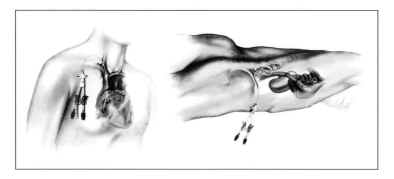

Fig. 1. Example of modern catheters for acute dialysis: the Ash Split catheter and the translumbar Split Cath.

during catheter insertion such as hemorrhage and pneumothorax, thrombosis, local and systemic infection represent a potential risk for the patient and should be given special attention.

Most DLHDCs used today are inserted with the Seldinger technique via venous access using jugular, subclavian and femoral veins. Standard noncuffed DLHDCs are generally indicated for temporary access. If a protracted treatment is foreseen, tunneled cuffed DLHDCs should be utilized for their low infection risk profile.

Characteristics of Catheters

The ultimate DLHDC must be biocompatible, easy to insert and use, be functional and durable, carry a low risk of infection and thrombosis and must be inexpensive [2]. Structurally it should be designed to optimize size, flexibility, strength and compliance. A compromise of maximal luminal diameter for maximal blood flow, with compact dimensions to minimize complications, is needed as well as a balance of flexibility and rigidity to maintain lumen patency (fig. 1). DLHDCs can be made from polyethylene, Teflon, silicone, polyurethane and polyurethane/polycarbonate copolymers. Each material has individual characteristics which have advantages and disadvantages. Polyethylene is more rigid compared to silicone. Silicone is softer and thus a more flexible material, but more difficult to insert through ligamentous or fibrotic tissues and more prone to early mechanical failure because of lumen compression. However, a major advantage of flexible catheters is that the tip of the catheter may be left in the right atrium without danger of cardiac perforation. Polyurethane is intrinsically strong, thus constructed with thin walls, preserving rigidity in the longitudinal axis while avoiding lumen collapse at high negative pressures. It also has thermoplastic properties, becoming softer at body temperature.

Finally different materials are subject to chemical disruption by various products which can affect material performance. Alcohols including isopropyl alcohol and ointments containing polyethylene glycol (mupirocin or Betadine ointment) can weaken polyurethane catheters considerably. Catheters created from copolymer materials are resistant to such chemicals and may be the principal material used for future DLHDCs.

Insertion Techniques

Insertion techniques have clearly improved contributing to reduced insertion-related complications and increasing catheter function duration. Insertion sites (jugular, subclavian and femoral veins) are dictated by the clinical situation. Subclavian cannulation is associated with a high incidence of stenosis and is contraindicated if the risk of chronic dialysis is foreseen [3]. Real-time ultrasound-guided cannulation is associated with less complications and has been strongly recommended by the DOQI committee on vascular access [4]. Such technology reduces the number of needle passes, failed placements, and insertion-related complications (fig. 2, 3). Inexperienced operators increase their success rate to 95% with the use of ultrasound guidance [5]. Ultrasound imaging is a valuable tool in caring for dialysis patients because about 30% have significant vein abnormalities, such as total occlusion, non-occlusive thrombus, stenosis and anatomic variation [6]. Postinsertion chest x-ray after internal jugular or subclavian insertion confirms the position of the catheter tip in the superior vena cava and allows evaluation for possible pneumothorax and hemothorax.

The length of time a catheter should be left in situ remains controversial. The rate of infection for internal jugular noncuffed catheters suggests that they should be used for no more than 3 weeks [4]. Femoral catheters left in place for 7–14 days did not develop any complications whereas the number of complications rose significantly in patients in whom femoral catheters were left in place for over 21 days [7].

Instructions on the technique of insertion of DLHDCs is beyond the scope of this review and can be found in various other texts [8].

Catheter Positioning

Based on opinion and DOQI guidelines, fluoroscopy or chest x-ray control of correct catheter position and tip location must be performed prior to any use.

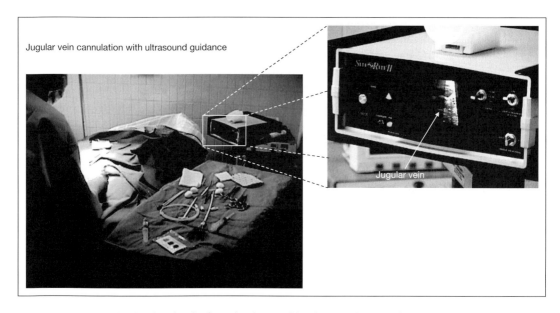

Jugular vein cannulation with ultrasound guidance

Jugular vein

Fig. 2. The site-rite is a simple portable ultrasound device for guidance of catheter placement.

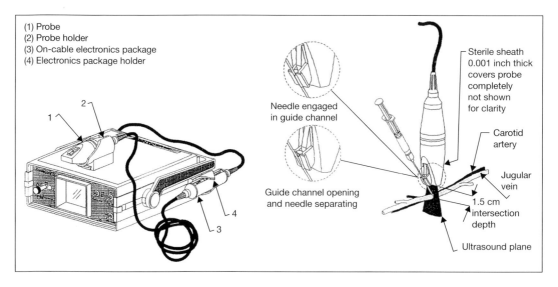

(1) Probe
(2) Probe holder
(3) On-cable electronics package
(4) Electronics package holder

Needle engaged in guide channel

Guide channel opening and needle separating

Sterile sheath 0.001 inch thick covers probe completely not shown for clarity

Carotid artery

Jugular vein

1.5 cm intersection depth

Ultrasound plane

Fig. 3. Pictorial view of an ultrasound-guided insertion of a catheter.

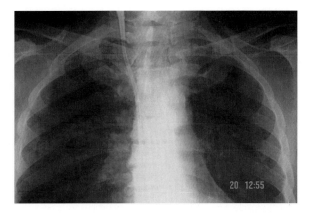

Fig. 4. Right internal jugular vein cannulation: ideal position of a jugular catheter controlled by x-ray.

Improper tip placement is a common cause of poor flow. The tip of a semirigid catheter should extend to the superior vena cava, 1–2 cm above the right atrium (fig. 4). Shorter catheters may be plagued by excessive recirculation and longer catheters risk atrial perforation. The optimal length for a right internal jugular catheter is approximately 15 cm. Femoral catheters should be longer in order to reach the inferior vena cava to minimize recirculation. The optimal orientation of the catheter tip is important for proper function and good flow. Silicone catheters allow higher blood flows when the distal tip is located in the right atrium. Fluoroscopy is required to optimize cuffed tunnelled catheter placement.

Catheter-Related Morbidity

Clinicians inserting acute catheters should be aware of the immediate and late complications of the procedure. The risk of insertion-related complications varies according to the skill of the operator, site of insertion, and use of imaging equipment such as ultrasound and fluoroscopy. Complications can be immediate or delayed. Early dysfunction is usually related to mechanical problems (e.g., inappropriate positioning or kinking), while late dysfunction (>2 weeks) is often caused by thrombotic problems such as partial or total obstructive thrombosis of the catheter lumen, thrombosis or stenosis of the cannulated vein, external sheath formation on the catheter distal end and internal catheter clotting. In the latter case, the partial or complete occlusion of the lumen and distal and/or lateral perforations greatly increase the extracorporeal resistances and reduce the effective blood flow accordingly.

Table 1. Immediate complications of catheter insertion

Jugular or subclavian
    Arterial puncture 4.4% (range 0–12%)
    Local bleeding 4.0% (range 0–16%)
    Pneumo/hemothorax
    Pneumo/hemomediastinum
    Right heart valve perforation
    Pleural damage
    Cervical hematoma compressing adjacent structures
    Phrenic nerve injury
    Thoracic duct injury (left subclavian vein)
    Horner's Syndrome

Femoral
    Groin, retroperitoneal or pelvic hematoma
    Peritoneal puncture
    Injury to the femoral nerve

Immediate Complications

These occur in the minutes or hours following catheter insertion. Severe immediate complications are almost entirely associated with use of the anatomic landmark technique (blind insertion technique). The success of the landmark-guided placement of the catheter assumes normal vascular anatomy, the vein being patent and of normal caliber. The average complications reported in the literature are listed in table 1. These risks are greater in critical care patients because of coexistent coagulopathies, thrombocytopenia, liver disturbances and drug-related bleeding problems. With insertion of a femoral catheter, bleeding is usually easily controlled unless severe deep damage to the arterial wall has occurred. Puncture of the femoral artery along its superficial path is rarely associated with more than a small hematoma, but heparin-free dialysis is advised for a minimum of 24 h. Severe femoral artery damage or rupture, particularly if deep to the inguinal ligament, may cause uncontrollable hemorrhage into the retroperitoneal space, requiring urgent surgical intervention. Both subclavian and internal jugular vein line insertions have a low risk of uncontrolled arterial bleeding in case of accidental arterial puncture. Visualization of the anatomy, with a hand held ultrasound device, prior to the procedure has further decreased the incidence of arterial puncture, although a small risk is still recognized. Hemostasis can usually be obtained by pressure over the puncture site when the carotid artery has been punctured by the finder or introducer needle. If the large bore dialysis catheter has been introduced into the arterial system, the catheter should not be removed until the surgical team is present, as bleeding is less easily controlled once the catheter has been removed. Subclavian artery damage is more difficult to control and is associated with hemothorax. Urgent exploration by a vascular surgeon with repair of the damaged vessel is required.

Local bruising is rarely troublesome unless the bleeding leads to the formation of a hematoma. This can become secondarily infected or, if the bleeding is arterial, form a false aneurysm. If during subclavian and internal jugular vein catheter insertion the patient complains of shortness of breath the procedure should be stopped and a chest x-ray obtained. Rarer complications include air embolism, damage to the superior vena cava, right common carotid artery fistula, right atrial thrombus, lymphorrhea, pericardial tamponade and arrhythmias occurring as a result of attempted catheterization (the latter is usually precipitated by the guidewire irritating the sinoatrial node or conducting tissues). The use of ultrasound-guided cannulation has resulted in a substantial decrease in procedural complications. Randolph et al. [5] performed a meta-analysis of the literature and concluded that ultrasound guidance decreased central venous catheter placement failure (relative risk of 0.32), decreased complications from catheter placement (relative risk of 0.22), and decreased the necessity of multiple catheter placement attempts (relative risk of 0.60) when compared to landmark cannulation techniques.

Other authors performed a meta-analysis with the aim of testing whether complications happen more often with the internal jugular or the subclavian central venous approach [9]. In six trials (2,010 catheters) they found significantly more arterial punctures with jugular catheters compared with subclavian ones (3.0 vs. 0.5%, RR 4.70). In six trials (1,299 catheters), there were significantly fewer malpositions with the jugular access (5.3 vs. 9.3%, RR 0.66). In ten trials (3,420 catheters), the incidence of hemo- or pneumothorax was 1.3 versus 1.5%. The authors concluded that there are more arterial punctures but less catheter malpositions with the internal jugular compared with the subclavian access, and that there is no evidence of a difference in the incidence of hemo- or pneumothorax. These data were from nonrandomized studies, and a selection bias cannot be ruled out. For rational decision-making, randomized trials are needed.

Long-Term Complications

These are frequently caused by thrombotic problems (fig. 5) such as partial or total obstructive thrombosis of the catheter lumen, thrombosis or stenosis of the cannulated vein, and catheter-related infections.

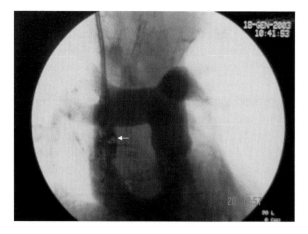

Fig. 5. Malfunction of the catheter is diagnosed by an angiographic technique. The arrow indicates mural thrombus of the arterial tip.

Thrombotic Occurrences

Thrombosis of cannulated veins is much more frequent than the clinical examination would suggest. The incidence of catheterized vein thrombosis varies from 20 to 70% according to the sites and diagnostic modalities used. Central vein stenosis and thrombosis are more common with subclavian catheter. Recently, in prospective studies, stenosis/thrombosis was found to complicate up to 28% of subclavian dialysis catheters, and infection further increased the risk [10]. For this reason, subclavian catheters should be avoided if possible. They are contraindicated if the patient is expected to require future permanent access on the same side as the catheter. Acute catheters in the jugular vein caused thrombosis/stenosis in only 2% of cases surveyed with ultrasound in one study [11]. Femoral venous catheterization is associated with a greater risk of thrombotic complication than subclavian catheterization in ICU patients [12]. Several factors contribute to the thrombogenicity on the catheter. Schematically, they are represented by the catheter type (material and composition, flexibility, aspect and surface treatment), insertion mode, host vein (including diameter, local hemodynamics), duration of use, hemorrheology and clotting status of the patient (hyperfibrinogenemia, inflammatory disease, thrombocytosis, previous thrombosis). The prothrombotic risk of a patient may be reduced by administering anticoagulants (e.g., low molecular weight heparin) and/or antiplatelet drugs. However, only rarely does one encounter a patient with a definable hypercoagulability state; most cases of thrombosis can only be attributed to activation of the contact coagulation cascade by a relatively bioincompatible device. Catheter-associated thrombosis can be classified as extrinsic when the thrombus forms outside the catheter and intrinsic when the thrombus is either intraluminal or attached to the surface of the device.

Extrinsic Thrombi

Mural thrombus, intra-atrial thrombus, and superior vena cava thrombosis are the principal types of extrinsic thrombosis.

Mural thrombus is attached to the wall of the vessel or the atrium at the point of catheter contact. It is presumed that movement of the catheter tip causes endothelial damage that results in thrombus formation. The tip of the catheter may become encased in this thrombus, which is generally not identified unless there is catheter malfunction, at which time it may be visualized angiographically (fig. 5). When the thrombus is recognized, removal of the catheter accompanied by 3 months of anticoagulation is indicated [13]. A large mural thrombus raises the risk of a significant embolism when the catheter is removed. Thus, these catheters are best removed under real time observation so that immediate lytic therapy can be employed if indicated.

Atrial thrombus may present as hemodialysis catheter malfunction, pulmonary or systemic emboli, or a mass within the right atrium (as observed angiographically or with an echocardiogram). This probably represents a variant of the mural thrombus and can at times be life threatening. Real time catheter removal with lytic therapy on standby in case a large pulmonary embolism develops is probably warranted. Treatment consists of removal of the catheter and anticoagulation. The progress of the thrombus should be followed by echocardiography.

The prevalence of catheter-related superior vena cava venous thrombosis is not clear. Authors report an incidence of 2–63.5% [13]. The reported frequency appears to depend on whether the thrombosis is searched for systematically or only when it becomes symptomatic. It is clear that symptomatic central vein thrombosis is not common, but when it does occur the symptoms can be dramatic. The patient generally presents with pain and tenderness in the base of the neck, the shoulder area, and swelling of the ipsilateral extremity. Embolization from this complication is unusual. Treatment of symptomatic patients consists of catheter removal and anticoagulation therapy. Oral anticoagulants can be started within 24 h with subsequent dose adjustments to achieve an international normalized ratio of 2.0–3.0 for a period of 1 month.

Intrinsic Thrombosis

Most catheter flow problems are related to intrinsic thrombosis. Intraluminal thrombus, catheter tip thrombus, and fibrin sheath thrombus are the principal types of intrinsic thrombosis.

Intraluminal thrombus usually occurs when an inadequate volume of heparin is instilled into the catheter after dialysis or when heparin escapes from the catheter lumen between dialysis sessions. Blood can enter into the catheter and form an intraluminal thrombus. When this occurs, the catheter may become completely occluded. Urokinase instillation characteristically resolves the thrombosis [4]. This type of thrombus in not very common because routine catheter maintenance techniques are generally sufficient to prevent the problem.

Many catheters have side holes at the tip of the arterial limb. Unfortunately, the portion of the catheter from the side holes to the tip does not retain heparin and thrombus can form. A tip thrombus may be occlusive or it may act as a valve. Preventive measures that are commonly used to avoid intraluminal thrombosis are largely subverted by the presence of the side holes. Urokinase instillation usually resolves this problem.

Fibrin sheath thrombus is the most common type of thrombus. The term 'fibrin sheath' refers to a sleeve of fibrin that surrounds the catheter starting at the point where it enters the vein. The fibrin sheath is only loosely attached to the catheter. As the sheath extends downward, it eventually closes over the tip of the catheter. It is probable that all central venous catheters become encased in a layer of fibrin within a few days of insertion. The incidence of catheter dysfunction secondary to fibrin sheath has been reported to be 13–57% [13]. The term 'fibrin' does not describe this sheath with complete accuracy; on close examination, the older portion actually appears fibrous or leathery in texture. There is experience to suggest that chronic systemic anticoagulation (e.g., warfarin) is beneficial [14].

Prevention of Catheter Thrombosis

Proper flushing and heparinization of the catheter with concentrated heparin following dialysis will serve to decrease but not eliminate the risk of thrombosis. As soon as the bloodline is disconnected from each side of the catheter, the catheter should be flushed with saline to remove any residual blood. The catheter must then be clamped prior to removal of the syringe to prevent blood from entering at the tip while the catheter is open. Each side of the hemodialysis catheter has a fill volume inscribed on the clear portion of the catheter just below the cap. This volume is different for both lumens. The venous volume is generally 0.1–0.2 ml greater than the arterial volume. However, a 0.1- to 0.2-ml overfill is recommended. Chronic anticoagulation with either warfarin or low molecular weight heparin has gained anecdotal support for preventing both lumen thrombus and fibrin sheath formation on hemodialysis catheters [14].

Treatment of Catheter Thrombosis

Appropriate treatment is dependent upon the types of the thrombosis. Although treatment types overlap, it is useful to think of treatment as primary and secondary. Thrombosed, noncuffed catheters can be exchanged over a guide wire or treated with urokinase.

Primary treatment of catheter malfunction refers to treatment that can be immediately applied in the hemodialysis facility. The first step when a catheter is suspected of being thrombosed is to flush the catheter (forceful flush). The flush should be performed with maximum force, the purpose being to dislodge the small piece of clot that is occluding the tip of the catheter. Once the flush has been delivered, aspiration of blood should be attempted. If this is possible, two or three additional forceful flushes should be made. If this is also unsuccessful, the procedure can be abandoned. Second step, numerous protocols for urokinase administration or urokinase catheter lock are in use. The urokinase protocol [4] is successful in resolving the thrombus in 70–90% of instances. This protocol should be attempted as the first procedure to resolve catheter thrombosis because it is the least invasive and least costly of all catheter salvage techniques. Tissue plasminogen activator (tPA) has been used with equal success. Fibrinolytic enzymes have been used in two ways for the treatment of catheter dysfunction – by instillation and by infusion. Urokinase catheter lock is not a good solution for the treatment of a fibrin sheathing. Thrombolysis only occurs within the catheter and at its tip. Additional data are emerging on the role of continuous thrombolytic therapy in the treatment of malfunctioning catheters. Evidence suggests that continuous infusion of 20,000–40,000 units or the higher dose of 125,000–250,000 units during the dialysis treatment may also be an effective treatment of fibrin sheath. Further studies of the use of continuous urokinase infusions are pending. tPA differs from urokinase in that it has a shorter half-life and appears to be somewhat more effective pharmacologically. Studies based on thrombosed central venous catheters used for chemotherapy have shown tPA to be more successful in restoring patency than urokinase. The dose of enzymes used was not large enough to result in systemic effects, and no complications were reported. Advantages of the use of a fibrinolytic enzyme are that it is safe, preserves the catheter, and is less expensive than either catheter exchange or fibrin sheath stripping. Since there is no systemic thrombolytic effect, however, one must assume that most of the fibrin sheath is not exposed to the enzyme. Mechanical treatment to remove the occluding thrombus using a guidewire, Fogarty catheter, or ureteral biopsy brush has been reported. The advantages of the mechanical technique are that it has a high success rate and produces no systemic effect, making it safe and relatively inexpensive. It has the disadvantage of not being a permanent solution to the problem, and usually a physician must perform the procedure. If a fibrin sheath is the cause of catheter malfunction, mechanical removal of the occlusion is not a long-term solution.

If primary treatments are unsuccessful or if the problem quickly recurs, a radiographic study using contrast should be performed based on the radiographic findings. Appropriate treatment generally requires catheter exchange. This technique can be effectively used to eliminate the problem of catheter thrombosis. It is important that the patient be checked for a fibrin sheath prior to insertion of the new catheter because it is possible to place the new catheter back into the retained sheath and have the same problem within a short time. If a fibrin sheath is present, it can be stripped using a snare catheter. The snare is introduced through the femoral vein and advanced up to the level of the dialysis catheter. The reported success of this procedure ranges from 92 to 98%. Fibrin sheath stripping generally results in asymptomatic embolization of the fibrin sheath. Advantages of this techniques include a good success rate, safety and preservation of the catheter with a patency duration that is reasonable. Disadvantages are the cost of the snare and the time required to accomplish the procedure, and the fact that it is not a permanent solution to the problem.

Catheter-Related Infections

Infectious complications represent one of the major recurrent risks of venous catheters for RRT modalities. Nontunnelled percutaneous catheters used as a short-term therapy carry a bacteremia risk estimated between 3 and 10% in ICU. Temporary catheters have higher rates of infection than tunnelled dialysis catheters (bacteremia 6.2/1,000 vs. 1.8/1,000 catheter-days and exit site infection 3.6/1,000 vs. 1.4/1,000 catheter-days in not cuffed or tunnelled catheters, respectively). A prospective study of 211 patients with acute catheters found the risk of catheter-related bacteremia (CRB) from acute catheters increased over time in an exponential fashion at both the femoral and internal jugular site [15].

While the risk of infection at the femoral site was always greater than at the internal jugular site, the instantaneous risk (hazard) of bacteremia at the femoral site increased after 1 week compared with 3 weeks at the internal jugular site. In addition, if an exit site infection occurred and the catheter was left in place, the risk of bacteremia rose from 2% at 24 h from onset of exit site infection to 13% at 48 h. These findings support the NKF-K/DOQI guidelines to limit acute dialysis catheter use in the femoral vein and internal jugular vein to 1 and 3 weeks, respectively, and to remove catheters immediately if an exit site infection occurs. Despite these recommendations, some centers manage patients for months to years with 'acute' dialysis catheters. One study reports a bacteremia rate of only 1.2/1,000 catheter-days with long-term use. This center uses povidone and mupirocin ointments with dry gauze dressings which have been shown to significantly reduce the risk of bacteremia from acute dialysis catheters in randomized controlled trials. Nontunnelled internal jugular access appears more prone to infections, notably in patients with a tracheotomy. Recently, authors concluded that femoral venous catheterization is associated with a greater risk of infectious complication than subclavian catheterization in ICU patients [12].

The prolonged use of a dialysis catheter in an acute patient carries an infectious risk that increases with time. This risk is known but unfortunately unavoidable. It must be alleviated through suitable nursing care. There are a number of risk factors for the development of catheter-related infections. These include skin and nasal colonization with staphylococcus, catheter hub colonization, duration of catheterization, thrombosis, frequency of catheter manipulation, diabetes mellitus, iron overload, immunoincompetence, use of a transparent dressing and the conditions of catheter placement.

Prevention of catheter-associated infection encompasses three aspects: the technique of catheter placement, daily catheter exit site care and catheter management in the hemodialysis facility. It is critically important that maximal barrier precautions be used when a catheter is placed. If not done in an operating room, the environment should simulate an operating room. Care given to the catheter after placement is of equal importance. The use of either mupirocin or povidone-iodine or another antibiotic ointment at the exit site until it is healed has been advocated. The use of a transparent occlusive dressing has been indicated as a risk factor for catheter-related infection, since it promotes skin colonization. The question as to whether it is best to use gauze or a plastic dressing remains unresolved and controversial. We adopted the approach of keeping the catheter exit site covered with sterile gauze at all times and using povidone-iodine or other antibiotic ointment, in accordance with the DOQI recommendations.

Infections can develop at the exit site, within the tunnel with tunnelled catheters and CRB. The therapeutic approach to each of these is somewhat different. Exit site infection is defined as localized infection of the skin and soft tissue around the exit site. Erythema, purulent discharge and local tenderness are typically present. Fever and other signs of systemic infection are absent. With a temporary catheter, removal of the catheter is warranted with replacement at an alternate site. With tunnelled dialysis catheters, bacteremia has not been shown to be clearly associated with exit site infection and CRB. It is plausible that the presence of infection in close proximity to the catheter tract and ports might increase the risk of bacteremia, with or without a subcutaneous cuff and tunnel. Recent reports of the incidence of exit site infection range from 1.2 to 2.2/1,000 catheter-days. Exit site infection may result from inadequate skin preparation at the time of DLHDC placement, incorrect suture material or technique, improper exit site care by dialysis clinic staff, or poor patient hygiene. The site should be cleaned with a disinfectant appropriate for the catheter material and a sterile dressing applied at each dialysis session until the site is fully healed, clean, and dry. Most exit site infections are caused by gram-positive organisms including *Staphylococcus aureus* and *Staphylococcus epidermidis*, although other bacteria can be involved. Exit site infection can usually be treated effectively with oral or intravenous antibiotics. In more severe cases or those that fail to respond to antibiotics, revision of the catheter with creation of a new exit site remote from the infected area may resolve the exit site infection. If these measures fail, the tunnelled catheter may ultimately need to be removed. Tunnel infections are invasive soft tissue infections that extend along the subcutaneous tunnel toward the vein. These typically involve the cuff and exit site, although in some cases they may appear only in the tunnel proximal to the cuff, with no drainage or communication to the exit site. Tenderness, swelling, and erythema along the catheter tract are typical, with purulent drainage from the exit site. Fever and other signs of systemic infection are often present, and bacteremia may occur. In most series, tunnel infection is relatively uncommon; a recent report showed an incidence of 0.12/1,000 catheter-days. Appropriate treatment consists of parenteral anti biotics according to culture results and catheter removal. The catheter should not be replaced at this site.

CRB from acute catheters should be treated with immediate catheter removal and appropriate antibiotics. The decision to remove a tunnelled catheter for suspected CRB must often be made clinically prior to blood culture results and individualized based on the severity of sepsis, comorbid illnesses, status of permanent arteriovenous access, and alternatives for venous access. *S. aureus* is the most common organism representing 33–80% of positive cultures. The prevalence of nasal carriage of *S. aureus* among patients undergoing hemodialysis has ranged from 30 to 60%. Reduction of nasal carriage of *S. aureus* has resulted in a decrease in yearly bloodstream infections due to *S. aureus*. The prolonged empiric use of vancomycin should be avoided because of the risk of inducing vancomycin-resistant enterococcus. Initial therapy with vancomycin and an aminoglycoside antibiotic (or a β-lactam with lactamase inhibitor or a quinolone) until culture results are available is prudent. Rapid conversion to appropriate antibiotics based on culture sensitivities is needed not only to prevent emergence of resistant organisms, but also to avoid ototoxicity. Antibiotic therapy should be continued for a minimum of 3 weeks. Blood cultures should be repeated a week following therapy to ensure that the infection has been eradicated. The presence of a biofilm on the inner or outer surface of the catheter may play an important role in catheter bacteremia. Authors demonstrated the presence of a biofilm on the surface of 100% of the central venous catheters removed from 26 ICU patients.

A major management dilemma is whether to attempt salvage of the tunnelled catheter if sepsis is controlled and alternative access is difficult. Recent reports show only 32–37% are salvageable. If significant symptoms persist beyond 48 h despite effective antibiotics the tunnelled catheter should be removed. The presence of biofilm on the catheter surface may prevent antibiotic penetration. Inadequate antibiotic levels within the catheter lumen may also be a factor. When the catheter is removed in the presence of CRB, DOQI guidelines recommend that a new permanent catheter should not be placed until the patient has negative cultures with antibiotic therapy and has been afebrile for 48–72 h.

The choice of initial antibiotics must be guided by a number of factors, including severity of clinical sepsis, patient comorbidities, known previous infections in that patient and the spectrum of infections in the dialysis unit. Lower-risk patients may be safely managed with relatively narrow spectrum antibiotics. In higher-risk patients with severe clinical sepsis, initial coverage must consider methicillin-resistant *S. aureus*, Enterococcus, and Pseudomonas. This may require vancomycin and a cephalosporin (e.g., ceftazadime or cefepime) or aminoglycoside. In these situations, it is potentially dangerous to rely entirely on an aminoglycoside for gram-negative coverage, given unpredictable peak levels (compounded by a tendency to underdose dialysis patients) and variable residual renal function potentially leading to subtherapeutic levels during the first 24–48 h of treatment [16].

Management of dialysis CRB would be simplified if it were possible to eradicate the source of the infection without having to replace the catheter. Instillation of concentrated antibiotic solutions into the lumen of silicone vascular catheters (antibiotic lock) in vitro eliminates the biofilm, representing a useful clinical application and studies in tunnelled DLHDCs have suggested that the biofilm can be eradicated by an antibiotic lock solution instilled into the catheter lumen, permitting bacteriologic cure without replacing the catheter. These studies have prompted a recent consensus panel to recommend the use of antibiotic locks for clinical management of uncomplicated bacteremia related to tunnelled DLHDCs. However, there are no large, prospective studies assessing the efficacy of this approach in treating hemodialysis patients. Recently, Krishnasami et al. [17] reported that the use of an antibiotic lock, in conjunction with systemic antibiotic therapy, can eradicate CRB while salvaging the catheter in about half of the cases.

Furthermore, this management approach offers clinical advantages over routine catheter exchange. Considering the high incidence of CRB and the multiple severe comorbidites frequently seen in dialysis patients, one would expect a large number of complications from CRB. Marr et al, reported a very high incidence of infectious complications from CRB (9 out of 41 episodes, 22%; with 6 patients developing osteomyelitis, four bacterial endocarditis and one septic arthritis). In contrast, other studies have reported few infectious complications, with bacterial endocarditis occurring in 1.6 to 3.5% of cases. It is important to consider bacterial endocarditis in all cases of CRB, especially those that involve *S. aureus* and prolonged or recurrent bacteremia and fever.

Catheter Performances and Recirculation

Blood flow through the catheter is directly proportional to the pressure generated by the blood pump across the catheter and inversely proportional to resistance in the catheter itself. Modern blood pumps have a limited capacity to generate pressure, and high pressures can be damaging to red cells, so a major goal of catheter design has been to reduce the resistance to flow as much as possible. The resistance to flow is directly related to length and inversely proportional to the fourth power of the catheter diameter. The viscosity of blood at body temperature is relatively constant and is not easily modified, but the manufacturer can optimize both the length and diameter of the catheter to reduce resistance.

Intermittent extracorporeal hemofiltration modalities requiring blood flows between 250 and 400 ml/min are much more dependent upon the catheter's physical characteristics compared to continuous RRT modalities, which require lower blood flows (150–200 ml/min). It is worth recalling that the immediate use of high flux catheters allows all RRT modalities to be performed without changing the venous site or catheter. The presence of lateral distal and circular catheters is essential to reduce the internal resistance, limit the risk of dysfunction through parietal suction and prevent its obstruction by the (internal or external) formation of a fibrin sleeve. The negative pressure recorded on the arterial side reflects resistance to blood suction. It depends on the blood flow applied, on the degree of venous collapse, blood pressure and on the patient's intravascular fluid status. Negative pressure should not exceed $-300\,mm\,Hg$ to prevent the risk of parietal vascular lesions and/or blood hemolysis. The positive pressure recorded on the venous side reflects resistance to venous return. It depends on the blood flow and the degree of obstruction of the venous catheter. With the catheters in use today, venous pressure approximates one half of that of the blood flow displayed (i.e., for a blood flow rate of 300 ml/min, venous pressure is close to 150–175 mm Hg). Thus, any change in arterial and/or venous blood pressures regimen must be indicative of catheter dysfunction that should be followed by suitable corrective actions. Oliver et al. [14] in patients with acute renal insufficiency demonstrated that early mechanical dysfunction of the catheter was more frequently associated with double-lumen catheters (nontunnelled) in the subclavian vein than with those inserted at other sites. Specific anatomic abnormalities (fibrous band, interosseous mobile zone) can create kinking or stricture along the subclavian pathway.

Catheter recirculation can reduce dialysis efficacy. It depends on the site of catheter insertion and blood flow prescribed. Recirculation is much less important in continuous RRT modalities since lower flows are required. Both chest and femoral central vessels are prone to recirculation. Femoral catheters, particularly short ones, exhibit a high recirculation rate averaging 20% (5–38%). Internal jugular and subclavian catheters have a much lower recirculation rate averaging 10% (5–15%). Catheter recirculation is increased by reversing connecting lines (blood recirculation rates reach 20–30%), but whether recirculation in catheters relates to poor cardiac output, valvular insufficiency, use of vasopressor, or other clinical states is not known. An extra 20–30 min of dialysis time was recommended to compensate for the adverse effect of reversing the catheters on solute kinetics. Cardiopulmonary recirculation is defined as the flow of dialyzed blood back through the dialyzer via the central blood circuit (heart and lungs) without equilibration with blood in the rest of the body. Cardiopulmonary recirculation accounts for much of the rebound in solute concentration following dialysis: approximately 30% of the total rebound of urea and less for other solutes. It might be speculated that in patients with isolated central venous catheters there is negligible cardiopulmonary recirculation, so the efficiency of dialysis could be slightly higher than that achievable with arteriovenous fistulas. This concept however still remains to be proven but it could partially offset the lower clearance achievable through catheters due to their lower blood flow rates.

Care and Maintenance of the Catheters

Dialysis catheters, like all intravenous lines, should be kept clean and covered at all times. To avoid bacterial contamination, the line should not be used for administration of medications, parenteral nutrition or accessed for blood sampling, except in an emergency. The use of dry gauze dressings and povidone-iodine and mupirocin ointment at the catheter exit site can reduce the incidence of exit site infections, especially in patients who have nasal carriage of *S. aureus*. In the patients with an allergy to povidone-iodine, alternate agents such as polyantimicrobial gel can be substituted. The glycol constituents of ointment should not be used on polyurethane catheters. Catheter placement near the patient's nose and mouth, as with subclavian or jugular vein catheters, exposes the catheter exit site to nasal drainage/discharge and infectious airborne droplets. A surgical mask worn by the patient and nurse at any time when the catheter is accessed reduces the spread of infectious droplets and reduces contamination of the catheter site. When not in use the lumens should be filled with 1 ml heparin (5,000 units/ml) mixed with 2 ml normal saline and heparin should always be removed and discarded prior to using the line. Antibiotic use and an anticoagulant lock of the catheter appear to be efficient ways to prevent endoluminal bacterial contamination in high-risk patients. Studies comparing silver or antibiotic-coated material with commonly treated catheter material have led to encouraging results in reducing the incidence of infection. However, the real benefits of such an approach have yet to be evaluated and deserve further studies. The catheter exit site should be covered at all times. Dry gauze dressings rather than transparent film dressings are recommended because transparent film dressings pose a greater threat of exit site colonization. Dressing should be changed at least twice weekly, or more frequently if any discharge or moisture is noted at the exit site. Antimicrobial ointments used at the exit site reduce the incidence of bacterial contamination but are associated with higher rates of fungal infection, and should be avoided, especially in the immunocompromised patient in ICU.

Conclusions

Double-lumen catheters are an essential and convenient way to allow various venovenous RRTs. Semirigid polyurethane catheters are the first choice for short-term use. Hemocompatible, flexible silicone catheters which are less damaging to blood vessels seem better suited for medium- and long-term use. All acute catheters should be placed in the femoral or internal jugular veins if possible. The subclavian vein site should be avoided to reduce overall catheter-related complications, particularly subclavian stenosis. Ultrasound should be used to survey local anatomy prior to insertion and/or it should be used in real time to reduce complications and increase the success rate of insertion. Despite the success of short- and long-term central venous catheterization, several improvements in catheter design are needed: improvement of biocompatibility and a reduction in the incidence of septic and thrombotic episodes, possibly by coating the material with bonded anticoagulant or antibiotic; reduction of arterial flow variability at high blood flow rates, possibly by modifying catheter tip design, and provision of a cuffless catheter for use in above- or below-average size patients to facilitate insertion.

References

1   Pisoni LR, Young EW, Dykstra DM, Greenwood RN, Hecking E, Gillespie B, Wolfe RA, Goodkin DA, Held PJ: Vascular access use in Europe and the United States: Results from DOPPS. Kidney Int 2002;61:305–316.
2   Ash SR: The evolution and function of central venous catheters for dialysis. Semin Dial 2001; 14:416–424.
3   Beenen L, van Leusen R, Deenik B, Bosch FH: The incidence of subclavian vein stenosis using silicone catheters for hemodialysis. Artif Organs 1994;18/4:289–292.
4   NKF-K/DOQI Clinical Practice Guidelines for Vascular Access: UPDATE 2000. Am J Kidney Dis 2001;37:S137–S181.
5   Randolph AG, Cook DJ, Gonzales CA, Pribble CG: Ultrasound guidance for placement of central venous catheters: A meta-analysis of the literature. Crit Care Med 1996;24:2053–2058.
6   Forauer AR, Gloockner JF: Importance of US findings in access planning during jugular vein hemodialysis catheter placements. J Vasc Interv Radiol 2000;11:233–238.
7   Weyde W, Wikiera I, Ginger M: Prolonged cannulation of the femoral vein is a safe method of temporary vascular access for hemodialysis. Nephron 1998;80/1:86.
8   McGee DC, Gould MK: Preventing complications of central venous catheterization. N Engl J Med 2003;348:1123–1133.
9   Ruesch S, Walzer B, Tramèr MR: Complications of central venous catheters: Internal jugular versus subclavian access – A systematic review. Crit Care Med 2002;30:454–460.
10 Hernandez D, Diaz F, Rufino M, Lorenzo V, Perez T, Rodriguez A, De Bonis E, Losado M, Gonzales-Posada JM, Torres A: Subclavian vascular access stenosis in dialysis patients: Natural history and risk factors. J Am Soc Nephrol 1998;9:1507–1510.
11 Oliver MJ: Acute dialysis catheters. Semin Dial 2001;14:432–435.
12 Merrer J, De Joughe B, Golliot F, Lefrant JY, Raffy B, Barre E, Rigaud JP, Casciani D, Misset B, Bosquet C, Outin H, Brun-Buisson C, Nitenberg G: Complications of femoral and subclavian venous catheterisation in critically ill patients. JAMA 2001;286:700–707.
13 Schwab SJ, Beathard G: The hemodialysis catheter conundrum: Hate living with them, but can't live without them. Kidney Int 1999;56:1–17.
14 Obialo CI, Conner AC, Lebon LF: Maintaining patency of tunneled hemodialysis catheters. Scand J Urol Nephrol 2003;37/2:172–176.
15 Oliver MJ, Callery SM, Thorpe KE, Schwab SJ, Churchill DN: Risk of bacteremia from temporary hemodialysis catheters by site of insertion and duration of use: A prospective study. Kidney Int 2000;58:2543–2545.
16 Mermel LA, Farr BM, Sherertz RJ, Raad II, O'Grady N, Harria JS, Crafen DE: Guidelines for the management of intravascular catheter-related infections. Clin Infect Dis 2001;32:1249.
17 Krishnasami Z, Carlton D, Bimbo L, Taylor ME, Balkovetz DF, Barker J, Allon M: Management of hemodialysis catheter-related bacteremia with an adjunctive antibiotic lock solution. Kidney Int 2002;61:1136–1142.

Claudio Ronco, MD,
Department of Nephrology, St. Bortolo Hospital,
Viale Rodolfi, IT–36100 Vicenza (Italy)
Tel. +39 0444 993869, Fax +39 0444 993949, E-Mail cronco@goldnet.it

Ronco C, Levin NW (eds): Hemodialysis Vascular Access and Peritoneal Dialysis Access.
Contrib Nephrol. Basel, Karger, 2004, vol 142, pp 178–192

....

Totally Implantable Subcutaneous Devices for Hemodialysis Access

John E. Moran[a]*, Frank Prosl*[b]

[a] Satellite Healthcare, Mountain View, Calif., and
[b] Biolink Corp., Mansfield, Mass., USA

The creation and maintenance of hemodialysis vascular access continues to be one of the major clinical issues that limits the delivery of adequate dialysis therapy in end-stage renal disease (ESRD) patients [1]. Guidelines from the National Kidney Foundation's Kidney/Dialysis Outcomes Quality Initiative (K/DOQI) recommend an increased utilization of arteriovenous (AV) fistulas for hemodialysis access and a reduced utilization of tunneled cuffed catheters as permanent access for ESRD patients [2]. These recommendations are based on the low complication rate and increased patency associated with AV fistulas.

Tunneled cuffed hemodialysis dialysis catheters are increasingly being used for dialysis access in ESRD patients [3]. Data from the Dialysis Outcomes and Practice Patterns Study (DOPPS) indicates that 61% of hemodialysis patients in the United States started dialysis using a catheter [4]. The rates of catheter use at the start of dialysis reported from the DOPPS study for the United Kingdom, Japan and the rest of Europe were 50, 31 and between 15 and 39%, respectively [4]. Clearly, catheters have an important role in delivering hemodialysis in certain patient populations; however, their use is associated with a number of clinical limitations and complications, including low blood flow rates, recirculation, thrombosis, occlusion, and high rates of infection and hospitalization [5–9]. These limitations and complications likely contribute to the higher mortality rate reported for ESRD patients utilizing catheters compared to other hemodialysis access options [10].

The limitations and associated complications inherent with the use of hemodialysis catheters have led to the recent development of a new dialysis access option, totally subcutaneous hemodialysis access systems. These devices have been designed to provide improved dialysis performance and decreased complications compared to tunneled cuffed hemodialysis catheters. Two totally subcutaneous hemodialysis access devices have undergone extensive clinical investigation, the Dialock® Hemodialysis Access System (Biolink, Inc., Mansfield, Mass., USA) and the LifeSite® Hemodialysis Access System (Vasca, Inc., Tewksbury, Mass., USA) [11–20].

The totally subcutaneous design of these new subcutaneous hemodialysis access systems addresses an important shortcoming of tunneled cuffed hemodialysis catheters, specifically, the need for a transcutaneous portion of the device to be externalized through the skin surface. The externalized portion of catheters is responsible in part for the high rates of infections and hospitalizations associated with these devices. The external portion of the catheter can also be affected by changes in body position during dialysis, leading to erratic performance and frequent alarms. The exposed catheter is also at risk of physical damage or contamination and reduces quality of life for patients who desire a more discreet access.

Historical Precursors to Totally Subcutaneous Access Devices

Efforts to develop alternative hemodialysis access options led to the development and availability of two unique devices in the 1980s. The Bentley DiaTAP button (American Bentley, Irvine, Calif., USA) and the Hemasite (Renal Systems, Minneapolis, Minn, USA) were designed to offer immediate, pain-free vascular access [21–26]. The DiaTAP consisted of a carbon-based access port and attached polytetrafluoroethylene (PTFE) graft that provided AV access. The PTFE graft was usually placed in the upper arm or leg in either a looped or straight configuration. A thin layer of Dacron velour was used to cover the port-PTFE graft junction. The access port was sealed with a replaceable conical polyethylene plug and a sterile, disposable polyethylene cap was used between dialysis sessions to keep the plug in place. Access to the device was achieved by removing the disposable cap and inserting a sterile needleless connector set. Insertion of the connector disengaged the plug and allowed for blood flow.

The Hemasite device consisted of an externalized button-shaped device, which was implanted with or without an accompanying PTFE vascular graft [24]. The device was usually placed in the upper arm or the thigh. The external portion of the device was separated from the circulation by a Silastic diaphragm. The device was accessed by removing an external cap and then inserting a specialized connector through the silastic diaphragm. Unlike newer subcutaneous hemodialysis access devices, both the Hemasite and the Bentley button required externalization of the device through the skin surface. This transcutaneous design contributed to their ultimate failure [26, 27].

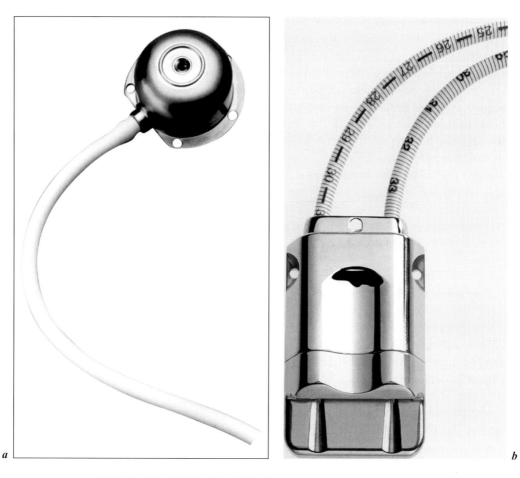

Fig. 1. a The LifeSite Hemodialysis Access System. *b* The Dialock System.

Complications associated with Hemasite and DiaTAP included blood leakage from the device, breakdown of the silastic diaphragm, local infections around the device, bacteremia, venous stenosis, and thrombosis [21–26].

Totally Subcutaneous Hemodialysis Access Devices

The LifeSite System (fig. 1a) and the Dialock System (fig. 1b) represent the first true totally subcutaneous hemodialysis access systems available for clinical use. While these two devices share some features with tunneled cuffed

Table 1. Differences between totally subcutaneous access devices and hemodialysis catheters

	Subcutaneous access devices	Tunneled catheters
Structural components	Subcutaneous valve and indwelling cannula	Indwelling catheter
Placement properties	Fully implantable	Transcutaneous
Subcutaneous cuff	No	Yes
Access technique	Dialysis needle	Luer lock connection
Placement location	Upper chest, thigh	Neck, thigh
Placement vein(s)	Internal and external jugular, subclavian, and femoral	Internal and external jugular, subclavian, and femoral

hemodialysis catheters, there are a number of physical differences (table 1). Both types of devices have internal portions that are inserted into the central venous system; however, the new totally implantable access devices also consist of a subcutaneous valve that opens and closes following the insertion or removal of an access needle. The uniqueness of these valves allows for the totally subcutaneous placement of these devices.

The LifeSite System valve is comprised of medical grade titanium, 316 series stainless steel, and silicone elastomers. The valve stem connects to a 12-French silicone cannula that is placed in the central venous circulation. The cannula can be inserted into the vein in either a side hole or no side hole configuration at the distal tip. Two LifeSite Systems are placed, one for blood draw and the other for blood return during hemodialysis. The LifeSite valve has an internal mechanism that isolates the fluid pathway of the device from the associated implanted cannula when not in use. The unique design of the valve allows blood access upon insertion of a manufacturer-approved 14-gauge cannulation set (fig. 2a). Removal of the needle from the device closes the valve's internal mechanism and prevents access to the fluid pathway. The tapered chamber of the valve allows the 14-gauge needles to be held in place as a result of a friction fit between the needle and the device. The valve's properties also allow for irrigation of the valve and access tract with an antimicrobial solution. A smaller 25-gauge needle is inserted into the valve to allow for antimicrobial irrigation without the activation of the valve's internal mechanism (fig. 2b). This prevents the entry of the antimicrobial solution into the LifeSite cannula and the patient's vasculature. The device is accessed through the same needle site for each dialysis session with the resultant development of a

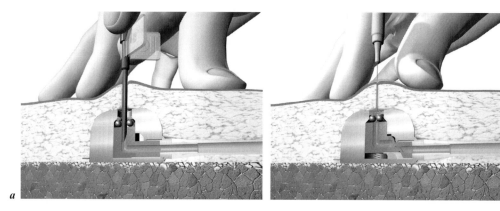

Fig. 2. a LifeSite valve mechanism. *b* Antimicrobial irrigation of the LifeSite valve.

pain-free fibrous tissue tract or 'buttonhole'. Periodic establishment of a new buttonhole site may be required if the access site is not aligned over the center of the valve.

The Dialock System consists of a titanium body which houses two internal access valves and two attached cannulas which are reinforced with nitinol. The device is accessed via separate insertion of two specially designed 15-gauge cannulation sets. Each cannulation set consists of a 15-gauge noncoring needle with attached extension tubing for making the bloodline connection and a separate stylet into which the needle is inserted while the access site is punctured. The stylet is used to puncture the skin and create the access pathway to the device through the subcutaneous tissue. The front of the valve has a trough-like design to guide the needles into the individual pathways. When the needles are inserted, the internal valve is forced open allowing for blood flow (fig. 3). The internal mechanism is also designed to prevent dislodgement of the needles during dialysis. Once the needles are inserted, the stylet is removed and the external hubs of the needles are locked together to increase device stability during dialysis. Removal of the needles from the device closes the internal valve mechanism and prevents access to the patient's bloodstream. Unlike the LifeSite System, only one Dialock System is required for dual-needle hemodialysis to be performed.

Device Placement

The proper placement of subcutaneous hemodialysis access systems is essential in order to optimize outcomes with these devices. Physicians placing

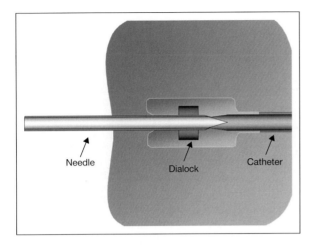

Fig. 3. Dialock System Internal Mechanism.

these devices should plan in advance the ideal placement in an individual patient basis, allowing for differences in body habitus and access history. Properly placed, these devices are easy for the dialysis staff to access. Improper placement of these devices may result in difficulty in cannulation with multiple needle sticks by dialysis staff and poor outcomes [28].

The procedure for placing both the LifeSite System and the Dialock System is usually performed under local anesthesia with conscious sedation. Patients should be clear of infections for a minimum of 2 weeks prior to device placement. The recommended placement location is the upper chest (fig. 4a, b) with the device cannulas inserted into a central vein (preferably the right internal jugular) using the Seldinger technique. These devices have also been placed in the upper thigh allowing for blood access via a femoral vein in patients with poor upper chest vasculature [19, 20, 29]. Upper chest placement of these devices is associated with improved outcomes compared to femoral placement [19]. The dual valve designed for the LifeSite System also allows for flexibility in device placement location including bilateral placement.

Following the achievement of venous access and insertion of the device cannulas into a central vein, a subcutaneous pocket is formed for the valve portion of the device. For the LifeSite System, two separate subcutaneous pockets should be created, one for each valve, to insure the stability of each device during dialysis. The pocket should allow for the device to be approximately 1–1.5 cm below the skin surface. This depth reduces the risk of skin erosion over the surface of the device and allows the device to be easily accessed by the dialysis staff. It is also important that the implanting physician

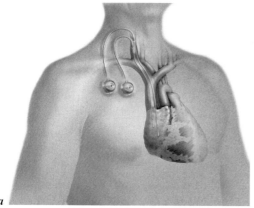
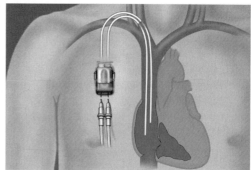

Fig. 4. a Typical placement of LifeSite system. *b* Typical placement of Dialock system.

insures meticulous pocket hemostasis after the pocket is formed. The use of cautery and/or tying off bleeding vessels is imperative to reduce the risk of postsurgical hematoma formation, which can lead to difficult cannulation and to infection.

Following creation of the subcutaneous pocket(s), the cannulas are then tunneled to the pocket(s) and attached to the valve(s). The valve(s) is then placed into the pockets and anchored with sutures to the muscle fascia following confirmation of correct placement of the cannula tips. Failure to adequately suture the device(s) into the pocket can result in valve migration and difficult cannulation. For optimal blood flow and reduced risk of recirculation, the distal tips of the cannulas should be placed in the right atrium with the return cannula being placed at least 2 cm deeper than the draw cannula. The system is accessed to check function, rinsed with saline and then the cannula is locked with heparin or an appropriate locking solution. To reduce the risk of overheparinization and bleeding when heparin is utilized as the locking solution, it is recommended that the concentration of heparin be no higher than 1,000 units/ml. An upright chest x-ray should be performed following the placement procedure to insure the correcting positioning of the cannula tips.

Clinical Outcomes

Numerous authors have reported on outcomes associated with the use subcutaneous hemodialysis access systems [11–20, 30, 31]. In general, these reports have shown the use of totally subcutaneous hemodialysis access system is associated with high blood flows, the delivery of adequate dialysis, excellent device survival and a low risk of device-related complications with several studies showing improved outcomes with these devices when compared to tunneled cuffed hemodialysis catheters [11, 17–20].

Clinical Studies with the LifeSite System

Numerous authors have reported on clinical outcomes associated with the use of the LifeSite System with several of these studies comparing the use of the LifeSite to the use of standard hemodialysis catheters [11, 12, 17–20]. Initial pilot studies with the device were performed with the use of 0.2% sodium oxychlorosene (Clorpactin®; United Guardian, Hauppauge, N.Y., USA) as the antimicrobial solution [11, 12]. Subsequent in vitro and clinical data have shown that the use of 70% isopropyl alcohol as an antimicrobial solution with the LifeSite System results in significantly better antimicrobial activity compared to oxychlorosene [12]. As a result of these findings, the only antimicrobial solution now recommended for use with the LifeSite System is 70% isopropyl alcohol.

Schwab et al. [11] reported on the 6-month outcomes associated with the use of the LifeSite System compared to the Tesio-Cath hemodialysis catheter. This prospective multicenter study documented the efficacy of using 70% isopropyl alcohol as the antimicrobial solution for irrigating the LifeSite System. Blood flow rates were significantly higher in the LifeSite group compared to the Tesio-Cath group (358.7 vs. 331.8 ml/min, $p < 0.001$ for machine-indicated blood flow of 400 ml/min). The device-related infection rate was significantly lower for the LifeSite IPA group compared to the Tesio-Cath group (1.3 vs. 3.3 events per 1,000 patient-days, $p < 0.05$). The need for thrombolytic infusions was also significantly lower in the LifeSite group versus the Tesio-Cath group (2.27 vs. 8.81 infusions per 1,000 patient-days, $p = 0.0295$). Device survival at 6 months after stratification by diabetic status and adjusting for age was significantly better in the LifeSite IPA group (89.9%) than in the Tesio-Cath group (69.1%, $p = 0.0292$).

Moran et al. [17, 18] recently reported the 12-month results from the above study. Patients in the LifeSite group experienced a lower rate of device-related infections compared to the Tesio-Cath group at 12 months (2.37 vs. 3.28 events per 1,000 patient-days, $p = 0.0535$). Twelve-month device survival was also better in the LifeSite group versus the Tesio-Cath group (67.1 vs. 48.0%). A subgroup analysis showed that among patients with a history of previous access the use of the LifeSite was associated with a significantly lower rate of device-related infection (2.63 vs. 4.58 events per 1,000 patient-days, $p = 0.05$). The same was true for patients who had diabetic ESRD (2.39 vs. 3.94 events per 1,000 patient-days, $p = 0.0237$).

Capling et al. [19] recently reported data from a retrospective study comparing device survival for 57 patients implanted with the LifeSite System versus 97 patients receiving tunneled hemodialysis catheters. The authors report that overall probability of device survival in the LifeSite patient group at 100 and 300 days was greater than the probability of device survival in the tunneled catheter group at the same time points (91 vs. 78 and 72 vs. 51%, respectively). A separate analysis limited to patients with jugular vein placement of the devices also showed an improved device survival in the LifeSite group at 100 and 300 days (96 vs. 82 and 88 vs. 53%).

Lamarche et al. [20] have recently reported the results of a retrospective analysis of 45 patients receiving the LifeSite System. Average blood flow rate and Kt/V associated with the use of the LifeSite System during the observation period was 347 ml/min and 1.46, respectively. The overall rate of device-related infections was 2.5 per 1,000 patient-days with a device-related bacteremia rate of 0.8 per 1,000 patient-days. Among patients with upper chest placement (internal jugular vein or subclavian vein) of the LifeSite System, the rate of device-related infections was 1.9 per 1,000 patient-days. Patients who were dialyzed with a catheter prior to receiving the LifeSite System (n = 28) showed an improvement in both average Kt/V (1.45 vs. 1.31, p = 0.07) and average blood flow (339.6 vs. 317.8 ml/min, p = 0.081).

Clinical Studies with the Dialock System

Several reports of preliminary studies with the Dialock System have been published to date [13–16, 31]. Limited prospective or retrospective data directly comparing outcomes with the Dialock versus tunneled cuffed catheters is available.

Levin et al. [13] have reported on the results from a pilot study of the Dialock System in a series of 10 hemodialysis patients. The mean duration of device use per patient in this study was 7.3 months. The average Kt/V exceeded 1.6 and the average blood flow rate was 326 ml/min. The overall bacteremia rate was 2.3 per 1,000 patient-days; however, no infections resulted in the need for device removal. The device was very well accepted by both patients and nursing staff. Canaud et al. [14] also reported initial clinical results with the Dialock System in 10 hemodialysis patients. The mean duration of device use in this series was 5.7 months. Average Kt/V was 1.36 with an average blood flow of 307 ml/min. The calculated bacteremia rate for patients reported in this series was 1.73 per 1,000 patient-days.

Canaud et al. [15] also reported on a combined experience with the Dialock System based on longer-term data from the above two pilot studies. The authors reported on a total of 23 patients implanted with the device for an average of 11 months. Device survival was 71% at 12 months and 65.3% at

18 months. Average delivered dialysis dose ranged from 1.48 to 1.8, and average blood flow for Dialock patients in this series from the United States was 348 ml/min compared to 311 ml/min for the patients in France. The calculated bacteremia rate for patients reported in this series was 2.43 per 1,000 patient-days.

Quarello and Rorneris [16] recently reported the results of a retrospective cohort analysis of 35 patients implanted with the Dialock System. Infection-related outcomes in these patients were compared to infectious outcomes in a concurrent series of 37 patients receiving dialysis via Tesio-Cath hemodialysis catheters. The average follow-up time for patients implanted with the Dialock System was 7.5 months compared to 12 months in the Tesio group. The overall device-related infection rate in the Dialock group was 0.97 per 1,000 patient-days compared to 4.75 per 1,000 patient-days for the catheter group. Analysis of the infection rate by location of infection showed that the Dialock group experienced a similar rate of device-related bacteremias compared to the catheter group (0.85 vs. 0.81 per 1,000 patient-days). The difference in the overall rate of device-related infections was due to the high rate of exit site infections in the catheter group (3.6 per 1,000 patient-days) compared to the rate of pocket infections in the Dialock group (0.12 per 1,000 patient-days).

Sodemann et al. [31] have recently reported outcomes in 70 patients implanted with the Dialock System in whom a novel catheter locking solution, taurolidine, was used in conjunction with the device. The mean patient device experience exceeded 12 months in this series of patients. The authors report that the overall device-related infection rate was 1.09 per 1,000 patient-days with the majority of these events being pocket infections. The rate of device-related pocket infections was 0.8 per 1,000 patient-days in this series compared to a device-related bacteremia rate of 0.29 per 1,000 patient-days.

Device-Related Complications

Complications associated with the use of subcutaneous hemodialysis access systems may result from an improper implant technique, improper nursing care, or poor patient hygiene. Strict conformance to manufacturer-recommended procedures for the implantation, use and maintenance of these devices is vital in minimizing the risk of device-related complications.

Insertion-Related Complications
Acute insertion-related complications associated with the placement of subcutaneous hemodialysis access devices are similar to those seen with the

placement of tunneled cuffed hemodialysis catheters. The appropriate use of ultrasound guidance and fluoroscopy during the implant procedure can be expected to significantly reduce the risk of these complications. Potential complications include puncture of the carotid artery, hemothorax, pneumothorax, hemopericardium and air embolism.

An improper implant technique can also increase the risk of chronic device-related complications. The formation of a pocket hematoma can result from the failure to obtain adequate hemostasis in a newly created pocket prior to device insertion or the use of a heparin concentration of greater than 1,000 units/ml for locking the device cannulas. If a pocket hematoma develops it should be evacuated immediately to prevent the development of a pocket infection [28]. Failure to place the device cannulas in the right atrium can lead to poor flows and an increased risk of clotting and fibrin sheath formation. Obtaining a postoperative upright chest x-ray to confirm proper placement of the distal tip of the cannula is mandatory. Poor flow or repeated need for thrombolytic infusions (greater than 3 infusions) suggests improper tip placement. Removal of the affected cannula and replacement with another cannula positioned correctly in the right atrium are recommended when the cannula is malpositioned.

Chronic complications can also result from poor placement location of the device. A valve implanted too deep may result in an increased risk of infection due to the increased difficulty nurses will encounter when trying to access the device. A shallow valve increases the risk of erosion over the top of the device and increases the risk of infection and the need for device removal. Placement of the valves in a position that increases the difficulty for accessing the device (e.g. near armpit, deep in breast tissue) should be avoided to insure the dialysis staff can easily access the device. Implanting physicians should take steps to identify a level body plane on the upper chest to allow for proper positioning and implant depth of the device prior to creating the valve pockets.

Care and Maintenance-Related Complications

Since some dialysis staff may be unfamiliar with these devices, it is important that they receive adequate training on how to access and care for the device prior to managing patients implanted with these subcutaneous systems.

The failure to adhere to strictly aseptic techniques can lead to the increased risk of infection. Dialysis staff accessing the device and the patient should wear a surgical mask covering both their nose and mouth during the insertion and removal of needles. Adequately scrubbing the access area for the appropriate length of time before and after accessing the device is also important towards reducing the risk of contamination. For the LifeSite System, it is important to complete the isopropyl alcohol irrigation step before insertion and after removal of the 14-gauge needle.

Bleeding-related complications can result from the use of improper needles when accessing the device or the failure to insure the needles are properly seated in the device prior to the initiation of hemodialysis. The use of the incorrect concentration or volume of heparin to lock the device cannulas can also lead to an increased bleeding risk [15]. Bleeding can result in the formation of pocket hematomas, and as discussed above, immediate evacuation of blood from the pocket and irrigation of the pocket with saline are required to reduce the risk of infection.

Infectious complications associated with the use of subcutaneous hemodialysis access systems can often be treated without the need for device removal [13–15, 31–33]. The use of systemic antibiotics in combination with antimicrobial or antibiotic locking solutions to treat bacteremias [31, 32] or the irrigation of the infected valve pocket with an antibiotic solution [31] have both proven effective in eradicating infections associated with these devices. An algorithm to treat bacteremias associated with the LifeSite System has also been developed [33]. This protocol involves daily irrigation of the LifeSite pockets with 70% isopropyl alcohol in combination with administration of intravenous antibiotics for 2 weeks. If a repeat culture taken 1 week after completion of antibiotics indicates that infection is still present, daily alcohol irrigation of the LifeSite pockets and administration of antibiotics for an additional 2 weeks is indicated in conjunction with the exchange of the affected LifeSite cannula(s). If cultures taken 1 week after completion of the second course of antibiotics are positive, it is recommended that the device be removed.

Patient Care and Maintenance-Related Complications

While the risk of patients contributing to complications with subcutaneous dialysis access systems is likely less than would be seen with externalized hemodialysis catheters, poor patient hygiene and care for the access area between dialysis sessions can lead to an increase in the risk of infection with these devices. Patients should be educated on the proper care of their access, to clean the access site on a regular basis, and to inspect the skin area around the access site for signs of infection daily [34]. Patients should also be told to communicate with their physician or dialysis staff if they observe any redness, swelling or discharge at the site. Since subcutaneous devices also allow patients to bath and swim, it is important that they follow proper care recommendations before and after entering the water. This includes the application of triple antibiotic ointment to the access site and covering the site with a waterproof bandage. Patients should also be warned to avoid activities that may irritate or traumatize the access site.

Other Devices

A newer transcutaneous device has recently been developed which provides for needle-free AV access. The Hemaport® (Hemapure AB, Uppsala, Sweden) is comprised of a percutaneous titanium housing connected to a PTFE graft. The device is placed in either the upper arm or the thigh [35]. Unlike the totally subcutaneous design of the Dialock and LifeSite Systems, the Hemaport has an externalized housing which remains in place and is covered by a disposable sealing plate between dialysis sessions. Blood continues to flow through the device when the sealing plate is in place. When blood access for dialysis is needed, the sealing plate is replaced by a specialized disposable dialysis lid using an applicator. After the dialysis session is complete, the dialysis lid is replaced by a new sealing plate.

Ahlmen et al. [35] recently presented preliminary data from a six-center study of the Hemaport. A total of 13 patients were implanted with an average per patient device experience of 5.5 months. Mean blood flow in these patients was 364 ml/min. Complications resulted in the removal of 6 devices to date with 5 patients being reimplanted with a Hemaport. Reasons for device removal were reported to be insufficient vascular flow, thrombosis and/or infection. Further clinical data is needed to determine whether this newer transcutaneous device can overcome the clinical challenges that limited the use and acceptance of the Hemasite and the DiaTAP.

Summary and Conclusions

Subcutaneous hemodialysis access systems represent a uniquely different hemodialysis access option. The ideal role for these devices is to help patients to achieve a functioning AV fistula by providing temporary access while patients are waiting for the creation or maturation of an AV fistula. An ideal bridge device would allow for immediate use following placement, provide blood flow rates sufficient to ensure adequate dialysis, have a low complication rate, and have sufficient length of technical survival to allow AV fistula development and maturation without the need for device replacement. Clinical data reported to date supports the use of subcutaneous hemodialysis access systems as a bridge device instead of a hemodialysis catheter [11, 12, 17–20]. The increased emphasis on AV fistula placements in patient populations who are at higher risk of having fistulas that fail to mature increases the need for a bridge device which provides improved outcomes during longer maturation periods especially in patients in whom more than one fistula attempt is made or for patients who are receiving upper arm fistulas [21, 36].

Several studies have also documented the utility of subcutaneous hemodialysis access systems in catheter-dependent patients who have exhausted other access options [12–15, 19, 20]. The hope offered for improved outcomes in this patient population should be tempered by realistic expectations for device performance especially in patients with significant morbidities, poor vasculature, a history of poorly performing hemodialysis catheters, or multiple catheter-related infections.

Totally subcutaneous hemodialysis access systems offer a unique option for ESRD patients. The development of these devices represent a key step towards improving dialysis delivery and hemodialysis vascular access-related outcomes. Following recommended procedures for implanting, accessing and maintaining these devices is key towards achieving optimal device performance.

References

1   Hakim R, Himmelfarb J: Hemodialysis access failure: A call to action. Kidney Int 1998;54: 1029–1040.
2   National Kidney Foundation: K/DOQI Clinical Practice Guidelines for Vascular Access, 2000. Am J Kidney Dis 2000;37(suppl 1):S137–S181.
3   Centers for Medicare & Medicaid Services: 2002 Annual Report, End State Renal Diseases Clinical Performance Measures Project. Baltimore, Department of Health and Human Services, Centers for Medicare & Medicaid Services, 2002.
4   Rayner HC, Pisoni RL, Gillespie BW, Goodkin DA, Akiba T, Akizawa T, Saito A, Young EW, Port FK: Creation, cannulation and survival of arteriovenous fistulae: Data from the Dialysis Outcomes and Practice Patterns Study. Kidney Int 2003;63:323–330.
5   Schwab SJ, Beathard G: The hemodialysis catheter conundrum: Hate living with them, but can't live without them. Kidney Int 1999;56:1–17.
6   Butterly DW, Schwab SJ: Catheter access for hemodialysis: An overview. Semin Dial 2001; 14:411–415.
7   Beathard GA: Catheter thrombosis. Semin Dial 2001;14:441–445.
8   Saad TF: Central venous dialysis catheters: Catheter-associated infection. Semin Dial 2001;14: 446–451.
9   Nassar GM, Ayus JC: Infectious complications of the hemodialysis access. Kidney Int 2001;60: 1–13.
10 Dhingra RK, Young EW, Hulbert-Shearon TE, Leavey SF, Port FK: Type of vascular access and mortality in U.S. hemodialysis patients. Kidney Int 2001;60:1443–1451.
11 Schwab SJ, Weiss MA, Rushton F, Ross JP, et al: Multicenter clinical trial results with the LifeSite hemodialysis access system. Kidney Int 2002;62:1026–1033.
12 Beathard GA, Posen GA: Initial clinical results with the LifeSite Hemodialysis Access System. Kidney Int 2000;58:2221–2227.
13 Levin NW, Yang PM, Hatch DA, Dubrow AJ, Caraiani NS, et al: New access device for hemodialysis. ASAIO J 1998;44:M529–M531.
14 Canaud B, My H, Morena M, Lamy-Lacavalerie B, Leray-Moragues H, et al: Dialock: A new vascular access device for extracorporeal renal replacement therapy. Preliminary clinical results. Nephrol Dial Transplant 1999;4:692–698.
15 Canaud B, Levin N, Ing T, My H, Dubrow AJ, Polashegg HD, Prosl FR: Dialock: Pilot trial of a new vascular port access device for hemodialysis. Semin Dial 1999;12:382–388.
16 Quarello F, Rorneris G: Prevention of hemodialysis catheter-related bloodstream infection using an antimicrobial lock. Blood Purif 2002;20–92.

17   Moran J, Pedan A, Patz M and the LifeSite Hemodialysis Access System Study Group: Device related infection rate: A comparison of the LifeSite Hemodialysis Access System versus the Tesio-Cath hemodialysis catheter (abstract). J Am Soc Nephrol 2002;12:228A.

18   Moran J, Pedan A, Patz M and the LifeSite Hemodialysis Access System Study Group: LifeSite Hemodialysis Access System versus the Tesio-Cath hemodialysis catheter: A comparison of one year device survivals (abstract). J Am Soc Nephrol 2002;12:228A.

19   Capling RK, Ziyad AAM, Gellens M, Bander SJ, Martin KJ: Clinical utility of LifeSite Dialysis Access Systems: Comparison of outcomes between LifeSites and tunneled catheters (abstract). J Am Soc Nephrol 2002;12:227A.

20   Lamarche MB, Zeik JC, Clark RV, Lebron AJ, Gupta AK, et al: High performance and low complication rates of a subcutaneous vascular access device-A retrospective analysis of the LifeSite® Hemodialysis Access System. Dial Transplant 2002;31:799–806.

21   Paul MD, Parfrey P, Marshall D, Aldrete V, Purchase L, Gault H: The outcome and complications of the DiaTAP bioCarbon button-graft vascular access device in haemodialysis patients: A two-year experience. Nephron 1986;44:96–102.

22   Alarabi AA, Wahlberg J, Danielson BG, Tufveson G, Wadstrom J, Wikstrom B: Experience with the Hemasite device in haemodialysis and haemofiltration patients with vascular access problems. Nephrol Dial Transplant 1990;5:508–512.

23   Reed WP, Moody MR, Newman KA, Light PD, Costerton JW: Bacterial colonization of Hemasite access devices. Surgery 1986;99:308–317.

24   Gault MH, Costerton JW, Paul MD, Parfrey PS, Purchase LH: *Staphylococcal epidermidis* infection of a hemodialysis button-graft complex controlled by vancomycin for 11 months. Nephron 1987;45:126–128.

25   Nissenson AR, Raible D, Higgin RE, Golding AL: No-needle (NND): Experience with the new carbon transcutaneous hemodialysis (HD) access device (CTAD). Clin Nephrol 1981;15:302–308.

26   Kapoian T, Sherman RA: A brief history of vascular access for hemodialysis: An unfinished story. Semin Nephrol 1997;17:239–245.

27   Megerman J, Levin NW, Ing TS, Dubrow AJ, Prosl FR: Development of a new approach to vascular access. Artif Organs 1999;23:10–14.

28   Webb M: Managing complications with the LifeSite Hemodialysis Access System; in Henry ML (ed): Vascular Access for Hemodialysis. Chicago, Access Medical Press, 2002, vol 8, pp 337–339.

29   Ross J: Subcutaneous implantation of the LifeSite Hemodialysis Access System in the femoral vein. J Vasc Surg 2001;2:91–96.

30   Ross J: Bridging to a high flow upper arm native fistula for hemodialysis with the LifeSite® Hemodialysis Access System. J Vasc Access 2001;2:139–144.

31   Sodemann K, Polaschegg HD, Feldmer B: Two year's experience with Dialock and CLS™ (a new antimicrobial lock solution). Blood Purif 2001;19:251–254.

32   Boorgu R, Dubrow AJ, Levin NW, My H, Canaud BJ, Lentino JR, Wentworth DW, et al: Adjunctive antibiotic/anticoagulant lock therapy in the treatment of bacteremia associated with the use of a subcutaneously implanted hemodialysis access device. ASAIO J 2000;46:767–770.

33   Moran J; LifeSite Hemodialysis Access System Study Group: Effectiveness of a treatment algorithm for treating through infections in patients implanted with LifeSite Hemodialysis Access System (abstract). J Am Soc Nephrol 2001;12:298A.

34   Wofford S: Care and maintenance of hemodialysis catheters and subcutaneous access devices: A nurse's perspective. Nephrol News Issues 2002;16:27–31.

35   Ahlmen J, Goch J, Wrege U, Larsson R, Honkanen E, Althoff P, Danielson BG: Preliminary results from the use of new vascular access (Hemaport) for hemodialysis (abstract). Hemodialysis Int 2003;7:74.

36   Allon M, Robbin ML: Increasing arteriovenous fistulas in hemodialysis patients: Problems and solutions. Kidney Int 2002;62:1109–1124.

John E. Moran, MD, Chief Scientific Officer,
Satellite Healthcare, 401 Castro St, Mountain View, CA 94041 (USA)
Tel. +1 650 404 3620, Fax +1 650 625 6020, E-Mail MoranJ@SatelliteHealth.com

Ronco C, Levin NW (eds): Hemodialysis Vascular Access and Peritoneal Dialysis Access.
Contrib Nephrol. Basel, Karger, 2004, vol 142, pp 193–215

....

Complications of the Vascular Access for Hemodialysis

Klaus Konner

Department of Internal Medicine I, Cologne General Hospital,
University of Cologne, Germany

Introduction

This chapter summarizes vascular access (VA) complications in patients using an arteriovenous fistula (AVF) or an arteriovenous graft (AVG) for maintenance hemodialysis therapy as well as complications with central venous catheters (CVC) and other types of prosthetic devices.

For better diagnosis and treatment of VA complications we should be aware of the fact that arteriovenous (AV) connections – fistulae and grafts – are unphysiological [1]. Vascular remodeling and adaptation to high-flow conditions as well as the effects of repeated cannulation play a pivotal role [2] in developing complications. Optimal conditions will result in a harmonious equilibrium of high flow in the setting of arterial and venous dilatation as well as low intravascular pressure. This is observed with the resulting shear stress being reduced to normal levels [3]. Complications of AV VA are nothing other than a disequilibrium of this idealized anatomical and functional status. CVC potentially give raise to additional problems resulting from any type of transcutaneous connection, here mainly exit site infections. Ports combine the benefit of subcutaneous placement and the risk of catheters, and are also prone to flow problems and thrombosis. Treatment of any thrombotic or flow complication aims at a restoration of optimal flow conditions. Four decades of hemodialysis therapy have shown that prevention is the best therapy for complications, when it can be achieved.

Surgical and interventional radiologic procedures will also be discussed. It is astonishing that studies comparing results obtained by surgery and by interventional procedures demonstrate mixed and often conflicting results in patients with AVF. It seems that local expertise and dedication are determining (and limiting) factors.

Complications

Differentiating between local and systemic complications of dialysis access is somewhat artificial since the two are interrelated. For example, correction of a severe central venous stenosis increases access blood flow rates with the potential risk of cardiac overload or onset of peripheral ischemia. Treating one complication may cause another complication: systemic, local, or both. Thus, complications will be described following the frequency of their clinical occurrence.

AVF and AVG

Thrombosis and Stenosis

Thrombosis, the by far most frequently observed complication of VA, is usually the final result of a process that is characterized by a reduction of blood flow progressing to a complete stop of circulation with clotting. In most patients the underlying mechanism is a downstream-located venous narrowing that develops into a stenosis over time often occurring as a relentless process. There is an interesting exception when a moderate stenosis in AVF is detected in a timely fashion; it has been observed that it can be widened by concentrating cannulations exactly to that venous segment resulting in relative dilation that can correct the underlying stenosis [4]. Hemodynamically relevant stenoses along the arterial inflow tract are observed in a small minority of patients as recently described by Guerra et al. [5]. So, the path from narrowing to stenosis and ultimately to thrombosis offers a wide array of opportunities for monitoring and surveillance of deteriorating AVF and AVG function. Although the optimal monitoring strategy is far from clear, and likely depends on many factors, monitoring and surveillance can lead to preemptive and elective surgical and/or interventional revision of the dysfunctional AVF or AVG. This strategy was demonstrated several years ago by Sands and Miranda [6] when they succeeded in lowering the rate of AVG thrombotic episodes from 3.6 to 1.1 per patient-year. Commonly accepted techniques for monitoring and surveillance are mentioned elsewhere.

Treating VA thrombosis involves a two-step procedure: simultaneous correction of the underlying arterial or – as most often observed – venous stenosis is an integral part of both surgical as well as interventional thrombectomy. To perform thrombectomy alone is a mistake since rethrombosis within a short time will be inevitable. So, treatment of thrombosis entails removing the thrombotic material and then treating the underlying stenosis.

Location of Stenoses in AVF

Stenoses of the feeding artery are rarely observed [5]. Most commonly stenoses are close to the AV anastomosis along the first venous segment. This is probably caused by the devascularization of the venous wall during dissection accounting for about 50% of all stenoses in AVF leading to reduced inflow. More cephalad located stenoses are observed within cannulation areas or venous segments in the upper arm, mainly causing elevated levels of venous outflow pressure [7]. The most difficult cases occur with stenoses along the subclavian vein or even with a more central location. Here, the leading clinical sign is arm edema.

Location of Stenoses in AVG

Stenoses along the inflow tract and the graft itself ('midgraft stenosis') are rarely seen. Predominantly, stenoses are seen in the outflow tract, usually as graft-vein stenosis. This is a frequent, but not yet solved problem of multifactorial origin. First, aspects of the surgical technique in creating these graft-vein anastomoses should be reconsidered. To create a well-functioning graft-vein anastomosis, the graft approaching the vein will preferably be in a parallel position forming an acute angle; the anastomosis is sutured at a length of 20–30 mm [8]. Unfortunately, no comparative study can confirm the benefit of this procedure, although it has proven successful in our institution for many years. The mechanisms of intimal hyperplasia and new options for therapy are an issue of intensive research.

At the present time, there are more questions than answers aimed at solving problematic neointimal hyperplasia [9].

Timing of Revision in the Case of VA Thrombosis

In native AVF, thrombectomy should be performed as early as possible. An upper limit may be 2 days since we know that interactions of the organizing thrombus and the intimal layer of the vein reduce the longevity of a mechanically successful thrombectomy. As observed in many cases with delayed referral after onset of thrombosis, waiting for revision often causes an appositional growth of the thrombus and a substantial loss of venous capital.

In AVG, thrombectomy can be done successfully even after a couple of months. Undoubtedly, an immediately scheduled procedure will be the preferred option. The more the proximal, central venous segment is involved, the earlier revision should be initiated.

Surgical Procedures in AVF

Thrombectomy

The incision is in any case placed parallel to the vein close to the palpable stenosis, mostly involving the cephalad end of the thrombosed venous segment. The thrombosed vein is opened transversally in a tiny, possibly still maturing vein; a dilated, aneurysmatic venous segment may be opened by a longitudinal incision for simultaneous partial resection of an aneurysmatic enlargement of the vein. First, thrombotic material is removed by digital massage of the vein, supported by repeated maneuvers with a Fogarty catheter of the appropriate size. Special attention is needed to completely remove the arterial plug at the 'arterial' end of the thrombus.

Treatment of Stenosis

Different surgical techniques are used depending on the length of the stenosis and on the diameter of the pre- and poststenotic vein. Short stenoses up to 1 cm can easily be resected; the venous stumps are reanastomosed in an end-to-end fashion after sufficient mobilization of the pre- and poststenotic venous segments. A clever procedure to repair a short stenosis particularly in ectatic veins is to open the stenotic segment longitudinally and to resuture transversally, which is absolutely simple and effective. In selected cases, a patch from a native vein can successfully enlarge the diameter of a narrowed vein. Stenoses at a length of 1–4 cm may be repaired by a long venous patch (if available!) or, more elegantly, by using a mobilized, transposed venous side branch as a local patch. Sometimes, the stenosis can be replaced completely by a segment of a dilated venous side branch. If a venous collateral with a sufficient lumen is not available, a new channel of adequate lumen is constructed using two venous segments with a single smaller lumen and inserted after resection of the stenosis, a time-consuming but effective procedure. Occasionally, a combination of these techniques is used successfully. Lacking these options using native veins, graft material will be an alternative in the repair of stenoses exceeding 4 cm in length, particularly in veins with an inner diameter exceeding 6 mm as experienced with stenoses along well-dilated cephalic or basilic veins in the upper arm.

In patients where local repair of a stenosis as described is not feasible or appropriate, a proximal AV reanastomosis will be the better option preferably in the wrist and forearm AVF. With an increasing use of subcutaneous superficialization of the basilic vein stenoses at the cephalad end of the mobilized vein are observed. This type and location of stenosis as well as more centrally located obstructions are favorably treated using interventional techniques. From time to time, case reports are published with successful surgical solutions even to the right atrium in desperate cases.

Surgical Procedures in AVG

As AVG usually clot far more frequently than AVF surgeons are more familiar with the therapy of graft thrombosis, a more uniform procedure when compared to the more individualized conditions in AVF. We know that in about 85% of graft thrombosis the stenosis is located at the graft-vein anastomosis or a few centimeters more proximal along the native vein [7].

Thrombectomy

The graft is exposed by one incision at the apex in a loop configuration or in the region of the two anastomoses in case of close proximity. The aim is the optimal accessibility of the arterial and venous anastomosis to start declotting. A series of Fogarty maneuvers are necessary to 'clean' the graft. Special attention is paid to the arterial plug and to the graft-vein anastomosis as well as the central part of the draining vein. Sensitive handling of the Fogarty catheter gives a reliable image of the inner conditions of the vessels prior to angiography. Angiography can be avoided in uncomplicated cases. Nevertheless, if there is clinical suspicion of an additional, more cephalad/central stenosis angiography is mandatory.

Treatment of Stenosis

A couple of techniques are in use. In our experience with the repair of graft stenoses, the patch techniques are less successful with regard to long-term results. The reason may be that the inner surface of the repaired section is still characterized by the presence of intimal hyperplasia. If the surgically initiated widening of the diameter is incomplete, intimal hyperplasia will relapse. So, the indications for patch angioplasty should be discussed again in the future. The insertion of a 'jump graft' as a bypass between the prestenotic graft and the poststenotic vein represents an alternative. It is easier to suture the graft-graft anastomosis in an end-to-end fashion, whereas the new graft-vein anastomosis is created terminolaterally at a length of 20–30 mm [8]. The stenostic area remains in situ. This technique provides a good result and a high fistula volume flow. Resecting the stenotic area completely with insertion of a segmental graft with two end-to-end anastomoses is repeatedly described as 'graft extension'. The preference of the technical procedure is determined by the local conditions (scar tissue, stenosis along the proximal draining vein, incomplete thrombectomy) and the expertise of the surgeon.

Midgraft stenoses are resected completely and replaced by a new graft segment with the same diameter.

Aiming at an optimal mechanical result, we abandoned the technique of surgical patch angioplasty for the therapy of graft-vein stenoses (as well as interventional angioplasty) for the preceding couple of years. Repeated thrombotic episodes due to restenosis contributed substantially to an increase in patients' overall morbidity, hospitalization and rising expenditures.

Percutaneous Interventional Procedures for Thrombosis and Stenosis in AVG and AVF

Turmel-Rodrigues et al. [10] stated in 2000 that declotting an AVF 'requires greater technical skill and experience than for arteriovenous grafts'. Furthermore, 'the technique of thrombus removal must be adapted to large vessels and large clots'. Similar to surgical strategies, the two-step procedure includes removal of the thrombotic material and treatment of the underlying stenosis.

Interventional Declotting Techniques

There are a variety of declotting techniques: including pharmacological, pharmacomechanical and mechanical approaches.

Pharmacological thrombolysis means injection of a thrombolytic agent into the thrombosed VA. Systemic effects of thrombolytic agents should be avoided. Pharmacomechanical techniques first perform pharmacological thrombolysis followed by mechanical maceration and removal of residual thrombotic material.

Mechanical declotting is achieved using different devices and approaches such as the percutaneous thrombectomy device by Trerotola et al. [11] where the thrombotic material from the AVG is pushed into the lungs. This has been discussed controversially in the literature since its publication. Results in AVF are not available.

The saline pulse-spray technique as described by Valji et al. [12] and Beathard et al. [13] was also predominantly used in AVG. In addition, declotting machines became available using rotating devices or the Venturi effect.

As mentioned with the pulse-spray technique the majority of the interventional declotting methods were introduced for treatment of thrombosed AVG. There is no commonly accepted criterion for a preference of one of the above described techniques. Personal expertise, skill and experience determine the results. Furthermore, remarkable differences exist in the expenditure for these devices.

A different aspect is given in AVF. In clotted native AVF, European interventional radiologists mostly use manual catheter-directed thrombaspiration [7] or use additional devices such as the hydrolyzer [14]. Even in this field, there is no complete consensus as demonstrated by a recently published discussion [15, 16]. For example, Haage et al. [17] attempted maceration of the thrombus by balloon angioplasty alone in cases of a very short plug-like thrombus selectively obstructing the anastomosis. Treatment of long-segment thrombosis was performed by mechanical thrombectomy with a series of different devices. Residual thrombus material was compressed locally by angioplasty. On more complicated clinical situations, atherectomy catheters and cutting balloons can solve special individual problems.

In any case of interventional thrombectomy, percutaneous transluminal angioplasty will follow to treat the underlying stenosis. This has become a standard strategy with some variations such as anticoagulation during and after the procedure, duration of the balloon inflation, or type of anesthesia. It seems that not all declotting techniques used for AVG can be successfully adapted for native AVF [10].

There is still much room for individual treatment variation and learning new techniques.

Stent Placement

Stents have become an important tool in the interventional armamentarium to treat stenosis in VA, particularly in stenosis that recoils ('elastic stenoses') or in case of early and repeated restenoses. There are experienced interventional radiologists hesitating to insert stents in the arm, particularly close to the AV anastomosis or along cannulation sites [14]. Covered stents are exclusively used in case of vessel rupture. There is consensus on the commonly accepted location of stent placement along stenoses of the central veins where surgery is time-consuming and risky. In case of restenosis within a stent an attempt is justified to perform percutaneous transluminal angioplasty. When inserting a stent, protrusion into one of the great draining veins (e.g. into the basilic, cephalic, internal jugular or superior caval vein) has to be avoided. This type of protrusion would compromise future surgery and/or interventional procedures.

For a couple of years, there has been a continuous yet open discussion in the literature on the superiority of surgery over interventional techniques and vice versa. This discussion reveals important aspects: interventional procedures and devices were once introduced for the treatment of the large number of thrombotic episodes in AVG. Results of both types of treatment were compared and interventional results seemed to be slightly better than surgery in the therapy of thrombosis and stenosis in AVG.

A new field emerged when interventional techniques were introduced for the therapy of thrombosis and stenosis in native AVF. Here, reliable comparative studies are much more difficult to perform because of the individual variation in the types of AVF and the types of complications. It is understandable that the community of VA surgeons complain about the absence of studies comparing surgical and interventional results in the treatment of thrombosis and stenosis in native AVF. Interventional radiology is dominated by a few dedicated experts providing excellent and exemplary results. Surgery is performed following many strategies, but in most institutions an analysis of the results is missing. Therefore, surgeons doing VA are asked worldwide to provide data for a fair comparison that reflects reality. As randomization is not possible, only a very large series of patients will provide reliable results. Furthermore, a consensus is needed on a common basis for statistical evaluation as recently proposed by Aruny et al. [18].

One additional aspect are expenditures: repeated catheter procedures are expensive. Obviously, the availability of catheters and other technical devices is limited in developing countries and in industrial countries at least subject to discussion.

A lot of work is still needed in the field of stenosis and thrombosis in VA.

Missing, Delayed Maturation

Delayed maturation is mostly a problem in wrist or forearm AVF and means that the arterialized vein cannot be cannulated soon enough after initial fistula placement. We observe a wide range of time between the first operation and the first cannulation. With optimal conditions such as early fistula placement, absence of catheter hemodialysis, a 'healthy' artery and a 'healthy' vein, first cannulation can be performed within 3 days after surgery, and in most patients with primary elbow AVF within week 1 or 2. In our practice we have learned that on the basis of ultrasound measurements cannulation can be performed successfully with a blood flow volume of about 500 ml/min and a reliably palpable vein.

In our experience with >2,000 consecutive native primary AVF, impaired arterial inflow due to poor quality of the artery involved is by far the leading cause of delayed fistula maturation: small arterial lumen, thickened and stiff wall with loss of distensibility, and in the worst cases calcifications [19]. Clinically, the arterialized vein is difficult to palpate, and auscultation provides a weak bruit that disappears with elevation of the arm above the level of the heart; in addition, elevation as described will result in a complete collapse of the vein. These clinical symptoms obtained at bedside within 1 min can be confirmed by ultrasound: dilatation of the radial artery from 2 to 3.5 mm is lacking and blood flow volume will be less than 500 ml/min, in most cases less than 300 ml/min.

The only therapeutic option is to create a new anastomosis at a more proximal location using a 'healthy' arterial segment. A 'healthy' artery can feed two or even three main veins. Are there tools to prevent this situation of a nonmaturing AVF?

In addition to the clinical examination, including palpating the arteries in the arm, preoperative ultrasonographic evaluation of the brachial artery with measurement of the diameter (4 mm) and flow volume (60–80 ml/min) as well as diagnosis of calcifications are helpful. Along the radial and ulnar artery orthograde flow should be found as a sign of a functioning palmar arch; the resistance index should be measured as a sign of sufficient arterial functional reserve [20]. During the initial operation, a special test can be performed: if the artery does not seem to be as suitable as expected, a few drops of a diluted solution of papaverine are applied onto the surface of the artery. A suitable artery will dilate substantially after 1 or 2 min. Otherwise, a more proximally located segment of the artery should be preferred to construct the AV anastomosis.

The case of a juxta-anastomotic venous stenosis preventing dilatation of the veins and maturation was mentioned above. Late diagnosis of stenosis of the feeding radial or ulnar artery can lead to percutaneous transluminal angioplasty.

One widespread misunderstanding should be mentioned in this context. A series of articles describe techniques 'to salvage nonmaturing AVF', mostly by interventional procedures [21, 22]. Pivotal interest is given to the ligation of venous side branches/collaterals to increase blood flow volume into the main draining vein. European opinion is certain about the fact that there is no pathophysiological hemodynamic rationale to support 'venous ligation' [23]. As we know, venography of a well-functioning, well-dilated vein with a high-flow volume but low intravascular pressure will never show the side branches [3]. In case of missing maturation, the underlying cause is impaired arterial inflow that cannot be cured by ligation of venous side branches. A venographically visualized venous side branch is an auxiliary draining vein due to a proximal stenosis of the main vein. Correction of this obstruction along the cephalad main draining vein will lead to the disappearance of the collaterals. Otherwise, ligation or embolization of the venous collaterals/side branches without revision of the proximal mainstream venous stenosis will result in venous hypertension, decrease of flow volume and finally in AVF thrombosis. A lot of time may be lost by neglecting some basic hemodynamic rules.

The phenomenon of missing or delayed maturation can be reduced substantially by paying attention to two aspects: (1) selecting a 'healthy' artery for initial creation of AVF by routine ultrasound evaluation and (2) testing the continuity and the diameter of the venous lumen during initial AVF placement of a simple venous catheter before construction of the anastomosis by introduction. Heparinized saline is injected against proximal digital occlusion of the main vein to dilate any segment of the vein.

The AV anastomosis is not the fistula!

Aneurysm and False Aneurysm

An aneurysm is defined as a local enlargement of the lumen, mostly a result of destruction of the venous wall by area cannulation and replacement by scar tissue with loss of elasticity [4]. Aneurysms with a thinned layer of skin are prone to a high risk of bleeding or rupture in case of infection; they should preferably undergo partial resection. The venous continuity can be preserved in most cases. The same procedure is recommended in case of parietal thrombosis that is prone to infection. Here, a single dose of antibiotic is indicated, preferably using a drug that covers *Staphylococcus aureus*.

As experienced in many patients, aneurysms are followed downstream by a stenosis. A rise in intravascular pressure increases the process of aneurysmatic enlargement of the venous lumen. Partial resection of the aneurysm is recommended and the resected tissue may be used as a patch to treat the stenosis – a simple but effective procedure. Ultrasound evaluation has proved to be an excellent tool in preoperative diagnosis, particularly in describing location and extent of stenosis and partial thrombosis as well as the measurement of fistula volume flow. A great variety of surgical procedures are in use, a challenge for the creativity of the surgeon involved.

In patients with a long history of hemodialysis treatment, calcifications in the wall of the venous aneurysm are observed as a product of intravascular pressure and disordered calcium-phosphorus homeostasis, thus limiting the surgical options when using the native venous material. Here, the use of prosthetic graft material is indicated.

A vein with a constant, but equal lumen of ~10 mm or more does not require surgical repair per se. An indication for a revision may result from high-flow conditions causing peripheral ischemia or cardiac overload.

Aneurysms in grafts were observed exclusively in the very early years from 1973 to 1975 in single cases. What we see nowadays are false aneurysms caused by area cannulation where the original graft wall is replaced by collagenous scar tissue often combined with partial thrombosis [4]. Similar to the risks in aneurysms in native veins, infection represents the main complication. False aneurysms along AVG are easily replaced by a new graft segment. Surgery done in time reduces the risk of infection.

Konner

Peripheral Ischemia, Steal Syndrome, Ischemic Monomelic Neuropathy

A moderate steal syndrome in wrist AVF with a reversal of blood flow direction along the distal radial artery, the digital and palmar arch arteries has been known since the late 1970s [24]. Sivanesan et al. [25] confirmed these early data recently when they demonstrated that immediately after placement of the AVF $26 \pm 15\%$ of the flow volume is provided by the distal limb of the radial artery versus $74 \pm 15\%$ by the proximal limb, meaning that one quarter of the fistula volume flow is drawn via the ulnar artery and the palmar arch. This is a 'physiological' phenomenon in AV connections in patients with a normal arterial anatomy, not a complication.

If the contribution of the distal arterial limb to the fistula flow volume is increasing over time parallel to an increasing high-flow fistula volume, the arterial supply of the hand and the retrograde inflow into the AV anastomosis cannot be provided by the ulnar artery. This deficit causes peripheral ischemia of differing degrees, in the worst cases resulting in necroses of the fingers. Amputations have been described [26]. If the palmar arch is open, a ligation of the artery distal to the anastomosis can be performed with wrist and forearm AVF; in elbow AVF, the technique of 'distal revascularization-interval ligation' is an option [27]. The results of reducing the diameter of the anastomosis or banding procedures as described in the past in many variations were unpredictable and disappointing.

In patients with a well-functioning AVF, particularly in the region of the elbow that drains into a dilated basilic as well into a cephalic upper arm vein, ligation of one of these veins can reduce fistula flow volume substantially and restore peripheral arterial supply to varying degrees depending on patient anatomy. It is mandatory to simulate venous ligation before surgery by digital compression using color-coded duplex ultrasonography. If a flow signal is found along the radial artery during compression of one of the great upper arm veins, this vein should be ligated. This procedure is by far more sensitive than to palpate for the recurrence of distal pulse. All these techniques have been used or are in use in high-flow AVF.

In 2003, the problem is more frequently peripheral ischemia than steal syndrome. Since diabetic, elderly and hypertensive patients count for the vast majority of new patients [28], symptoms of peripheral ischemia are observed in many patients before initial access operation or after the placement of first access even with a marginally low-flow fistula volume of ~300 ml/min. Obstruction of the palmar arch is a routine finding in these patients. Here, closure of the anastomosis is the only option. These patients are candidates for an atrial catheter. Skilled and experienced access surgeons may succeed in constructing an AV bridge graft between the axillary or subclavian artery and a suitable vein. This is major surgery and not an option in all patients with advanced arterial disease and extensive comorbidities.

A potential cause of peripheral ischemia are central arterial stenoses. The combination of low access volume flow and peripheral ischemia will prompt angiographic evaluation. Interventional or surgical options should be considered depending on the local expertise with a clear preference of angioplasty as the first therapeutic choice.

Ischemic Monomelic Neuropathy

Ischemic monomelic neuropathy is a complication of VA observed almost exclusively in diabetic patients with preexisting peripheral neuropathy and/or peripheral vascular disease as described in detail by Riggs et al. [29] in 1989: acute pain, weakness, and paralysis of the muscles of the forearm and hand developing immediately, within minutes to hours, after the placement of an AV access preferably in the region of the elbow using the brachial artery as a feeding artery. Sudden diversion of the blood supply to the nerves of the forearm and hand results in damaging nerve fibers without necrosis of other tissues.

Diagnosis of ischemic monomelic neuropathy is a clinical diagnosis and includes weakness or paralysis of the entire or most of the forearm and hand muscles and paresthesia and numbness of all three forearm nerves. The hand is usually found to be warm without a diagnosis-related change in the quality of the radial pulse. Electromyography reveals acute, predominantly distal denervation of all upper limb nerves. Involvement of a single upper limb nerve excludes the diagnosis of ischemic monomelic neuropathy and focusses on local nerve compression, e.g. hematoma caused by access surgery or cannulation.

To prevent severe and irreversible neurologic injury, immediate access closure is required [30]. Doing this, the outcome is not predictable and varies. Delay in diagnosis and treatment will reduce the chance of improvement. Nephrologists and VA surgeons should be familiar with this clinical entity and dialysis staff should be trained thoroughly as they are in the best position for the early recognition of potentially serious problems.

In addition, we should not forget that in most patients the underlying peripheral arterial occlusive disease will progress during the period of dialysis therapy, thus contributing to a substantial reduction of life expectancy in this group of dialysis patients [31].

Cardiac Overload

The risk of cardiovascular disease in patients with end-stage renal disease results from the additive effect of multiple factors, including hemodynamic overload and several metabolic and endocrine abnormalities typically found in uremia [32]. Foley [33] describes that at least half of all patients starting dialysis therapy have overt cardiovascular disease. Left ventricular hypertrophy, ischemic heart disease and cardiac failure are commonly found, but clinically compensated in most patients.

Nevertheless, cardiac decompensation caused by an AVF with normal flow is uncommon except in rare patients with underlying cardiac disease [34]. Since there is no commonly accepted consensus on the amount of AVF flow that will cause cardiac symptoms, the patients' individual conditions will determine the outcome. A volume flow exceeding 1,000–1,500 ml/min can be suspicious. Day-by-day clinical experience teaches us that severe cardiac failure, mostly combined with a hypotensive state, per se prevents pathological high-flow fistulae.

In the very rare case of high-flow conditions, surgical procedures should be initiated to reduce AV flow volume. There are a series of technical options such as banding procedures by incomplete ligation of the main draining vein (risky!), interposition of a short 4-mm graft segment, reducing the diameter of the AV anastomosis and others. In any case, the result is not predictable. A more challenging technique in elbow and upper arm AVF is the distal arterial distension by replacing the arterial inflow from the brachial to the radial artery; a flow reduction of more than 50% is achievable [35]. Preoperative and postoperative flow measurement is mandatory.

An AVF remaining functional after successful renal transplantation may support left ventricular hypertrophy and hypertension [19]. Here, ligation of the AVF will be beneficial. In any of these procedures there should be an option for the future placement of a new access preferably at the ipsilateral side.

Experienced VA surgeons reduce the diameter of the anastomosis when constructing more cephalad located AV connections. This means that an anastomosis to the brachial artery should not substantially exceed the diameter of the artery, 4–6 mm being the optimal length.

Infection

Arteriovenous Fistulae
For the last couple of years, infections in AVF have been rarely observed. Training of medical doctors, staff and patients in aseptic techniques in the care for AVF has reduced infection rates. Standardized cannulation techniques contribute to this welcome development.

If infection occurs, conservative therapy is the first option: the arm should be fixed in a neutral position, cannulation is avoided along the infected venous segment, and antibiotic therapy is initiated. This procedure will cure the vast majority of infections.

Surgery is needed in case of a paravenous abscess. There is a wide range of potential techniques from simple drainage to a new AV anastomosis in the same extremity. Segmental replacement of an infected naive vein using graft material is risky and should be avoided whenever possible.

Arteriovenous Grafts

As outlined by Minga et al. [36] graft infection results in substantial morbidity, prolonged dependence on dialysis catheters, and multiple VA procedures. AVG are correlated with an increased mortality risk when compared with AVF often due to infectious complications with a risk ratio of 2.47 [37].

The conservative strategy is the same as in AVF but not as successful. Surgical options are quite different. In case the region of an anastomosis is involved the graft has to be removed completely as soon as possible. Neglecting this rule may cause major complications such as clinical sepsis, septic arthritis, epidural abscess, endocarditis, osteomyelitis and even death. After removal of an infected graft, patients were catheter dependent for a median of 3.8 months; during the period of catheter dependence, patients required a mean of 9.7 access procedures, as reported in detail by Minga et al. [36].

Midgraft infection can first be treated conservatively. Segmental resection of the graft and replacement by a new graft is a risky option; isolating the infected graft segment and insertion of a graft bypass far away from the infected area is another technique. Obviously, comparative studies are not possible. For this reason, all decisions are based on the surgeon's and the center's expertise.

Special attention has recently been given to occult infection of old non-functioning AVG. The risk of prosthetic AVG infection does not end when the graft is no longer in use [38, 39]. If these patients have a fever of uncertain origin, an indium scan will be helpful to diagnose silent graft infection. This is particularly important in patients after renal transplantation. Furthermore, patients with an old, nonfunctioning AVG should not be considered as candidates for organ transplantation unless silent AVG infection has been excluded. The best protection against complications is complete removal.

In any case, an infected AVG is a major risk for the patient with a poorly predictable outcome. A timely and aggressive surgical approach is mandatory in most cases. Presumably, there will be no essential difference in the outcome between different graft materials. Prosthetic devices may have the advantage theoretically of an unlimited availability for future access operations.

The greatest benefit for the patient is avoiding the use of AVG (and CVC) in favor of native AVF. In addition, all non-AV graft-related infections should to be treated promptly [40].

CVC and Subcutaneous Devices

The Dialysis Outcomes and Practice Patterns Study (DOPPS) data describe in detail the widespread use of CVC in hemodialysis patients [37, 40]. In Europe, for example, despite the aging of the dialysis population and the increasing proportion of diabetics, the number of patients with synthetic grafts has decreased in recent years at the expense of a rising proportion of CVC [19].

It is time to accept that permanent catheters are not permanent [41]. Untunneled catheters are commonly used for short-term use; otherwise, tunneled catheters are the preferred choice. Unfortunately, it is not clear which material and design are the best choice for catheters used in hemodialysis therapy. Furthermore, in case of emergency hemodialysis treatment, the femoral vein is advantageously used for the placement of an untunneled catheter. The right internal jugular vein is reserved, whenever possible, for early implantation of a tunneled cuffed catheter predominantly for bridging the maturation period of an AV access. This seems to be conclusive. In contrast, in the US, the subclavian vein and the internal jugular vein were the most commonly used sites for untunneled CVC each with 46% whereas tunneled catheters were placed predominantly in the internal jugular vein (62%) and the subclavian vein (36%) [42]. Cannulation of the subclavian vein with a high risk of stenosis or obstruction should become an obsolete procedure in all patients where an AV access is planned in the future [43]. Undoubtedly, a significantly higher complication rate is observed in untunneled and tunneled catheters as compared with AVF and even AVG. This means an increased risk in morbidity and even mortality [37, 40].

Unfortunately, no reliable data are available from the literature on the percentage of patients who for cardiovascular reasons are candidates for the exclusive long-term use of a tunneled CVC as VA [17].

This section refers to complications of placement, catheter-related infections and thrombotic complications.

Complications of Placement of CVC

Various types of acute complications with catheter placement have been described, most of them occurring rarely. The formation of hematomas is the main complication caused by femoral as well as subclavian and jugular vein cannulation by accidental injury of the adjacent artery rarely resulting in pseudoaneurysm and AVF; injury of the femoral artery can lead to life-threatening retroperitoneal hematomas.

Preoperative ultrasound evaluation of the femoral and internal jugular vein has become a commonly accepted preventive tool for safe and successful catheter placement. Ultrasound-guided cannulation has proven to be an effective technique to reduce this main type of complications during the insertion of the catheter [44].

Careful handling of guidewires and introduction devices in a sterile setting is mandatory. Fluoroscopic/angiographic control of the catheter during and at the end of the placement confirms the correct catheter position, absence of kinking and other types of malposition. In addition, endocavitary electrocardiography allows accurate location of the catheter tip [45]. Skill and experience of the surgeon or the interventionalist are an essential contribution to success and safety leading to a substantial reduction of early complications as exemplarily demonstrated by Work [46].

Catheter-Related Infections

As CVC are foreign bodies permanently crossing the integument, they represent an unphysiological phenomenon prone to infectious complications. Catheter-related bacteremia remains the most common and serious CVC complication, mostly caused by gram-positive organisms such as *S. aureus* and *Staphylococcus epidermis*. Potential mechanisms for infection are external contamination from hands and breath of health care personnel, contaminated solutions or poorly managed dressings as well as internal colonization such as fibrin sleeve formation, intramural thrombi and inadequate tunnels [47].

Any infectious episode has the potential risk of metastatic infection via hematogenous dissemination: endocarditis, vertebral osteomyelitis, spinal dural abscess and spinal cord compression as severe 'complication of complication'. Severe comorbidity and immunotherapy favor hematogenous dissemination.

Although therapeutic tools are manifold, optimal management of CVC infection is still controversial: antibiotics alone do not seem to be sufficient. New locking solutions such as gentamycin sodium citrate or taurolidine citrate are said to reduce the endoluminal biofilm, thus reducing one of the most risky factors for CVC infections including hematogenous dissemination. CVC catheter care should be done in the same way as caring for peritoneal dialysis catheters.

Exit site infection in tunneled catheters can be healed in most cases by intensified application of external disinfecting agents (chlorhexidine, povidone-iodine or alcohol) and sterile dressings until the exit site is dry and clean combined with parenteral or enteral antibiotics directed at gram-positive organisms. Untunneled catheters with exit site infection will be removed.

Tunnel infection requires immediate catheter removal in any case. No time should be lost.

Since catheter-related bacteremia is established and proven by blood cultures an antibiotic therapy is to be initiated to avoid sepsis. Hemodynamic and respiratory instability as observed in comorbid and elderly patients requires hospitalization. In many cases, the decision to remove a catheter based on the clinical situation prior to blood culture results is very difficult and can only be made considering the individual patients' conditions. This depends on factors such as severity of sepsis and comorbidity as well as alternative VA options. Guidewire exchange has been described repeatedly; the decision has not become easier with the knowledge of these data [48]. Furthermore, there is no consent on the efficacy of antibiotic locking solutions in this situation of acute infection.

Prevention of catheter-related bacteremia starts with the proper handling by the dialysis staff. Thorough training and control are indispensable to establish a strategy that is the same in any patient at any time. Here, uniformity is the key to a successful prevention policy.

Thrombotic Complications

CVC malfunction due to poor flow is a common problem. Technical reasons such as catheter kinking account for early episodes of malfunction, whereas late occurrence is mostly caused by thrombus formation. Treatment should be initiated at an early point, otherwise inadequate dialysis therapy will result.

Beathard [49] proposed to classify the types of thrombosis into extrinsic thrombi (mural and atrial thrombi, central vein thrombosis) and intrinsic thrombi (intraluminal and catheter tip as well as fibrin sheath thrombi).

Mural Thrombi

Mural thrombus: The mural thrombus at the tip of the CVC with adherence to the wall of the central vein at the atrium as a result of an assumed interaction between the pulse-dependent movement of the catheter tip causes catheter malfunction. Diagnosis is conformed angiographically. In case of large thrombus formation, transesophageal echocardiography will be helpful. In any case, removal of the CVC is the therapy of choice. In patients with a large thrombus, anticoagulation should be initiated for a period of 1 month.

Atrial thrombus: An atrial thrombus may cause manifold symptoms ranging from simple catheter malfunction, pulmonary or (paradoxically) systemic emboli to a mass within the right atrium as diagnosed angiographically or by echocardiography. Atrial thrombosis can develop life-threatening symptoms. Anticoagulation is indicated until disappearance of the thrombotic material as controlled advantageously by echocardiography.

Central vein thrombosis: The rates reported range from 2% [50] to 63.5% [51], presumably dependent on the intensity of initiating diagnostic angiography and paying attention to clinical symptoms mostly represented by local pain and tenderness. In other patients, central vein thrombosis caused by a CVC develops and appears silent, without any dramatic symtomatology unless an AV access is created ipsilaterally. Once diagnosis is confirmed, removal of the catheter is indicated except in desperate cases. In any case anticoagulation should be started for at least 1 month.

Intrinsic Thrombi

Intrinsic thrombi localized intraluminally at the tip of the CVC or as a fibrin sheath account for the majority of catheter flow problems during hemodialysis sessions.

Intraluminal thrombi: In case of an inadequate or incomplete heparin lock or when heparin escapes from the lumen during the dialysis interval, the entering blood can clot either blocking the lumen incompletely or in an occlusive fashion.

Catheter tip thrombi: They are observed mostly at the level of side holes where heparin can be washed out easily. The result can be a complete occlusion; sometimes the thrombus appears like a ball valve. These events should initiate considerations on number, size and configuration of side holes, a wide field for future investigations.

Fibrin sheath thrombi: There is a consent that fibrin sheath formation is the most frequent type of tunneled catheter thrombosis. Morphologically, a sleeve of fibrin is found that surrounds the catheter starting from the entrance into the vein proceeding over time to the tip of the catheter, thus closing the side holes as well as the opening at the tip; here, a flap valve mechanism can be established that allows exclusively injection of fluid and prevents aspiration of blood.

Therapy of CVC Thrombosis

Forceful flush: After an incomplete attempt to aspirate the locking solution, in the clinical setting of a dialysis room, therapy of a malfunctioning catheter starts with a powerful injection of saline. A 10-ml syringe is advantageously used. No more than two or three attempts are recommended. Once aspiration of blood is successful, dialysis treatment can be started as usual.

Intraluminal thrombolysis: For effective thrombolysis, urokinase can be used or tissue plasminogen activator. The agents can be instilled locally into the catheter or given systematically via infusion during the dialysis session or during the dialysis interval. The use of this kind of thrombolysis has become a widely accepted procedure around the world.

Mechanical therapy: It seems hazardous to treat intraluminal CVC thrombosis with manipulations using a guidewire, a Fogarty catheter or a brush. Otherwise, in case of an emergency, such procedures may be justified to provide life-saving dialysis therapy.

If these techniques are not successful or thrombosis occurs repeatedly, there is an indication for diagnostic angiography. In most cases, exchange of the catheter will be the best solution. A fibrin sheath can be stripped by use of a snare catheter introduced into the femoral vein resulting in an asymptomatic embolization of the fibrin sheath [52]. Due to limited duration of patency ranging from 20 to 90 days with the need of repeated time-consuming and expensive procedures, this technique cannot be recommended.

Prevention of Thrombosis

Beathard [49] recommends the use of a thrombosis prevention protocol similar to the infection prevention protocol. Proper flushing and heparinization techniques are mandatory carefully respecting the filling volumes. Unfortunately, there are no reliable data available on the systemic anticoagulation to prevent CVC thrombosis. Furthermore, potential adverse effects may play a role in deciding whether to use these agents in many patients with CVC.

Subcutaneous Ports

As an initially welcomed alternative to 'permanent' CVC two types of subcutaneously implantable port systems became available several years ago, the LifeSite® Hemodialysis Access System (Vasca, Inc., Tewksbury, Mass., USA) and the Dialock Hemodialysis System (Biolink Corp., Norwell, Mass., USA). Theoretically, they were considered to reduce the risk of infection inherent in tunneled CVC due to their subcutaneous position, the skin barrier thus remaining intact and undergoing cannulation comparable to AVF and AVG.

Initially encouraging results were published [53, 54]. The LifeSite Hemodialysis Access System is currently the only device that is commercially available for hemodialysis patients in the United States. In Germany and France, for example, initial enthusiasm disappeared in face of an increasing infection rate and problems with reimbursement.

A recently published study by Schwab et al. [55] revealed the superiority of the LifeSite Hemodialysis Access System compared to Tesio catheters with regard to blood flow and infection rates as long as 70% isopropyl alcohol was used as the antimicrobial agent for the LifeSite valve. No differences in infection rates were observed when oxychlorosene was used as the antimicrobial locking solution.

In summary, the results that are available at present are still preliminary in nature. The absolute number of implantations is limited, and too small to allow any comparison. A final conclusion is not justified. Nevertheless, future developments for both devices should include a reduction in their size and a decrease in the rate of infection based on improvements in design and methods in use [56].

Closing Remarks

The best treatment of complications is prevention. Care for VA for hemodialysis therapy is enhanced by respecting a few recommendations: careful preoperative diagnosis, preferably using ultrasonographic techniques; timely creation of VA during the predialysis period; meticulous, creative surgical technique; continuous monitoring and surveillance of VA by dialysis staff and nephrologists; early diagnosis of access dysfunction aiming at elective repair of the failing, not the failed access; absolute priority to native AVF; restricted use of grafts, untunneled/tunneled catheters and other devices; there should be no competition between surgical and interventional techniques but they should be used according to local expertise and dedication; reduction of infectious and thrombotic complications by proper implantation techniques and adequate staff training; documentation of strategies and analysis of complications and results aim at quality control and quality improvement; and care for VA is best provided by a multidisciplinary team, ideally directed by a VA coordinator.

References

1   Beathard GA: Improving dialysis vascular access. Dial Transplant 2002;31:210–219.
2   Konner K, Nonnast-Daniel B, Ritz E: The arteriovenous fistula. J Am Soc Nephrol 2003;14: 1669–1680.
3   Corpataux J-M, Haesler E, Silacci P, Ris HB, Hayoz D: Low-pressure environment and remodelling of the forearm vein in Brescia-Cimino haemodialysis access. Nephrol Dial Transplant 2002;17:1057–1062.
4   Krönung G: Plastic deformation of Cimino fistula by repeated puncture. Dial Transplant 1984;13:635–638.
5   Guerra A, Raynaud A, Beyssen B, Pagny JY, Sapocal M, Angel C: Arterial percutaneous angioplasty in upper limbs with vascular access devices for haemodialysis. Nephrol Dial Transplant 2002;17:843–851.
6   Sands JJ, Miranda CL: Prolongation of hemodialysis access survival with elective revision. Clin Nephrol 1995;44:329–333.

7   Turmel-Rodrigues L, Pengloan J, Baudin S, Testou D, Abaza M, Dahdah G, Mouton A, Blanchard D: Treatment of stenosis and thrombosis in haemodialysis fistulas and grafts by interventional radiology. Nephrol Dial Transplant 2000;15:2029–2036.

8   Konner K: The anastomosis of the arteriovenous fistula – Common errors and their avoidance. Nephrol Dial Transplant 2002;17:376–379.

9   Morice MC, Serruys PW, Sousa E, Fajadet J, Hayashi EB, Perin M, Colombo A, Schuler G, Barragan P, Guagliumi G, Molnàr F, Falotico R: A randomized comparison of a sirolimus-eluting stent with a standard stent for coronary revascularization. N Engl J Med 2002;346: 1773–1780.

10   Turmel-Rodrigues L, Pengloan J, Rodrige H, Brillet G, Lataste A, Pierre D, Jourdan J-L, Blanchard D: Treatment of failed native arteriovenous fistulae for hemodialysis by interventional radiology. Kidney Int 2000;57:1124–1140.

11   Trerotola SO, Vesely TM, Lung GB, Soulen MC, Ehrman KO, Cardella JF: Treatment of thrombosed hemodialysis access grafts: Arrow-Trerotola percutaneous thrombolytic device versus pulse-spray thrombolysis. Radiology 1998;206:403–414.

12   Valji K, Bookstein JJ, Roberts AC, Oglevie SB, Pittman C, O'Neill MP: Pulse-spray pharmaco-mechanical thrombolysis of thrombosed hemodialysis access grafts: Long-term experience and comparison of original and current techniques. Am J Roentgenol 1995;164:1495–1500.

13   Beathard GA, Welch BR, Maidment HJ: Mechanical thrombolysis for the treatment of thrombosed hemodialysis access grafts. Radiology 1996;200:711–716.

14   Vorwerk D: Non-traumatic vascular emergencies: Management of occluded hemodialysis shunts and venous access. Eur Radiol 2002;12:2644–2650.

15   Turmel-Rodrigues L: Comments on Vorwerk: Non-traumatic vascular emergencies: Management of occluded hemodialysis shunts and venous access. Eur Radiol 2003;May 7.

16   Vorwerk D: Reply. Eur Radiol 2003;May 7.

17   Haage P, Vorwerk D, Wildberger JE, Piroth W, Schürmann K, Guenther RW: Percutaneous treatment of thrombosed primary arteriovenous hemodialysis access fistulae. Kidney Int 2000;57: 1169–1175.

18   Aruny JE, Lewis CA, Cardella JF, Cole PE, Davis A, Drooz AT, Grassi CJ, Gray RJ, Husted JW, Jones MT, et al: Quality improvement guidelines for percutaneous management of the thrombosed or dysfunctional dialysis access. Standards of Practice Committee of the Society of Cardiovascular & Interventional Radiology. J Vasc Interv Radiol 1999;10:491–498.

19   Dikow R, Schwenger V, Zeier M, Ritz E: Do AV fistulas contribute to cardiac mortality in hemodialysis patients? Semin Dial 2002;15:14–17.

20   Malovrh M: Native arteriovenous fistula: Preoperative evaluation. Am J Kidney Dis 2002;39: 1218–1225.

21   Beathard GA, Settle SM, Shields MW: Salvage of the nonfunctioning arteriovenous fistula. Am J Kidney Dis 1999;33:910–916.

22   Arnold WP: Improvement in hemodialysis vascular access outcomes in a dedicated access center. Semin Dial 2000;13:359–363.

23   Turmel-Rodrigues L, Pengloan J, Bourquelot P: Interventional radiology in hemodialysis fistulae and grafts: A multidisciplinary approach. Cardiovasc Intervent Radiol 2002;25:3–16.

24   Anderson CB, Etheridge EE, Harter HR, Codd JE, Graff RJ, Newton WT: Blood flow measurements in arteriovenous fistulas. Surgery 1977;81:459–461.

25   Sivanesan S, How TV, Bakran A: Characterizing flow distributions in AV fistulae for haemodialysis access. Nephrol Dial Transplant 1998;13:3108–3110.

26   Levine MP: The hemodialysis patient and hand amputation. Am J Nephrol 2001;21:498–501.

27   Knox RC, Berman SS, Hughes JD, Gentile AT, Mills JL: Distal revascularization-interval ligation: A durable and effective treatment for ischemic steal syndrome after hemodialysis access. J Vasc Surg 2002;36:250–256.

28   Konner K, Hulbert-Shearon TE, Roys EC, Port FK: Tailoring the initial vascular access for dialysis patients. Kidney Int 2002;62:329–338.

29   Riggs JE, Moss AH, Labosky DA, Liput JH, Morgan JJ, Gutmann L: Upper extremity ischemic monomelic neuropathy: A complication of vascular access procedures in uremic diabetic patients. Neurology 1989;39:997–998.

30   Miles AM: Vascular steal syndrome and ischaemic monomelic neuropathy: Two variants of upper limb ischaemia after haemodialysis access surgery. Nephrol Dial Transplant 1999;14:297–300.

31   Konner K: Primary vascular access in diabetic patients: An audit. Nephrol Dial Transplant 2000; 15:1317–1325.

32   London GA: Cardiovascular disease in chronic renal failure: Pathophysiologic aspects. Semin Dial 2003;16:85–94.

33   Foley RN: Clinical epidemiology of cardiac disease in dialysis patients: Left ventricular hypertrophy, ischemic heart disease, and cardiac failure. Semin Dial 2003;16:111–117.

34   London GM, Marchais SJ, Guerin AP, Fabiani F, Metivier F: Cardiovascular function in hemo-dialysis patients; in Grünfeld JP, Bach JF, Funck-Brentano JL, Maxwell MH (eds): Advances in Nephrology. St Louis, Mosby-Year Book, 1991, vol 20, pp 249–273.

35   Bourquelot P: High flow – Surgical treatment. Blood Purif 2001;19:130–131.

36   Minga TE, Flanagan KH, Allon M: Clinical consequences of infected arteriovenous grafts in hemodialysis patients. Am J Kidney Dis 2001;38:975–978.

37   Dhingra RK, Young EW, Hulbert-Shearon TE, Leavey SF, Port FK: Type of vascular access and mortality in U.S. hemodialysis patients. Kidney Int 2001;60:1443–1451.

38   Nassar GM, Ayus JC: Clotted arteriovenous grafts: A silent source of infection. Semin Dial 2000; 13:1–3.

39   Nassar GM, Fishbane S, Ayus JC: Occult infection of old nonfunctioning arteriovenous grafts: A novel cause of erythropoietin resistance and chronic inflammation in hemodialysis patients. Kidney Int 2002;61(suppl 80):S49–S54.

40   Combe C, Pisoni RL, Port FK, Young EW, Canaud B, Mapes DL, Held PJ: Dialysis outcomes and practice pattern study: Data on the use of central venous catheters in chronic hemodialysis (in French). Néphrologie 2001;22:379–384.

41   Mickley V: Central venous catheters: Many questions, few answers. Nephrol Dial Transplant 2002;17:1368–1373.

42   Pisoni RL, Young EW, Dykstra DM, Greenwood RN, Hecking E, Gillespie B, Wolfe RA, Goodkin DA, Held PJ: Vascular access use in Europe and the United States: Results from the DOPPS. Kidney Int 2002;61:305–316.

43   Schillinger F, Schillinger D, Montagnac R, Milcent T: Postcatheterization vein stenosis in haemodialysis: Comparative angiographic study of 50 subclavian and 50 internal jugular accesses. Nephrol Dial Transplant 1991;6:722–724.

44   Farrell J, Gellens M: Ultrasound-guided cannulation versus landmark-guided technique for acute haemodialysis access. Nephrol Dial Transplant 1997;12:1234–1237.

45   Galli F, Efficace E, Villa G, Salvadeo A, Criffo A, Paroni G, Serafini G: Endocavitary electrocar-diography (EC-ECG) in monitoring central venous cannulation for vascular access in haemodial-ysis. Nephrol Dial Transplant 1993;8:480–481.

46   Work J: Chronic catheter placement. Semin Dial 2001;14:436–440.

47   Mandolfo S, Piazza W, Galli F: Central venous catheter and the hemodialysis patient: A difficult symbiosis. J Vasc Access 2002;3:64–73.

48   Beathard G: Management of bacteremia associated with tunneled-cuffed hemodialysis catheters. J Am Soc Nephrol 1999;10:1045–1049.

49   Beathard G: Catheter thrombosis. Semin Dial 2001;14:441–445.

50   Agrharkar M, Isaacson S, Mendelssohn D, Muralidharan J, Mustafa S, Zevallos G, Besely M, Uldall R: Percutaneously inserted silastic jugular hemodialysis catheters seldom cause jugular vein thrombosis. ASAIO J 1995;41:169–172.

51   Karnik R, Valentin A, Winkler WB, Donath P, Slany J: Duplex sonographic detection of internal jugular venous thrombosis after removal of central venous catheters. Clin Cardiol 1993; 16:26–29.

52   Brady PS, Spence LD, Levitin A, Mickolich CT, Dolmatch BL: Efficacy of percutaneous fibrin sheath stripping in restoring patency of tunneled hemodialysis catheters. Am J Roengenol 1999;173:1023–1027.

53   Levin NW, Yang PM, Hatch DA, Dubrow AJ, et al: Initial results of a new access device for hemodialysis. Kidney Int 1998;54:1739–1745.

54   Beathard GA, Posen GA: Initial clinical results with the LifeSite® hemodialysis access system. Kidney Int 2000;58:2221–2227.
55   Schwab SJ, Weiss MA, Rushton F, Ross JP, Jackson J, Kapoian T, et al: Multicenter clinical trial results with the LifeSite® hemodialysis access system. Kidney Int 2002;62:1026–1033.
56   Moran JE: Subcutaneous vascular access devices. Semin Dial 2001;14:452–457.

Klaus Konner, MD,
Medical Faculty University of Cologne,
Department of Internal Medicine I,
Cologne General Hospital Merheim Medical Center
Ostmerheimerstrasse 200, D–51109 Cologne (Germany)
Tel. +49 221 89070, Fax +49 221 899 11 44,
E-Mail klaus.konner@uni-koeln.de, klaus.konner@kfh-dialyse.de

Ronco C, Levin NW (eds): Hemodialysis Vascular Access and Peritoneal Dialysis Access.
Contrib Nephrol. Basel, Karger, 2004, vol 142, pp 216–227

....

Monitoring Techniques of Vascular Access

Jonathan H. Segal, William F. Weitzel

Department of Internal Medicine, University of Michigan Health System,
Ann Arbor, Mich., USA

The National Kidney Foundation guidelines, as well as many researchers and clinicians, have advocated access surveillance as a means to improve patient care and reduce access-related costs. The rationale for surveillance is grounded in what has been termed the 'dysfunction hypothesis' and states that stenosis causes graft dysfunction and this dysfunction reliably precedes and accurately predicts thrombosis [1]. Therefore, if a particular surveillance technique is to be successful at predicting access thrombosis, several assumptions of this dysfunction hypothesis must be true. Specifically, the measurements must be reproducible, stenosis should progress slowly enough so that there is time to intervene before thrombosis, and other factors outside of stenosis, such as hypercoagulability, should not abrogate or appreciably confound the surveillance technique's prediction of thrombosis. An ideal access monitoring test would predict nearly all patients who will thrombose (i.e. be highly sensitive), without falsely predicting thrombosis in those who do not have access dysfunction (i.e. be highly specific).

Most monitoring techniques that have been developed rely on detecting the hemodynamic dysfunction that results from an access stenosis, rather than detecting the stenosis itself. Unfortunately, there are few randomized controlled trials from which to draw conclusions about the benefit of surveillance with subsequent intervention to prevent thrombosis, and there are no randomized controlled trials to date that compare a control group receiving no monitoring with an intervention group that receives a particular method of surveillance. Nevertheless, several hemodynamically based techniques have been developed that may allow thrombosis risk assessment and therefore may have utility in access surveillance.

Venous Pressure Measurements

Using pressure measurements as a method for detecting access dysfunction was first described in a study that correlated venous drip chamber pressures with findings at venography [2]. This protocol involved the measurement of the venous dialysis pressure during the first 30 min of dialysis with a blood flow rate of 200 ml/min through 16-gauge needles. Patients with elevated venous dialysis pressures, defined as >150 mm Hg, who underwent venography and intervention had thrombosis rates that were similar to patients with normal venous pressures. Patients who had elevated venous pressures who did not undergo intervention had a 10-fold higher rate of thrombosis. Although this study has several limitations, such as the lack of a randomized control group, it was the first report that a surveillance technique might be able to reduce vascular access morbidity and stimulated the nephrology community to further investigate the utility of access surveillance in guiding intervention.

Some of the drawbacks to dynamic venous pressure monitoring include labile measurements from needle placement difficulties, different size needles, or variable systemic blood pressures. To avoid these problems, Besarab et al. [3] evaluated the predictive accuracy of static venous pressure measurements, that is pressure measurements at a blood flow rate of 0 ml/min. This method involved a stopcock-transducer system that was inserted between the venous return needle and dialyzer venous return bloodline. When the venous pressure at zero blood flow (VP_0) was expressed as a ratio with the systemic systolic blood pressure, values greater than 0.4 were found to have positive and negative predictive values of 92 and 84%, respectively, in detecting a 50% stenosis in AV grafts. Using this criterion for referral for intervention, a 70% decrease in thrombosis rate was obtained. This method was then simplified by eliminating the stopcock-transducer system, but required measuring the height difference between the vascular access and the venous drip chamber [4]. A strong correlation was found between the pressure measured from the venous drip chamber and the pressure measured directly from the access. In addition, when the VP_0 was expressed as a ratio with the mean arterial blood pressure, and a ratio of >0.5 was used as the threshold for intervention, the sensitivity was 86% with a specificity of 92% for detecting a 50% stenosis.

While these results are encouraging, static venous pressure measurements have not been replicated with the same degree of success. Other investigators have evaluated the value of static venous pressure monitoring in determining the predictive accuracy of AV graft thrombosis as opposed to stenosis. A static venous pressure ratio of >0.4 was found to have a sensitivity of only 73% and a specificity of 47% for thrombosis at 1 month [5]. Even with up to 4 months of follow-up, and evaluating an increase in static venous pressure ratio over

Table 1. Relative risk of access thrombosis with venous pressure monitoring

	Blood flow ml/min	Threshold	Relative risk
Static	0	VP/MAP > 0.5	10.3[a]
Low flow	50	VP/MAP > 0.6	20.0
Traditional	200	>150 mm Hg	10
High flow	400	>230 mm Hg	1.28[b]

VP = Venous pressure; MAP = mean arterial pressure.
[a]Relative risk is for detecting a stenosis >50%.
[b]Relative risk is for each 10 mm Hg increase in pressure above 230.

time, optimal test characteristics were not found. These results suggest that the decrease in thrombosis rate that has been reported with elective repair of stenosis comes at the cost of performing procedures in some patients who may derive no benefit.

Measuring venous pressure at slow blood flow rate may combine the ease of measurement of dynamic venous pressure monitoring while avoiding the difficulties related to needle size and positioning. A prospective, observational study evaluated the predictive value of measuring the venous pressure at a Qb of 50 ml/min, expressed as a ratio with the mean arterial blood pressure, in determining the risk of thrombosis [6]. Ratios greater than 0.6 were found to be predictive of thrombosis, with a sensitivity of 88%, specificity of 97%, positive predictive value of 90%, and a negative predictive value of 96%. Additional studies are required in different patient populations to confirm this degree of predictive power.

Other investigators hypothesized that measuring venous pressures at a higher blood flow rate might prove to be a more sensitive indicator of outflow stenosis [7]. A venous pressure over 230 mm Hg at a blood flow rate of 400 ml/min was the most efficient criteria for predicting thrombosis. There was substantial variability noted in venous pressures over time, but this variability was less when pressures were monitored at higher, as compared to lower, blood flows. The risk of access thrombosis as it relates to different venous pressure monitoring techniques is presented in table 1.

Measuring venous pressures as a surveillance method is attractive because it does not require expensive equipment or a significant amount of time from the dialysis unit nursing staff. Thus, it has the potential to be one of the most cost-effective methods for access surveillance. However, measuring venous pressures in autologous AV fistulae is less predictive of thrombosis and access failure when compared to measurements made in prosthetic AV grafts. This difference stems from the inherently lower resistance and pressure within the native vein fistula as well as the development of collateral veins that drain an AV fistulae with a stenosis and prevent an increase in venous pressure [8]. Furthermore, in prosthetic grafts, venous pressure measurements only reflect the amount of resistance in the outflow tract, which typically increases in the presence of stenosis, and does not detect arterial inflow or midgraft stenosis. Thus, a stenosis at the arterial anastomosis will lower venous pressure measurements and will go undetected by this screening technique. Monitoring pressures from the arterial needle within the graft may help solve some of the detection problems related to inflow and midgraft stenoses. However, venous outflow resistance is only one component of vascular access blood flow and, not surprisingly, venous pressure measurements have not been shown to correlate with access blood flow [9]. Specifically, high venous pressure does not always correlate with low graft flow, and not all grafts with low flow have high venous pressures. Lastly, venous pressure measurements are dependant on needle size, tubing diameter, type of dialyzer and machine characteristics, so that these variables also need to be considered when evaluating venous pressure measurements.

Access Blood Flow

Duplex Ultrasound

Duplex ultrasound with Doppler color flow imaging has been used to evaluate both anatomic features of the vascular access as well as to measure access blood flow. Using this technique in patients with prosthetic grafts, stenosis of >50% or an access volume flow of <500 ml/min has been found to be correlated with thrombosis within 6 months [10]. While many investigators have found that low access blood flow as measured by Doppler imaging is correlated with the risk of thrombosis [11, 12], it does not appear that the degree of stenosis itself is as valuable a predictor. In a study where patients with a 50% stenosis detected on duplex ultrasound were randomized to either observation or angiography with intervention, no difference in patency rates at either 6 or 12 months was detected between groups [13]. Thus, using ultrasound to screen for stenosis, without simultaneous blood flow measurement, does not appear to be an effective method to prevent access thrombosis.

Although using Doppler ultrasound to measure access blood flow was initially considered the 'gold standard', there are several challenges with this methodology. First, a cross-sectional area measurement of the vessel is required, and small variations in this measurement can lead to a large change in volume flow calculations, since the area varies with the square of the radius.

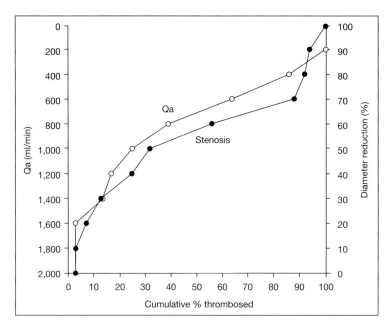

Fig. 1. Proportion of access thrombosis relative to both blood flow and stenosis [reprinted from 1].

Second, accurate knowledge of the Doppler signal beam angle is required to calculate the velocity in duplex volume flow determinations and is a potential source of error. Lastly, it is not practical to obtain measurements in the dialysis unit while the patients are receiving their treatment. As a result, duplex ultrasound has proven to be of greater value in assessing patients with suspected graft dysfunction, as opposed to routine screening for dysfunction.

Indicator Dilution Methods

Ultrasound dilution is the most commonly used method for determining access blood flow. This technique relies on the change in ultrasound velocity when blood is diluted with a bolus of normal saline at a known dialyzer blood flow rate (Qb). To measure the access blood flow (Qa), an ultrasound sensor is placed on the arterial and venous bloodline, after the lines have been reversed. With a Qb of 300 ml/min, and no ultrafiltration, a bolus of saline is given in the venous line. The change in velocity of blood through the tubing is detected by the sensors and the fraction of recirculated blood (R) entering the arterial line is measured. Qa can then be calculated by the relationship:

$$Qa = Qb(1 - R)/R$$

This technique, originally described by Depner and Krivitski [14], correlates well with Qa measurements done by Doppler ultrasound, as well as magnetic resonance angiography [15].

Several studies have demonstrated that low blood flow, as measured by ultrasound dilution, correlates with an increased risk of graft thrombosis. In one of the largest prospective studies of ultrasound dilution, with 172 prosthetic grafts [16], an access blood flow of <650 ml/min was associated with a relative risk of thrombosis of 1.67 within 12 weeks. When flow was <300 ml/min, the risk increased to 2.39. Interestingly, in this study dynamic venous pressure monitoring was not found to correlate with access thrombosis, although static venous pressure monitoring did. Similar results were reported in two smaller prospective studies with prosthetic grafts where the relative risk of thrombosis was between 3.1 and 7.2 for access blood flows of <500–600 ml/min [17, 18]. The relationship between low access blood flow, stenosis, and thrombosis is depicted in figure 1.

However, not all studies have found that low blood flow is associated with increased graft thrombosis. In a prospective cohort study by Paulson et al. [19], no difference in access blood flow was found between patients who had an access thrombosis when compared to those that did not. Furthermore, in a meta-analysis that combined data from 10 studies evaluating graft outcome, a single measurement of Qa was found to be a poor predictor of thrombosis. For example, to achieve a sensitivity of 80% in predicting thrombosis, the false-positive rate would be 58%, because many grafts with low flow continue to function. There was significant heterogeneity between studies, which could not be accounted for by chance alone, so that the benefit of a low Qa in predicting graft failure in some studies was negated by the lack of an association in others.

As vascular stenosis progresses, access blood flow will progressively decrease and, if detected, should predict impending thrombosis. One of the first studies [20] to examine this hypothesis was a prospective cohort study of 95 vascular accesses that had three consecutive access blood flow measurements that were 6 months apart over an 18-month period. The accesses that thrombosed had approximately a 20% decrease in flow in the first 6 months, and a 40% decrease in flow in the subsequent 6-month period. When accesses with no decrease in flow were considered as a reference range, there was an exponential increase in the risk of thrombosis for each blood flow decrement, so that a 25% decrease in flow was associated with a 7-fold increase in the risk of thrombosis at 12 weeks of follow-up, while a 50% decrease in flow had a 35-fold increase in risk (fig. 2).

However, when other investigators studied serial measurements performed more frequently (i.e. 1-month intervals), a change in access blood flow was not

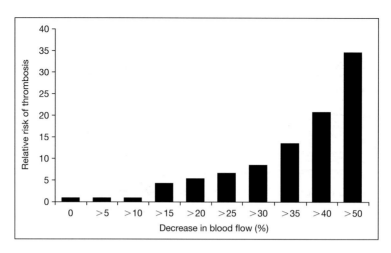

Fig. 2. Relative risk of thrombosis within 12 weeks by changes in access blood flow at 6-month intervals measured by ultrasound dilution [reprinted from 20].

found to be more predictive of thrombosis than a single low Qa measurement [21]. Even when the access blood flow was adjusted for the mean arterial pressure, the predictive accuracy was not improved. Thus, setting a threshold for serial access blood flow measurements to give a sensitivity of 80% would be at the cost of a false-positive rate of 30%. While this degree of combined sensitivity and specificity may be a helpful adjunct in deciding who should be referred for intervention, it is clear that factors in addition to flow play a role in thrombosis risk. It is not entirely clear whether the decrease in access blood flow that precedes thrombosis is too rapid to be detected by monthly screening, whether variable hemodynamics during dialysis impairs predictive accuracy, or if other patient- or operator-dependent factors influence thrombosis risk.

Other Methods of Determining Access Blood Flow

Hematocrit dilution is a technique that relies on the continuous monitoring of hematocrit that is possible with the use of an optical sensor. Dilution of the hematocrit with a saline bolus is used as an indicator to calculate access blood flow with a commercially available product, the Crit-Line III monitor (HemaMetrics, Kaysville, Utah, USA). This device requires a small blood chamber to be inserted between the arterial line and the dialyzer, and an optical sensor is applied to this chamber. Although the initial comparison with the Transonic ultrasound dilution technique [22] showed that the Crit-Line monitor overestimated access blood flow, subsequent models have improved accuracy. Despite improvements in this device, the technique relies on the dialysis machine Qb, which may be inaccurate, and can lead to errors in the calculation of access blood flow. Also, like other indicator dilution techniques, the Crit-Line III requires temporary reversal of the bloodlines during dialysis.

To overcome the reliance on the dialysis machine Qb, an alternative technique using the Crit-Line monitor has been described that uses abrupt changes in ultrafiltration rate [23]. Changes in the arterial hematocrit are measured, after a change in the ultrafiltration rate, with the dialysis lines in the normal and reversed positions. The advantage to this technique is that it does not require an assessment of the dialyzer blood flow rate, although it is time consuming to perform. This methodology has also been compared to the ultrasound dilution technique and found to have good correlation.

A transcutaneous device (TQA Sensor Pad; HemaMetrics) that uses hematocrit dilution has also been reported as a method for determining access blood flow [24]. An optical sensor with a light-emitting diode and a complementary photodetector is placed over the vascular access downstream from the venous needle. A 20-ml bolus of saline is injected into the venous line, reducing the hematocrit beneath the sensor, and the access flow rate is determined using indicator dilution principles. This device correlates well with ultrasound dilution, does not require reversal of the dialysis bloodlines, and is independent of the dialyzer blood flow rate. In addition, access flow measurements can be done independently of dialysis. However, care must be taken to inject a given amount of saline over a specified time interval, and careful placement of the sensor over the access is required.

Other methods have been developed that are based on indicator dilution principles with dialysis line reversal to calculate access blood flow. One method uses magnetic principles to measure differential conductivity so that access recirculation can be calculated. The device (Hemodynamic Monitor; Gambro Healthcare, Lakewood, Colo., USA) uses a noninvasive sensor that is clamped around the arterial and venous bloodlines. The sensor contains two magnetic cores: an excitation core that induces a magnetic field across the blood tubing and a sense core that detects the inductive reactance of blood within the tubing set. Access recirculation is measured by injecting a 1-ml bolus of hypertonic saline into the venous bloodline, causing a positive change in the differential conductivity of the venous bloodline with respect to the arterial bloodline. Using the dialyzer blood flow rate, access blood flow can then be calculated [25]. Measurement of Qa by this method correlates well with measurements by ultrasound dilution [22], but again is dependent on the accuracy of Qb from the dialyzer and requires temporary reversal of the dialysis bloodlines.

Dialysance conductivity makes ingenious use of changes in the dialysate conductivity with the bloodlines reversed to calculate dialysis access flow [26].

This technology has been incorporated into the dialysis machine itself (Fresenius Medical Care, Lexington, Mass., USA) to simplify the procedure. Thermodilution, a technique also incorporated into the Fresenius dialysis machine as the Blood Temperature Monitor, relies on a bolus of blood cooled to 35°C by reducing the temperature of the dialysate. Recirculation of the cooled blood into the arterial line is detected by a thermal sensor and, with Qb from the dialysis machine, access flow is calculated. Although cardiopulmonary recirculation of the cooled bolus of blood is also measured with this technique, access flow measured by the blood temperature monitor is consistent with the ultrasound dilution technique [27].

An additional surveillance method that does not rely on indicator dilution techniques has been described using Doppler ultrasound. It has been recognized that the dialysis pump induces a change in blood flow between the arterial and venous needles causing a change in the corresponding Doppler signal between the needles. The variable flow (VF) Doppler measurement uses this dialysis pump-induced change in signal to determine the dialysis access blood flow without duplex imaging and without line reversal [28]. Unlike duplex imaging, which requires accurate knowledge of the Doppler signal beam angle, the VF Doppler method uses any Doppler signal proportional to the volume flow and thereby corrects itself for Doppler beam angle variance, making the measurement insensitive to this source of error. Also, the Doppler signal used to calculate volume flow by this method changes more dramatically with variable pump speeds when an access has low volume flow, making this method inherently most accurate in patients with lower access flow rates who are at greater risk of access thrombosis. This technique appears reproducible and yields comparable to ultrasound dilution and duplex measurements [29]. Furthermore, additional observations have been made about abnormal flow patterns using this method, specifically reversed flow during diastole, that may be specific indicators of access pathology [30]. While the technique can be performed using conventional directional Doppler devices, no commercial device dedicated to this measurement method is currently available.

Access Recirculation

Most of the indicator dilution techniques rely on inducing vascular access recirculation by transposing the arterial and venous bloodlines. When access recirculation occurs while the bloodlines are in their proper configuration, the blood pump has exceeded the access flow and significant access dysfunction is likely to exist. Access recirculation can be measured by the classic urea-based method, indicator dilution methods, or differential conductivity. The methodology and clinical implications are discussed in depth in subsequent chapters.

Conclusions

Even though vascular access monitoring appears to predict progression of access stenosis, and allow for timely intervention to prevent thrombosis, there are some patient populations where either access flow or venous pressure monitoring seems to lack sufficient accuracy to aid the access monitoring process. There may be many patient- and population-dependent variables that influence access thrombosis in addition to access blood flow. In addition, the duration of the follow-up period for any surveillance technique will have a profound influence on the predictive accuracy of monitoring. Thus, additional study is needed to determine how best to use access flow or access pressure monitoring in conjunction with other patient-dependent factors.

Since factors independent of flow or pressure may affect the risk of thrombosis, it is likely that different patient populations would require monitoring at different intervals in order to achieve desirable sensitivity and specificity. There may be some groups where access flow or pressure monitoring is not helpful. Most nephrologists have encountered patients who thrombose repeatedly despite correcting structural abnormalities and maintaining adequate access flow or pressure. At the other extreme, there are some patients with grafts who have not thrombosed in years and yet maintain a relatively low access flow or marginal pressure and may be at lower risk of thrombosis for reasons that are not yet clear. While monitoring may be helpful for this latter group to ensure they receive adequate dialysis, caution must be used to avoid unnecessary procedures for these patients. It is clear that hemodynamically based monitoring strategies do help stratify thrombosis risk and can help guide clinical decision making to plan interventions. It is also clear that a better understanding of non-hemodynamic-related risk factors for thrombosis is needed in order to use these hemodynamically based monitoring tools optimally.

References

1   Paulson WD: Blood flow surveillance of hemodialysis grafts and the dysfunction hypothesis. Semin Dial 2001;14:175–180.
2   Schwab SJ, Raymond JR, Saeed M, Newman GE, Dennis PA, Bollinger RR: Prevention of hemodialysis fistula thrombosis. Early detection of venous stenoses. Kidney Int 1989;36: 707–711.
3   Besarab A, Sullivan KL, Ross RP, Moritz MJ: Utility of intra-access pressure monitoring in detecting and correcting venous outlet stenosis prior to thrombosis. Kidney Int 1995;47:1364–1373.

4   Besarab A, Al-Saghir R, Alnabhan N, Lubkowski T, Frinak S: Simplified measurement of intra-access pressure. ASAIO J 1996;42:M682–M687.
5   Dember LM, Holmberg EF, Kaufman JS: Value of static venous pressure for predicting arteriovenous graft thrombosis. Kidney Int 2002;61:1899–1904.
6   Sirken GR, Shah C, Raja R: Slow-flow venous pressure for detection of arteriovenous graft malfunction. Kidney Int 2003;63:1894–1898.
7   Agarwal R, Davis JL: Monitoring interposition graft venous pressures at higher blood-flow rates improves sensitivity in predicting graft failure. Am J Kidney Dis 1999;34:212–217.
8   Bosman PJ, Boereboom FTJ, Eikelboom BC, Koomans HA, Blankestijn PJ: Graft flow as a predictor of thrombosis in hemodialysis grafts. Kidney Int 1998;54:1726–1730.
9   Bosman PJ, Boereboom FTJ, Smits HFM, Eikelboom BC, Koomans HA, Blankestijn PJ: Pressure of flow recordings for the surveillance of hemodialysis grafts. Kidney Int 1997;52: 1084–1088.
10 Strauch BS, O'Connell RS, Geoly KL, Grundlehner M, Yakub YN, Tietjen DP: Forecasting thrombosis of vascular access with Doppler color flow imaging. Am J Kidney Dis 1992;19: 554–557.
11 Sands JJ, Young S, Miranda C: The effect of Doppler flow screening studies and elective revisions on dialysis access failure. ASAIO J 1992;38:M524–M527.
12 Bay WH, Henry ML, Lazarus JM, Lew NL, Ling J, Lowrie EG: Predicting hemodialysis access failure with color flow Doppler ultrasound. Am J Nephrol 1998;18:296–304.
13 Lumsden AB, MacDonald MJ, Kikeri D, Cotsonis GA, Harker LA, Martin LG: Cost efficacy of duplex surveillance and prophylactic angioplasty of arteriovenous ePTFE grafts. Ann Vasc Surg 1998;12:138–142.
14 Depner TA, Krivitski NM: Clinical measurement of blood flow in hemodialysis access fistulae and grafts by ultrasound dilution. ASAIO J 1995;41:745–749.
15 Bosman PJ, Boereboom FTJ, Eikelboom BC, Bakker CJ, Mali WPT, Blankestijn PJ, Koomans HA: Access flow measurements in hemodialysis patients: In vivo validation of an ultrasound dilution technique. J Am Soc Nephrol 1996;7:966–969.
16 May RE, Himmelfarb J, Yenicesu M, et al: Predictive measures of vascular access thrombosis: A prospective study. Kidney Int 1997;52:1656–1662.
17 Wang E, Schneditz D, Nepomuceno C, Lavarias V, Martin K, Morris AT, Levin NW: Predictive value of access blood flow in detecting access thrombosis. ASAIO J 1998;44:M555–M558.
18 Bosman PJ, Boereboom FTJ, Eikelboom BC, Koomans HA, Blankestijn PJ: Graft flow as a predictor of thrombosis in hemodialysis grafts. Kidney Int 1998;54:1726–1730.
19 Paulson WD, Ram SJ, Birk CG, Work J: Does blood flow accurately predict thrombosis or failure of hemodialysis synthetic grafts? A meta-analysis. Am J Kidney Dis 1999;34:478–485.
20 Neyra NR, Ikizler TA, May RE, Himmelfarb J, Schulman G, Shyr Y, Hakim RM: Change in access blood flow over time predicts vascular access thrombosis. Kidney Int 1998;54:1714–1719.
21 Paulson WD, Ram SJ, Birk CG, Zapczynski M, Martin SR, Work J: Accuracy of decrease in blood flow in predicting hemodialysis graft thrombosis. Am J Kidney Dis 2000;35:1089–1095.
22 Lindsay RM, Bradfield E, Rothera C, et al: A comparison of methods for the measurement of hemodialysis access recirculation and access blood flow rate. ASAIO J 1998;44:62–67.
23 Yarar D, Cheung AK, Lindsay RM, et al: Ultrafiltration method for measuring vascular access flow rates during hemodialysis. Kidney Int 1999;56:1129–1135.
24 Steuer RR, Miller DR, Zhang S, Bell DA, Leypoldt JK: Noninvasive transcutaneous determination of access blood flow rate. Kidney Int 2001;60:284–291.
25 Lindsay RM, Blake PG, Malek P, Posen G, Martin B, Bradfield E: Hemodialysis access blood flow rates can be measured by a differential conductivity technique and are predictive of access clotting. Am J Kidney Dis 1997;30:475–482.
26 Gotch FA, Buyaki R, Panlilio F, Folden T: Measurement of blood access flow rate during hemodialysis from conductivity dialysance. ASAIO J 1999;45:139–146.
27 Schneditz D, Wang E, Levin NW: Validation of haemodialysis recirculation and access blood flow measured by thermodilution. Nephrol Dial Transplant 1999;14:376–383.
28 Weitzel WF, Rubin JM, Swartz RD, Woltmann DJ, Messana JM: Variable flow Doppler for hemodialysis access evaluation: Theory and clinical feasibility. ASAIO J 2000;46:65–69.

29 Weitzel WF, Rubin JM, Leavey SF, Swartz RD, Dhingra RK, Messana JM: Analysis of variable flow Doppler hemodialysis access flow measurements and comparison with ultrasound dilution. Am J Kidney Dis 2001;38:935–940.
30 Weitzel WF, Khosla N, Rubin JM: Retrograde hemodialysis access flow during dialysis as a predictor of access pathology. Am J Kidney Dis 2001;37:1241–1246.

William F. Weitzel, MD,
Division of Nephrology, University of Michigan Health System,
Simpson Building – Room 312, 101 Observatory Street,
Ann Arbor, MI 48109–0725 (USA)
Tel. +1 734 615 3994, Fax +1 734 615 4887, E-Mail weitzel@umich.edu

Ronco C, Levin NW (eds): Hemodialysis Vascular Access and Peritoneal Dialysis Access.
Contrib Nephrol. Basel, Karger, 2004, vol 142, pp 228–237

Hematocrit-Based Measurements of Vascular Access Flow Rate

David A. Bell, Songbiao Zhang

HemaMetrics, Kaysville, Utah, USA

Introduction

Existing methods for determining the vascular access flow rate (Q_a) are based on devices that measure physicochemical properties of blood, such as ultrasound velocity [1, 2], temperature [3], conductivity [4–6], glucose concentration [7] or hematocrit [8, 9]. The detection of changes in these properties downstream from an injection of saline (or other intervention) within the access allows the use of indicator dilution principles to determine Q_a. To perform such measurements entirely within the extracorporeal circuit, it is often necessary to reverse the bloodlines to permit easy injection of an indicator such as saline upstream of the measuring device.

The development of methods for measuring hematocrit in flowing blood [10] has led to the use of the Crit-Line device (HemaMetrics, Kaysville, Utah., USA) in various methods for assessing Q_a. In all such applications, measured values of Q_a are inversely proportional to the induced change in hematocrit relative to its absolute magnitude or $\Delta H/H$, that is

$$Q_a \propto \frac{1}{\Delta H/H} = \frac{H}{\Delta H}$$

Thus, the accuracy of these determinations of Q_a is intrinsically dependent on accurate resolution of small percent changes in hematocrit. Crit-Line technology is particularly well suited to such applications because of the accuracy with which small changes in hematocrit can be resolved in real time. We review below the application of methods for determining Q_a using hematocrit measurements during the ultrafiltration method and the newly developed transcutaneous (TQA) method.

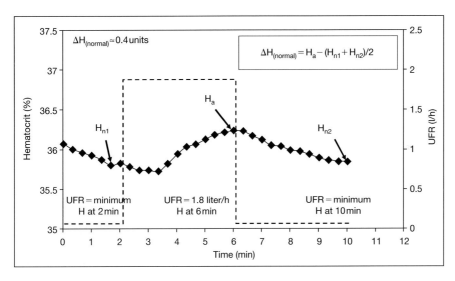

Fig. 1. Changes in the hematocrit ($\Delta H_{(normal)}$) induced by changing ultrafiltration with lines in the normal mode according to the UFR control sequence indicated by dashed lines.

Ultrafiltration Method

The majority of methods for determining Q_a within the extracorporeal hemodialysis circuit require the injection of saline with the bloodlines reversed. Several years ago, we developed an approach for determining Q_a without the need for saline injections [8]. When using this approach, termed either the ultrafiltration or Delta-H method, changes in arterial hematocrit are measured after abrupt changes in the ultrafiltration rate with the dialysis bloodlines in the normal and reversed configurations. Using this method, hematocrit in the extracorporeal circuit is acutely altered by rapidly removing plasma water rather than by intravenous injection of saline. As illustrated in figure 1, in the normal line configuration, the hematocrit changes as ultrafiltration is set to minimum for 2 min, stabilizing at H_{n1}. Ultrafiltration is then increased to 1.8 liter/h for 4 min and predictably the hematocrit increases to H_a. Ultrafiltration is reset to minimum and H_{n2} is determined at the 10th minute. $\Delta H_{(normal)}$ is then computed according to the indicated formula. Dialysis lines are reversed and a similar sequencing of the ultrafiltration produces a more pronounced change in $\Delta H_{(reversed)}$ as indicated in figure 2. The respective changes in hematocrit for both line modes are combined with maximum ultrafiltration rate (UFR) and the

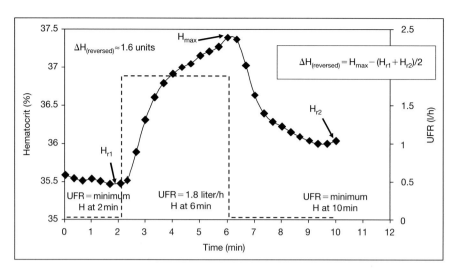

Fig. 2. Changes in the hematocrit ($\Delta H_{(reversed)}$) induced by changing ultrafiltration with lines in reversed mode according to the UFR control sequence indicated by dashed lines.

maximum hematocrit value observed in the reverse line mode ($H_{max(reversed)}$) to yield a precise intradialytic Q_a value:

$$Q_a = UFR \cdot \frac{H_{max(reversed)}}{\left(\Delta H_{(reversed)} - \Delta H_{(normal)}\right)}$$

This method was first tested in studies on 65 chronic hemodialysis patients from three separate dialysis programs in the United States as shown in figure 3 [8]. It was shown that the change in hematocrit with the bloodlines in the normal configuration was small (0.3 ± 0.2 H or hematocrit units, mean $\pm$ standard deviation) and was due to cardiopulmonary recirculation and blood volume depletion during the abrupt increase in the ultrafiltration rate. (Thus the effect of cardiopulmonary recirculation over the measurement time domain is accounted by the normal mode result, $\Delta H_{(normal)}$.) When the bloodlines were reversed to induce recirculation, however, the abrupt change in the hematocrit was 1.6 ± 1.0 H units. These changes in hematocrit are likely only detectable using an in-line monitor because the errors involved in blood sampling would likely overwhelm the accuracy of the measuring device. Using these measurements, Q_a was reported as $1,050 \pm 460$ ml/min, slightly higher than that determined using the reference method of ultrasound dilution of 950 ± 400 ml/min (HD01 Monitor, Transonic Systems, Ithaca, N.Y., USA). The measured bias was small ($16 \pm 25\%$), and there was a strong correlation between Q_a values

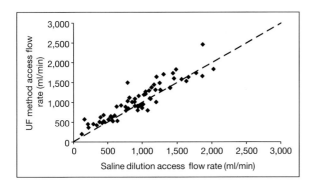

Fig. 3. Relationship between vascular access blood flow rate determined by the ultrafiltration (UF) method compared with those determined by saline dilution using an ultrasound flow sensor. The dashed line is the identity line. The best fit regression line (not shown) was Y = 0.96 ($\pm$0.05) X + 140 ($\pm$50); R = 0.92; N = 65.

measured using the ultrafiltration and ultrasound dilution methods. Furthermore, the averaged coefficient of variation from duplicate measurements of Q_a on the same patients using the ultrafiltration method was approximately 10% when assessed on either the same dialysis session or consecutive sessions.

There are both advantages and disadvantages of the ultrafiltration method over the ultrasound dilution method. In addition to a lack of a need for saline injections when using the ultrafiltration method, there is no need to accurately measure the dialyzer blood flow rate as required when using the ultrasound dilution method. When using the ultrafiltration method, the measurement accuracy of Q_a depends directly on the accuracy of the ultrafiltration rate that is precisely known during routine hemodialysis sessions using volume-controlled hemodialysis machines. The main disadvantage when using the ultrafiltration method is the time required (approximately 20 min) for performing the described measurements. Such requirements will be less important when devices for reversing the configuration of bloodlines can be performed automatically by the dialysis machine to permit this method to be fully automated. The accuracy of the ultrafiltration method has recently been validated in a pilot study by Besarab et al. [11]. In their study, Q_a values determined by the ultrafiltration method were 870 $\pm$ 672 ml/min, not significantly different from those determined using the ultrasound dilution method (HD02 Monitor, Transonic Systems) of 884 $\pm$ 606 ml/min. Moreover, the individual values were highly correlated (R = 0.95). Thus, Q_a values determined using the ultrafiltration method are equivalent to those determined using ultrasound dilution.

Two clinical trials have been performed to assess the usefulness of the ultrafiltration method for assessing vascular access function during routine hemodialysis. Roca-Tey et al. [12] determined Q_a in 50 hemodialysis patients using the ultrafiltration method. Ninety percent of these patients had a native arteriovenous fistula, whereas 10% had a synthetic graft. Mean Q_a was 1,147 ± 511 ml/min; mean (median) coefficient of variation for duplicate measurement was 4.9% (4.2%). All 11 patients whose Q_a was less than 700 ml/min showed arterial or venous arteriovenous fistula stenosis by angiography (≥80% in 10 patients and = 50% in the 11th). These workers recommended that Q_a less than 700 ml/min be used as a criterion for further investigation for vascular access stenosis during routine hemodialysis. More recently, Santos et al. [13] prospectively examined the use of Q_a determined using the ultrafiltration method and dynamic venous pressure measurements [14] for monitoring the function of arteriovenous synthetic (polytetrafluoroethylene) grafts. Seventy-one grafts in 69 hemodialysis patients were monitored monthly and angioplasty was triggered by either (1) a Q_a less than 600 ml/min, (2) decrease in Q_a of 25% during the past month with a Q_a value less than 1,000 ml/min or (3) dynamic venous pressure above 150 mm Hg confirmed in three consecutive dialysis treatments. During follow-up of 9 ± 3.4 months, this graft monitoring protocol identified 57 poorly functioning grafts, 41 of which were successfully angio-plastied with an increase in Q_a following the procedure. During this study, 23 thrombotic episodes occurred. Nine of these episodes were identified by the monitoring protocol, but the grafts clotted before the angioplasty could be performed. These trials indicate the clinical usefulness of routine monitoring of Q_a using the ultrafiltration method.

The recent clinical case history by Roca-Tey et al. [15] showed how routine vascular access monitoring using the ultrafiltration method can identify patients with excessively high Q_a. Left cardiac failure, secondary to volume overload, caused by excessive Q_a was significantly improved by banding the access site which reduced Q_a from 2,988 to 1,270 ml/min.

TQA Method

Virtually all existing devices for determining Q_a can only perform measurements within the extracorporeal circuit; thus, Q_a can only be determined using these devices during the hemodialysis procedure. The recent development of the TQA method for evaluating hematocrit in flowing blood within the access has opened new possibilities for Q_a measurements since these determinations can be made either within the extracorporeal circuit or directly at any time.

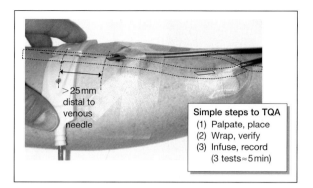

Simple steps to TQA
(1) Palpate, place
(2) Wrap, verify
(3) Infuse, record
   (3 tests ≈ 5 min)

>25 mm
distal to
venous
needle

Fig. 4. Placement of the TQA transdermal sensor distal to arteriovenous needle cannulation site on native fistula following palpation of the site and in preparation for wrapping and saline infusion. Sensor is positioned at least 25 mm distal to the tip of the nearest needle. Preferred infusion site for a 20-ml bolus delivered in approximately 4 s is the arterial needle.

Development of the TQA method for determining Q_a was made possible by the novel construction of a device which can measure relative changes in hematocrit in blood flowing underneath the skin [9]. The TQA method involves the use of a flexible sensor pad which is placed directly over the access distal (downstream) of a cannulated needle or needle set, depending on whether the measurement is to be taken intra- or predialysis. The sensor is positioned across the access following palpation of the site, and placement is guided by sensor-derived feedback on the TQA monitor. Figure 4 illustrates positioning of the TQA sensor on a lower arm native fistula.

The sensor technology for assessing TQA hematocrit is based on that developed for assessing hematocrit in blood flow within the extracorporeal of hemodialysis circuits (Crit-Line); however, it differs in several respects. First, the TQA optical sensor measures the absorbance and scattering of light due to the presence of hemoglobin and underlying tissues. The amount of light detected by the sensor is related to a parameter termed α which is reflective of the amount of blood flowing through the skin. Maximizing this parameter can therefore be used to detect blood flowing within the access site and can help to guide placement of the sensor directly over the access site. Second, in order to resolve the signal due to blood flowing within the access from that due to blood flowing within adjacent native vessels, it is necessary to normalize the signal. Thus, the sensor signal is proportional to changes in hematocrit in blood flowing through the access, and is obtained by comparing α values taken by sensor centerline elements positioned directly over the access site with α values

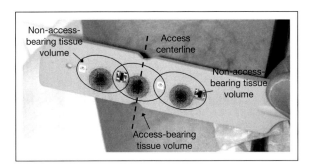

Fig. 5. Anterior side of the TQA sensor showing output regions for each of the three sensor emitter-detector combinations used to monitor the access (centerline combination) and the nonaccess tissue regions on either side of the access.

obtained in adjacent tissue regions not containing the access. (see Fig. 5). Third, it is important to note that the TQA optical sensor used in this application is only able to accurately assess relative changes in hematocrit, not the absolute hematocrit. The anterior side of the TQA transdermal sensor (placed firmly against the skin) is shown in figure 5 and describes the alignment of the emitter-detector combinations responsible for monitoring the access, as well as the non-access-bearing tissue on either side of the access. Note that the output of the TQA optical sensor is largely independent of skin melanin content or the depth of the access below the skin. The application of indicator dilution techniques for determining Q_a is different with the use of the TQA optical sensor than with the ultrafiltration method. First, it is not necessary to reverse the bloodlines when using TQA. This simplifies the procedure and allows it to be performed rapidly. Second, the accuracy of Q_a measurements with the TQA method is determined by the volume of the saline injection, not on its rate of injection as long as it occurs within a few seconds. Thus, care must be taken to accurately inject the required volume of saline during application.

The accuracy and precision of TQA was originally assessed from 72 measurements in 59 patients [9]. Q_a values determined by TQA were not different from those determined using ultrasound dilution (HD01 Monitor); the difference between the individual values (71 ± 62 ml/min) was not statistically significant. The precision of Q_a measurements using TQA (coefficient of variation of 10.5 ± 6.8%) was very similar to that when using the HD01 monitor (coefficient of variation of 8.9 ± 9.5%). In the original evaluation of the TQA method, measurements of Q_a were made primarily within the extracorporeal circuit [9]; however, the technology can be used without an intact extracorporeal circuit. Figures 6 and 7 plot Q_a values determined using the TQA method

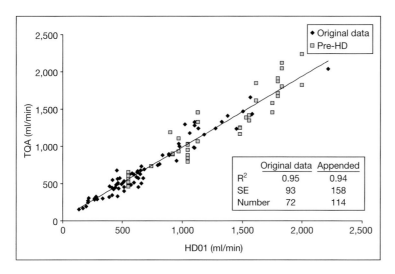

Fig. 6. Regression analysis comparison of vascular access blood flow rates determined using the TQA method with those determined using ultrasound dilution (HD01 Monitor, Transonic Systems). ◆ = Intradialytic data previously published [9]; ▫ = new data where the TQA method was exclusively measured predialysis.

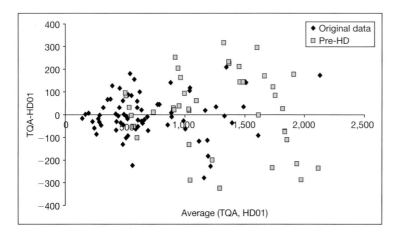

Fig. 7. Bland-Altman analysis of vascular access blood flow rates determined using the TQA method versus those determined using ultrasound dilution (HD01 Monitor, Transonic Systems) as described in figure 6. The Bland-Altman data format of the differences between reported values vs. the means of the reported data pairs (TQA and HD01) for the two systems demonstrates relatively little bias between the instruments.

during hemodialysis [9] and those determined before the patient was connected to the hemodialysis circuit versus those determined using ultrasound dilution technology. Excellent agreement was obtained using both procedures with Q_a values determined during hemodialysis using ultrasound dilution. These data demonstrate that Q_a can be accurately determined using the TQA method even when the patient is not undergoing a hemodialysis procedure.

Several investigators have reported clinical success when using the TQA method for determining Q_a. For example, von Albertini et al. [16] determined Q_a values by TQA either before or after hemodialysis. Q_a values were $1,411 \pm 431$ ml/min in 16 patients with native arteriovenous fistulas and $1,199 \pm 607$ ml/min in 7 patients with synthetic grafts. The precision of duplicate measurements of Q_a was excellent with a coefficient of variation of 8% [16]. Ronco et al. [17] have subsequently shown that Q_a values determined in 18 patients with native arteriovenous fistulas using TQA were not different when measured before or after the hemodialysis procedure (780 ± 312 vs. 919 ± 411 ml/min, respectively). Recent work by von Albertini et al. [18] showed that monthly changes in Q_a can be tracked using the TQA method similar to monthly changes in Q_a determined using ultrasound dilution. Finally, Besarab et al. [11] have recently shown in a pilot study of 5 patients that Q_a values determined using TQA were $16 \pm 47\%$ higher than those determined using either the ultrafiltration or ultrasound dilution methods. These data demonstrate that the TQA method for determining Q_a is more flexible than ultrasound dilution technology, yet comparable results are obtained with both technologies.

References

1   Krivitski NM: Theory and validation of access flow measurement by dilution technique during hemodialysis. Kidney Int 1995;48:244–250.
2   Krivitski NM: Novel method to measure access flow during hemodialysis by ultrasound velocity dilution technique. ASAIO J 1995;41:M741–M745.
3   Schneditz D, Fan Z, Kaufman A, Levin NW: Measurement of access flow during hemodialysis using the constant infusion approach. ASAIO J 1998;44:74–81.
4   Lindsay RM, Blake PG, Malek P, Posen G, Martin B, Bradfield E: Hemodialysis access blood flow rates can be measured by a differential conductivity technique and are predictive of access clotting. Am J Kidney Dis 1997;30:475–482.
5   Mercadal L, Hamani A, Béné B, Petitclerc T: Determination of access blood flow from ionic dialysance: Theory and validation. Kidney Int 1999;56:1560–1565.
6   Gotch FA, Buyaki R, Panlilio F, Folden T: Measurement of blood access flow rate during hemodialysis from conductivity dialysance. ASAIO J 1999;45:139–146.
7   Magnasco A, Alloatti S, Martinoli C, Solari P: Glucose pump test: A new method for blood flow measurements. Nephrol Dial Transplant 2002;17:2244–2248.
8   Yarar D, Cheung AK, Sakiewicz P, Lindsay RM, Paganini EP, Steuer RR, Leypoldt JK: Ultrafiltration method for measuring vascular access flow rates during hemodialysis. Kidney Int 1999;56:1129–1135.

9   Steuer RR, Miller DR, Zhang S, Bell DA, Leypoldt JK: Noninvasive transcutaneous determination of access blood flow rate. Kidney Int 2001;60:284–291.

10 Steuer RR, Bell DA, Barrett LL: Optical measurement of hematocrit and other biological constituents in renal therapy. Adv Ren Replace Ther 1999;6:217–224.

11 Besarab A, Lubkowski T, Frinak S, Afolabi D: Comparison of transcutaneous vascular access blood flow measurements (TQA) and dilution techniques for measurement of access flow (abstract). 3rd Int VAS Congress, Lisbon, 2003.

12 Roca-Tey R, Samon R, Ibrik O, Viladoms J: Study of vascular access blood flow rate (Q_A) during hemodialysis (HD) in 64 patients by the ultrafiltration method (abstract). Nephrol Dial Tranplant 2001;16:A151.

13 Santos C, Oliveira C, Carvalho D, Ponce P: Prospective monitoring of intra-access blood flow with hematocrit dilution technique for venous stenosis detection (abstract). J Am Soc Nephrol 2002;13:235A.

14 Schwab SJ, Raymond JR, Saeed M, Newman GE, Dennis PM, Bollinger RR: Prevention of hemodialysis fistula stenosis. Early detection of venous stenosis. Kidney Int 1989;36:707–711.

15 Roca-Tey R, Olivé S, Samon R, Ibrik O, García-Madrid C, Viladoms J: Monitorización no invasiva de fístula arteriovenosa (FAVI) humeral con repercusión hemodinámica. Nefrología 2003;23: 73–75.

16 von Albertini B, Berger J, Pereira O, Bringolf M, Wauters J-P, Haynie M: Optical transdermal vascular access blood flow measurements in patients off hemodialysis (abstract). J Am Soc Nephrol 2001;12:306A.

17 Ronco C, Brendolan A, Crepaldi C, D'Intini V, Sergeyeva O, Levin NW: Noninvasive transcutaneous access flow measurement before and after hemodialysis: Impact of hematocrit and blood pressure. Blood Purif 2002;20:376–379.

18 von Albertini B, Berger J, Marchland C, Wauters J-P, Pereira O: Utility and limitations of access blood flow monitoring for vascular access failure (abstract). J Am Soc Nephrol 2002;13:236A.

David A. Bell, PhD,
HemaMetrics,
Kaysville, UT 84037 (USA)
Tel. +1 801 451 9000, Fax +1 801 451 9007, E-Mail dbell@hemametrics.com

Ronco C, Levin NW (eds): Hemodialysis Vascular Access and Peritoneal Dialysis Access.
Contrib Nephrol. Basel, Karger, 2004, vol 142, pp 238–253

....

Hemodynamics of the Hemodialysis Access: Implications for Clinical Management

William D. Paulson[a], Steven A. Jones[b]

[a]Interventional Nephrology Section, Division of Nephrology and Hypertension, Department of Medicine, Louisiana State University Health Sciences Center, Shreveport, La., and [b]Biomedical Engineering, Louisiana Tech University, Ruston, La., USA

Introduction

Optimum prevention and management of access complications require an understanding of access hemodynamics. The hemodialysis access is unique in that it creates a low resistance shunt between the arterial and venous circulations. Thus, it is unlike the arterial synthetic graft used in atherosclerotic vascular disease in which the arterioles continue to provide the main source of resistance and blood flow regulation. This chapter describes access hemodynamics for nephrologists, interventionists, surgeons, and others who are involved in the management and preservation of the hemodialysis access. It develops a hemodynamic model that provides insight into access complications and management. Definitions and units of measurement are listed in the Appendix.

Basic Fluid Mechanics

Energy is required to drive flow in the access vascular circuit [1–3]. The total fluid energy per unit volume equals potential energy plus kinetic energy. Potential energy per unit volume exists as pressure (P), which is the force (F) exerted by fluid against an area A (F/A). Pressure is produced by ejection of blood from the left ventricle, by the force of elastic vessels pressing against the blood, and by differences in blood height. Kinetic energy per unit volume is defined as $\rho v^2/2$ where ρ is blood density and v is blood velocity.

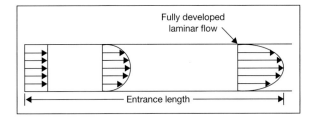

Fig. 1. Development of laminar flow in a tube. Length of arrows indicates velocity. Velocity of lamina immediately adjacent to tube wall is 0.

In the absence of friction, total fluid energy remains constant. This concept is known as Bernoulli's equation:

fluid energy/volume $= P + \rho v^2/2 =$ constant

For example, as blood enters a stenosis, velocity increases and pressure drops (ΔP), indicating energy has been converted from potential energy to kinetic energy. In reality, friction causes dissipation of energy as blood flows through the access circuit. Thus, the fluid energy in the inflow artery is greater than in the outflow vein. Energy loss within a circuit is conventionally approximated as the ΔP between entry and exit from the circuit.

It is important to characterize the type of flow in the access circuit. Laminar flow is organized motion in which fluid travels as a series of cylindrical laminae parallel to the wall of a tube. The lamina in contact with the wall is stationary, whereas each successive lamina slides against the friction of adjacent lamina. As fluid enters a perfectly cylindrical tube, these parallel laminae gradually develop a parabolic velocity profile in that the lamina closest to the wall remains motionless whereas the lamina in the center has the highest velocity (fig. 1). A minimum 'entrance length' is required for laminar flow to fully develop. Before this length is reached, the velocity profile is blunted. For most large arteries in the normal systemic circulation, the entrance length approaches the length of the artery, so that laminar flow is usually not fully developed. In these situations, laminar 'entry-flow' models are used to characterize flow [4].

The concepts of shear rate and shear stress are needed in order to define fluid friction in the access circuit [2, 3]. Shear rate is the change in flow velocity (Δv) per change in distance (Δx) perpendicular to the direction of flow:

shear rate $= \Delta v/\Delta x$

In figure 1, the shear rate near the wall is lowest for fully developed laminar flow because the difference in velocity of adjacent laminae is small in this parabolic profile. In contrast, the shear rate is extremely high at the tube entrance where the velocity abruptly increases from 0 at the wall to the velocity indicated by the blunt profile.

Shear stress is the force that is necessary to move a layer of fluid of area A across another layer of fluid (or vessel wall) of equal area:

shear stress = F/A

An increase in friction between fluid layers will increase the amount of force needed to move the fluid.

Viscosity connects the concepts of shear rate and shear stress, and is a measure of friction between contiguous layers of fluid [2, 3]. Dynamic viscosity (η) is defined as the ratio of shear stress to shear rate:

η = (shear stress)/(shear rate), or shear stress = η(shear rate)

Thus, if more force is required to move layers of fluid across each other at a given shear rate, then η is higher. Alternatively, for a given η, a higher shear rate indicates a higher shear stress is applied to overcome friction. This is the friction that causes dissipation of energy in the access circuit.

Poiseuille's law describes the ΔP caused by viscous losses in fully developed laminar (nonpulsatile) flow in a rigid tube with constant luminal radius (r) [2, 3]:

$$\Delta P = 8\eta LQ/\pi r^4$$

L is length along the tube and Q is flow.

Poiseuille's law provides an expression for estimating vascular resistance (R), which is defined as $\Delta P/Q$:

$$R = \Delta P/Q = 8\eta L/\pi r^4 = 128\eta L/\pi D^4$$

where D is luminal diameter. This equation shows that for a given ΔP, a smaller R will result in a larger Q. R increases linearly with η and L, but D has by far the largest influence since R is proportional to $1/D^4$. Thus, reductions in diameter can cause very large increases in R. Poiseuille's law is based on several assumptions that are generally not completely satisfied in the access circuit [2], so that it usually underestimates ΔP and R. Nevertheless, it is a valuable tool for illustrating hemodynamic principles.

Turbulent flow is characterized by random irregular motion rather than the organized motion of laminar flow. Sometimes flow is disturbed and has both laminar and turbulent characteristics. In models of turbulent or disturbed flow, ΔP is proportional to Q^2 and Q raised to other powers such as $Q^{7/4}$ [4]. This indicates that turbulent and disturbed flow cause a higher ΔP and R than predicted by Poiseuille's law. In these models, R is not constant but rather is a function of Q. Thus, an increase in Q causes an increase in R.

One of the most important predictors of whether flow is laminar or turbulent is the Reynolds number (Re) [2, 3]:

$$Re = 2\rho r v / \eta$$

In classical fluid mechanics, as Re increases above 2,000, laminar flow makes a transition to turbulent flow. Nevertheless, 2,000 is not a strict threshold. Turbulent flow may occur with Re as low as 1,000 and laminar flow may persist for Re above 3,000, depending on conditions.

Re can be rewritten in terms of Q rather than v. Note that $Q = vA = v\pi r^2$, in which A is vessel cross-sectional area. It follows that:

$$Re = 2\rho r Q / \pi r^2 \eta = 2\rho Q / \pi r \eta$$

when the variables are expressed in consistent units (ρ in g/cm³, Q in ml/s, r in cm, and η in g/cm·s). In clinical practice, Q is usually expressed in ml/min, which must be converted to ml/s by dividing by 60. Thus, when Q is in ml/min, the equation takes various forms:

$$Re = 2\rho Q / 60\pi r \eta = \rho Q / 30\pi r \eta = \rho Q / 15\pi D \eta$$

This equation illustrates that when fluid passes through smaller and larger vessels at the same Q, the smaller vessels have higher Re and thus are more prone to turbulence. Additional conditions that promote turbulence include wall irregularities, abrupt changes in tube dimensions, and disturbed flow upstream to the region of interest.

Consider the example of an access with $\rho = 1.056$ g/cm³, Q = 1,600 ml/min, D = 0.5 cm, and $\eta = 0.035$ poise [corresponding to hematocrit (Hct) = 33%]. It follows that Re = 2,049. Thus, Re is at the transition threshold, and flow may be laminar, turbulent, disturbed, or alternate between types of flow. Because resistance is higher in turbulent than laminar flow, these transitions contribute to variations in Q.

Stenoses may occur along the access circuit in a manner analogous to resistances in series in an electrical circuit [3]. Provided these stenoses are a minimum distance apart [5], the total vascular resistance equals the sum of the individual resistances:

$$R_{total} = R_1 + R_2 + R_3 + ... = \Sigma R_i$$

At the entrance to a stenosis, flow accelerates and pressure falls (recall the Bernoulli equation). The conversion of pressure (potential energy) into kinetic energy is efficient, so that there is minimal energy loss at the entrance to the stenosis. However, as blood exits the stenosis and decelerates, there is frictional energy loss because the conversion of kinetic energy back into pressure is less efficient [5].

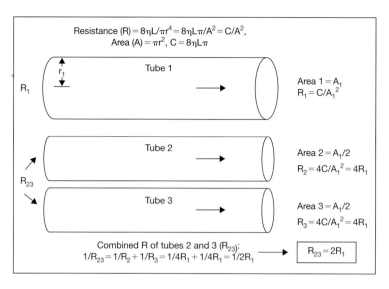

Fig. 2. Although luminal cross-sectional area of tube 1 (A_1) equals total cross-sectional area of tubes 2 and 3, resistance of tube 1 (R_1) is 1/2 combined resistance of tubes 2 and 3 (R_{23}). L is length along tube, r is radius, η is dynamic viscosity.

Because of this frictional loss, ΔP just downstream of the stenosis exit is greater than ΔP within the stenosis (where frictional loss is induced by wall shear stress). Thus, a single stenosis with length L has less resistance than two stenoses that both have length L/2 because the two stenoses contribute two larger exit ΔPs. This suggests that correcting two short stenoses may yield a better result than correcting a single longer stenosis.

Continuing the analogy with electrical circuits, resistances can also be in parallel [3]. A clinical example is outflow from an autogenous arteriovenous (AV) fistula that is carried in two veins rather than in a single vein. For parallel resistances, the total R is given by the equation:

$$1/R_{total} = 1/R_1 + 1/R_2 + 1/R_3 + \ldots = \Sigma(1/R_i)$$

Recall that from Poiseuille's law, $R = 8\eta L/\pi r^4$. It follows that if two tubes have a total luminal cross-sectional area equal to that of a single larger tube, then the total R of the two tubes is twice that of the single tube (fig. 2). Four of the smaller tubes would be needed to provide R as small as the larger tube. Thus, a fistula with two outflow veins has a higher R than a fistula with one outflow vein of an equal overall cross-sectional area. It follows that a single outflow vein may provide an adequate Q whereas two outflow veins may not.

Dilatation in Access Vascular Circuit

Creation of an access activates mechanisms that cause dilatation of the inflow artery and outflow vein. Q initially increases because the new circuit has a low resistance. This increase in Q causes a high shear stress on the endothelial surface. The shear stress can be estimated from Poiseuille's law [2]:

shear stress $= 4\eta Q/\pi r^3$

Because shear stress is proportional to $1/r^3$, small increases in diameter can offset the effect of an increase in Q.

Arteries adjust their diameters to maintain shear stress between 10 and 20 dyn/cm^2 [6, 7]. Although dilatation of the outflow vein has been attributed to increased pressure, it is possible that the vein also dilates in response to high shear stress [8]. This mechanism may explain why procedures that occlude accessory veins promote AV fistula maturation. Since these veins divert part of the outflow, occlusion increases Q through the small main outflow vein, thereby increasing shear stress. A larger diameter fistula is then produced when dilatation causes shear stress to return to normal.

The mechanism of acute dilatation is primarily endothelial release of nitric oxide, which relaxes smooth muscle [9]. Over a longer period, remodeling of the vascular wall changes its cellular and matrix composition [10, 11].

Model of Graft Vascular Circuit

The access circuit is a low resistance shunt between the arterial and venous circulations. The mean ΔP that drives flow in this shunt is the same as in the normal systemic circulation: mean arterial pressure (MAP) minus central venous pressure (CVP). Since $\Delta P = QR$, it follows that the large reduction in R must be matched by a large increase in Q. In addition, pressure must fall rapidly in the large arteries and veins of the access circuit so that CVP is reached by the time flow reaches the vena cava. This large ΔP contrasts with the normal systemic circulation in which up to 60% of ΔP is in the arterioles and 15% is in the capillaries, but only approximately 10% is in the arteries and 15% is in the veins [2].

Thus, the access vascular circuit has unique hemodynamic properties that must be taken into account when managing access problems. A model of the circuit can provide valuable insight into these properties. The engineering literature provides pressure-flow equations for hydrodynamic elements that are analogous to elements in the access circuit. We have applied these equations to a model of the synthetic graft vascular circuit in the upper extremity.

Table 1. Dimensions of segments in model of synthetic graft vascular circuit

Segment	Length cm	Luminal diameter, cm
Artery	40.0	0.5
Graft	30.0	0.5
Stenosis at venous anastomosis	1.0	0–0.5
Vein	40.0	0.7

The circuit can be modeled as a series of ΔPs. The total ΔP equals the sum of ΔPs from each segment:

$$\text{total } \Delta P = MAP - CVP = \Delta P_A + \Delta P_{AA} + \Delta P_G + \Delta P_{VA} + \Delta P_S + \Delta P_V$$

The subscripts indicate: A = artery, AA = arterial anastomosis, G = graft, VA = venous anastomosis, S = stenosis at venous anastomosis, V = vein. This model includes the stenosis that commonly occurs at the venous anastomosis. Given that flow is normally pulsatile, calculations of Q and pressure in the model should be considered time-averaged. The model ignores special circumstances, such as vessel elasticity, tapering or tortuous vessels, and variable diameters.

Dimensions of model segments and stenosis are shown in table 1. The luminal diameters are similar to values we have measured in our patients [12]. In the graft, the inflow artery usually has a smaller diameter than the outflow vein. In contrast, in the AV fistula, the two diameters are generally approximately equal. Thus, the fistula differs from the model in that the inflow and outflow resistances are approximately equal.

We modeled each segment with an appropriate ΔP equation (table 2). These equations are more complex than Poiseuille's law, and involve Q raised to various powers. Since R is defined as ΔP/Q, it is clear that resistance is not constant, but rather increases with Q. The inflow artery and graft have luminal diameters that may yield Reynolds numbers above and below the 2,000 transition (recall that Re is proportional to 1/D). Thus, we considered both laminar entry flow and fully developed turbulent flow in these segments [4]. In the outflow vein, we considered only laminar entry flow because the vein has a larger diameter that should yield a lower Re. The ΔPs of the two anastomoses were modeled with a T junction equation [13]. A T junction treats ΔP across the junction of two tubes, which is analogous to the anastomoses. Viscosity was adjusted for Hct [14].

Table 2. Equations used to model pressure drop (ΔP) at each segment of graft vascular circuit

---

Inflow artery and graft

    Shah's laminar entry-flow equation (for Reynolds No. <2,000) [4]

$$\Delta P_A = h_1 Q^{3/2} + (h_2 Q + h_3 Q^2 + h_4 Q^{3/2})/(1 + h_5 Q^2)$$

    Blasius's fully developed turbulence equation (for Reynolds No. >2,000) [4]

$$\Delta P_A = (0.0665 \rho^{3/4} L \eta^{1/4} / \pi^{7/4} r^{4.75}) Q^{7/4}$$

Arterial anastomosis: T junction equation [13]

$$\Delta P_{AA} = (8 \rho K_l / \pi^2 D_A^4) Q^2$$

Venous anastomosis: T junction equation [13]

$$\Delta P_{VA} = (8 \rho K_l / \pi^2 D_G^4) Q^2$$

Stenosis at venous anastomosis: Young's equation [5]

$$\Delta P_S = (8 K_t \rho / \pi^2 D^4)[(D_V/D_S)^2 - 1]^2 Q^2 + (4 K_V \eta / \pi D_V^3) Q$$

Outflow vein: Shah's laminar entry-flow equation [4]

$$\Delta P_A = h_1 Q^{3/2} + (h_2 Q + h_3 Q^2 + h_4 Q^{3/2})/(1 + h_5 Q^2)$$

D_A, D_G, D_S, D_V = Luminal diameters of artery, graft, stenosis, and vein, respectively; L = length of circuit segment; h = variables that depend upon viscosity, density, length of tube or circuit segment, and luminal diameter. K_l depends on luminal diameter; K_V depends on luminal diameters of vein and stenosis, and length of stenosis.

The ΔP equation for the entire circuit is a function of Q and the other variables and constants that characterize the circuit (table 2):

$$MAP - CVP = f(Q, Q^Z, X_i, C_i)$$

in which Z indicates various powers of Q, and X_i and C_i represent variables and constants. We assumed MAP = 100 mm Hg (1.33 × 10⁵ dyn/cm²) and CVP = 0 mm Hg.

Quantitative Predictions of Model

Figure 3 shows the predicted ΔPs for circuits with and without stenosis (percent reduction in luminal diameter). Laminar entry flow was assumed for the inflow artery and graft. The figure demonstrates the unique hemodynamics of the access circuit. In the normal systemic circulation, ΔP from the ascending aorta to the origin of the arterioles is normally small. In the access circuit,

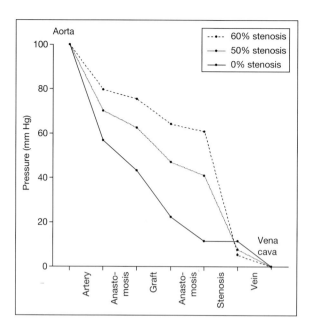

Fig. 3. Pressure drops (ΔPs) across each segment in model of graft vascular circuit. Total ΔP is MAP $-$ CVP. MAP $= 100$ mm Hg, CVP $= 0$ mm Hg, Hct $= 33\%$.

however, the high Q is accompanied by a large dissipation of energy so that a large ΔP occurs before flow reaches the graft. This agrees with the in vivo observation that the pressure in the arterial limb of a graft is 45% of MAP [15]. Because of the relatively small luminal diameter of the inflow artery [12], the stenosis ΔP does not match the artery ΔP until stenosis is $>$50%.

We also computed the inverse of the ΔP equation: Q $=$ f(ΔP_i, X_i, C_i). Figure 4 shows the solution for Q as a function of stenosis and MAP. The curve is sigmoid, so that it is initially relatively flat. As stenosis increases, however, the rate of decrease in Q accelerates. The slope is greatest at approximately 50% stenosis, where the risk of thrombosis becomes significant. The sigmoid (rather than linear) relation is important because it reduces the time interval during which Q monitoring can warn of impending thrombosis. Figure 4 also shows that MAP has a large effect on Q. Thus, a stable and reproducible Q measurement requires hemodynamic stability. Discontinuity in Q is shown because the model assumes transition from turbulent to laminar entry flow occurs as the Reynolds number falls below 2,000. Because resistance is lower in laminar flow, Q increases at this transition.

Figure 5 shows Q as a function of stenosis and Hct. Laminar entry flow was assumed for the inflow artery and graft. Hct influences Q because viscosity increases with Hct [14]. The influence is substantial at low stenosis, but

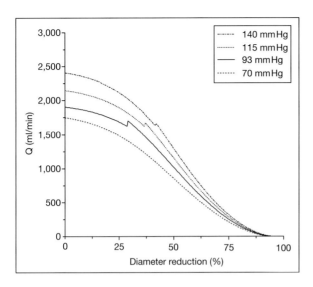

Fig. 4. Effect of MAP and stenosis on Q in model of graft vascular circuit. Hct is 35%.

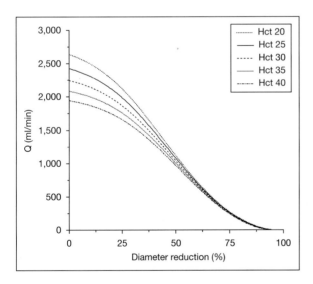

Fig. 5. Effect of Hct and stenosis on Q in model of graft vascular circuit. MAP is 100 mm Hg.

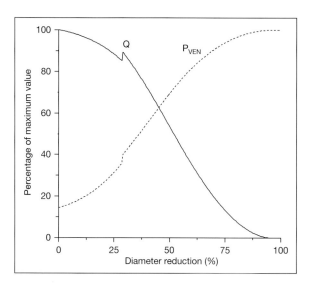

Fig. 6. Effect of stenosis on Q and intragraft pressure (P_{VEN}) in model of graft vascular circuit. Pressure is just upstream to stenosis at venous anastomosis. MAP is 100 mm Hg, Hct is 35%.

decreases as stenosis progresses. Thus, Hct should not have a significant effect on Q when stenosis is severe. Hct should have a lesser effect on Q in turbulent flow because viscous effects are reduced (not shown).

Venous drip-chamber pressure is also used to detect stenosis [16]. By turning off the dialysis blood pump, the drip-chamber pressure becomes equal to intra-access pressure (the pressure must be adjusted for the height relative to the graft). Figure 6 compares Q with intragraft pressure just upstream to the stenosis at the venous anastomosis. Pressure is largely the inverse of Q, indicating that venous pressure monitoring should, in principle, be equivalent to Q monitoring. Q has an advantage, however, in that it does not depend on the location of stenosis. For example, a stenosis that is upstream to the venous dialysis needle will not cause an increase in venous drip-chamber pressure. As in figure 4, discontinuities in curves are due to transition from turbulent to laminar entry flow.

Clinical Correlations

It is widely recommended that surveillance programs be used to detect access dysfunction so that stenosis can be corrected before thrombosis [17]. Grafts are most likely to benefit from such programs because they have a higher failure rate than established AV fistulae. The most popular surveillance method has been monthly Q measurements. Although low Q and decrease in Q are

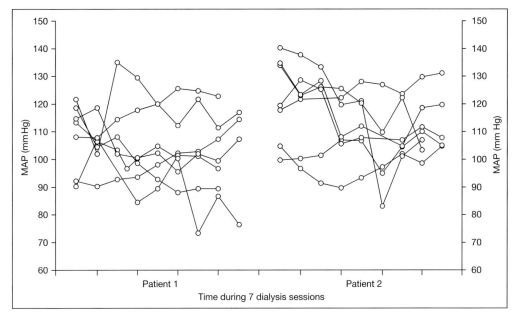

Fig. 7. MAPs of two representative patients during 7 consecutive dialysis sessions [reproduced with permission of the National Kidney Foundation, 22].

important risk factors for graft thrombosis, we and others have shown that Q has a poor predictive accuracy [18–21]. This result is consistent with the model, which predicts that variable hemodynamic conditions will strongly impair the relation between Q and stenosis.

Several studies have documented that variable hemodynamic conditions are indeed present during dialysis, when Q is usually measured [22–24]. The wide MAP range of 70–140 mm Hg in figure 4 is similar to the range we observed in 51 patients during 7 dialysis sessions [22]. The pooled within-patient MAP SD was 13.7 mm Hg, so that the average range within individual patients was approximately ±27 mm Hg. Figure 7 shows MAPs from two representative patients [22].

Resistance also varies widely during dialysis (fig. 8). Much of this variation is probably caused by changes in constriction of vessels that carry blood to and from the graft [25]. Transitions between laminar and turbulent flow may also contribute. Since $Q = (MAP - CVP)/R$, it follows that wide variation in MAP and R should cause considerable variation in Q.

Several studies have confirmed that Q varies widely within a single dialysis session [22–24]. For example, figure 9 shows changes in Qa and MAP between the first 30 and 90 min of a session [24]. Twenty-four percent of patients

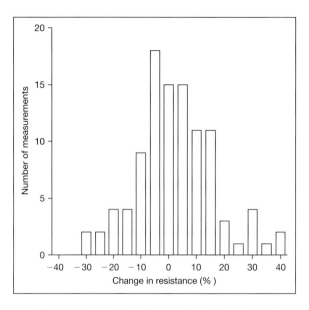

Fig. 8. Percent change in vascular resistance during dialysis in 51 patients with grafts. Data were obtained from a study of DeSoto et al. [22]. Changes in resistance were computed between first and middle thirds, and first and last thirds, of dialysis session. Resistance was defined as (MAP − CVP)/Q, with CVP set equal to 0.

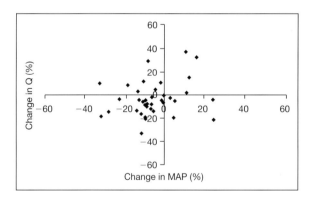

Fig. 9. Percent change in Q vs. percent change in MAP from 30 to 90 min after start of a dialysis session. Twenty patients had grafts, 12 had AV fistulae [reproduced with permission of the National Kidney Foundation, 24].

had changes in Q of at least 18%. Changes in Hct may also contribute to Q variation over a period of weeks or months. Measuring Q early at the same time in a session will not improve Q reproducibility because most of MAP variation is already present with the first MAP measured at the beginning of dialysis [22].

The foregoing illustrates the challenge in using access function to predict risk of thrombosis or failure. Access hemodynamics are unstable and subject to rapid changes during dialysis, when function is most commonly assessed. Measurement of Q more frequently than the standard monthly protocol would improve recognition of trends. However, this is generally impractical at this time and will probably have to await availability of easy and accurate on-line Q measurements.

There are other lessons to be drawn from hemodynamics of the access circuit. For grafts, the most severe stenoses usually occur at the venous anastomosis or outflow vein. However, because luminal diameters are usually largest in the vein [12], stenosis must be severe before it dominates resistance in the circuit. On the other hand, stenoses do commonly occur upstream to the venous anastomosis. Given the narrower luminal diameters in the upstream segments, it follows that even mild stenoses can have a significant impact on resistance. Thus, the interventionist has many issues to consider when treating stenoses with angioplasty. Not only must relative luminal diameters be considered, but as previously discussed, two or more short stenoses may have a greater influence on resistance than a single longer stenosis.

Access circuit hemodynamics can also be an important cause of complications, such as the steal syndrome. Consider a forearm graft anastomosed to the proximal radial artery. As figure 3 shows, low resistance causes a high Q with large ΔP before flow reaches the graft. Thus, the pressure in the radial artery distal to the graft is much lower than in the normal circulation. This low pressure induces retrograde flow from the digital and palmar arch arteries through the radial artery back to the graft. Reduced hand perfusion may result in ischemia, especially if arterial vascular disease is present in the hand [26]. A common method of preventing the high Q steal syndrome is to ligate the radial artery distal to the access.

Conclusion

The access vascular circuit has unique hemodynamic properties that can be analyzed according to principles of fluid mechanics. Concepts such as vascular resistance and shear stress help explain access function and maturation. The model of the graft circuit describes the factors that influence Q and pressure measurements, and explains why graft surveillance often fails to predict graft thrombosis and failure. The large ΔP in the access circuit plays an essential role in circuit hemodynamics and explains reduced distal perfusion in the steal syndrome. Consideration of hemodynamic principles can help in planning an optimum approach to preventing and treating access problems.

Appendix: Definitions and Units of Measurement

A	Cross-sectional area of tube or access (cm^2)
CVP	Central venous pressure ($1\,mm\,Hg = 1{,}333\,dyn/cm^2$)
D	Luminal diameter (cm)
ΔP	Pressure drop across part of access vascular circuit ($1\,mm\,Hg = 1{,}333\,dyn/cm^2$)
L	Length of tube or circuit segment (cm)
MAP	Mean arterial pressure ($1\,mm\,Hg = 1{,}333\,dyn/cm^2$)
η	Dynamic viscosity ($1\,poise = 1\,dyn\cdot s/cm^2 = 1\,g/cm/s$)
P	Pressure, defined as force exerted by fluid against an area A ($1\,mm\,Hg = 1{,}333\,dyn/cm^2 = 1{,}333\,g\cdot cm/s^2\cdot cm^2$)
ρ	Density of blood ($1.056\,g/cm^3$)
Q	Rate of flow $= vA = v\pi r^2$ ($1\,cm^3/s = 1\,ml/s = 60\,ml/min$)
R	Vascular resistance [1 peripheral resistance unit (PRU) $= 1\,mm\,Hg/ml/min = 8 \times 10^4\,dyn\cdot s/cm^5$]
r	Luminal radius (cm)
Re	Reynolds number, defined as ratio of inertial to viscous forces $= 2\rho rv/\eta = \rho Q/30\,\pi r\eta$ (dimensionless)
Shear rate	$\Delta v/\Delta x$ (s^{-1}) $=$ change in fluid velocity (Δv) per change in distance (Δx) perpendicular to the direction of flow
Shear stress	F/A (dyn/cm^2) $=$ force needed to move two layers of fluid of equal area A across each other
v	Mean cross-sectional velocity of fluid (cm/s)

References

1   Burton AC: Physiology and Biophysics of the Circulation. Chicago, Year Book Medical Publishers, 1972, pp 97–103.
2   Nichols WW, O'Rourke MF: McDonald's Blood Flow in Arteries: Theoretical, Experimental and Clinical Principles, ed 4. New York, Oxford University Press, 1998, pp 11–53.
3   Sumner DS: Essential hemodynamic principles; in Rutherford RB (ed): Vascular Surgery, ed 5. Philadelphia, Saunders, 2000, pp 73–120.
4   White FM: Viscous Fluid Flow, ed 2. Boston, McGraw-Hill, 1991, pp 291–293, 421–424.
5   Young DF: Fluid mechanics of arterial stenoses. J Biomech Eng 1979;101:157–175.
6   Kamiya A, Togawa T: Adaptive regulation of wall shear stress to flow change in the canine carotid artery. Am J Physiol 1980;239:H14–H21.
7   Zarins CK, Zatina MA, Giddens DP, Ku DN: Shear stress regulation of artery lumen diameter in experimental atherogenesis. J Vasc Surg 1987;5:413–420.
8   Corpataux JM, Haesler E, Silacci P, Ris HB, Hayoz D: Low-pressure environment and remodelling of the forearm vein in Brescia-Cimino haemodialysis access. Nephrol Dial Transplant 2002;17: 1057–1062.

9   Guzman RJ, Abe K, Zarins CK: Flow-induced arterial enlargement is inhibited by suppression of nitric oxide synthase activity in vivo. Surgery 1997;122:273–279.

10   Masuda H, Zhuang YJ, Singh TM, Kawamura K, Murakami M, Zarins CK, Glagov S: Adaptive remodeling of internal elastic lamina and endothelial lining during flow-induced arterial enlargement. Arterioscler Thromb Vasc Biol 1999;199:2298–2307.

11   Sho E, Sho M, Singh TM, Nanjo H, Komatsu M, Xu C, Masuda H, Zarins CK: Arterial enlargement in response to high flow requires early expression of matrix metalloproteinases to degrade extracellular matrix. Exp Mol Pathol 2002;73:142–153.

12   Ram SJ, Magnasco A, Barz A, Zsom L, Jones SA, Swamy S, Paulson WD: In vivo validation of glucose pump test for measurement of hemodialysis access blood flow. Am J Kidney Dis 2003;42:752–760.

13   White FM: Fluid Mechanics. Boston, McGraw-Hill, 1999, pp 367–375.

14   Cokelet GR, Merrill EW, Gilliland HS, Shin H, Britten A, Wells RE: The rheology of human blood – Measurement near and at zero shear rate. J Rheol 1963;7:303–317.

15   Sullivan KL, Besarab A, Bonn J, Shapiro MJ, Gardiner GA, Moritz MJ: Hemodynamics of failing dialysis grafts. Radiology 1993;186:867–872.

16   Besarab A, Frinak S, Sherman RA, Goldman J, Dumler F, Devita MV, Kapoian T, Al-Saghir F, Lubkowski T: Simplified measurement of intra-access pressure. J Am Soc Nephrol 1998;9:284–289.

17   National Kidney Foundation K/DOQI Clinical Practice Guidelines for Vascular Access. Am J Kidney Dis 2001;37(suppl 1):S137–S181.

18   Paulson WD, Ram SJ, Birk CG, Work J: Does blood flow accurately predict thrombosis or failure of hemodialysis synthetic grafts? A meta-analysis. Am J Kidney Dis 1999;34:478–485.

19   Paulson WD, Ram SJ, Birk CG, Zapczynski M, Martin SR, Work J: Accuracy of decrease in blood flow in predicting hemodialysis graft thrombosis. Am J Kidney Dis 2000;35:1089–1095.

20   McDougal G, Agarwal R: Clinical performance characteristics of hemodialysis graft monitoring. Kidney Int 2001;60:762–766.

21   Arbabzadeh M, Mepani B, Murray BM: Why do grafts clot despite access blood flow surveillance? Cardiovasc Intervent Radiol 2002;25:501–505.

22   DeSoto DJ, Ram SJ, Faiyaz R, Birk CG, Paulson WD: Hemodynamic reproducibility during blood flow measurements of hemodialysis synthetic grafts. Am J Kidney Dis 2001;37:790–796.

23   Schneditz D, Fan Z, Kaufman A, Levin NW: Stability of access resistance during haemodialysis. Nephrol Dial Transplant 1998;13:739–744.

24   Rehman SU, Pupim LB, Shyr Y, Hakim R, Ikizler TA: Intradialytic serial vascular access flow measurements. Am J Kidney Dis 1999;34:471–477.

25   Alfrey AC, Lueker R, Goss JE, Vogel JHK, Faris TD, Holmes JH: Control of arteriovenous shunt flow. JAMA 1970;214:884–888.

26   Miles AM: Upper limb ischemia after vascular access surgery: Differential diagnosis and management. Semin Dial 2000;13:312–315.

William D. Paulson, MD,
Department of Medicine,
Louisiana State University Health Sciences Center,
1501 Kings Highway, Shreveport, LA 71130 (USA)
Tel. +1 318 675 5911, Fax +1 318 675 5913, E-Mail wpauls@ lsuhsc.edu

Ronco C, Levin NW (eds): Hemodialysis Vascular Access and Peritoneal Dialysis Access.
Contrib Nephrol. Basel, Karger, 2004, vol 142, pp 254–268

······················

Vascular Access Recirculation: Measurement and Clinical Implications

Daniel Schneditz, Nikolai Krivitski

Department of Physiology, Karl-Franzens University Graz, Graz, Austria;
Transonic Systems, Inc., Ithaca, N.Y., USA

Introduction

The occurrence of recirculation has two major implications for hemodialysis. Recirculation significantly impairs the efficiency of the hemodialysis treatment [1, 2]. It can also be a sign of a pending access problem. Access recirculation detected in a peripheral access indicates impaired access blood flow [3] putting this access at high risk of failing because of thrombosis. The detection of access recirculation may lead to the finding of vessel stenosis, which may be correctable by intervention such as angioplasty and this may prolong the useful life of that particular access [4, 5].

The vascular access is the structure required for an efficient hydraulic connection between the cardiovascular system and the extracorporeal circulation during hemodialysis. The vascular access can be characterized by an upstream inlet part, a mid section, and a downstream outlet part where upstream and downstream refer to the direction of unperturbed intra-access blood flow. Depending on the type of access the hydraulic connection is established by placing catheters or access needles into the lumen of the vascular access. With dual line devices enabling continuous blood treatment it is important to draw blood from the access without dilution by cleared blood returned to the access as the efficiency of the treatment is significantly compromised under such circumstances [2].

Efficient use of the access is achieved with the following measures. (1) Access blood flow (Q_a) is larger than extracorporeal blood flow (Q_b). (2) Blood is drawn from the upstream and returned to the downstream part of the access. (3) Removal and return sites are separated from each other by a certain distance. These considerations are of importance when the hydraulic connections to the extracorporeal

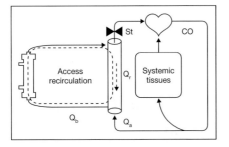

Fig. 1. Access recirculation. Scheme of access recirculation developing with an outflow stenosis. Q_b = Extracorporeal blood flow; Q_a = access blood flow; Q_r = recirculating blood flow; St = outflow stenosis; CO = cardiac output.

circulation are placed in the same branch of the vascular tree. However, under certain conditions processed blood returned to the access finds its way to the arterial line without systemic equilibration by recirculation (R). 'Recirculation' refers to the reflux of dialyzed blood from the venous return back into the arterial line [6].

Components of Recirculation

Recirculation may have different reasons, often resulting from violation of the basic requirements described above. However, it is not always due to real access problems. Thus, to identify access recirculation and to exclude false-positive results one needs to be aware of the situations which may affect and contaminate the recirculation measurement [7].

Local Recirculation

Recirculation is a local effect in the venovenous or central venous access [8]. In this type of access recirculation occurs when one or more conditions that cause admixture of cleared blood such as inadequate access flow, reversed and close placement of bloodlines are met.

Access Recirculation

Access recirculation into the arterial line is defined as the fraction of cleared extracorporeal blood flow (Q_r) that returns to the inlet of the extracorporeal bloodline taking the short connection between the access needles (fig. 1). In this type of recirculation there is retrograde flow in the vessel in which the access needles have been placed.

$$R = \frac{Q_r}{Q_b}$$
Eq. 1

With local recirculation a fraction of cleared blood returns to the inlet of the extracorporeal circulation without leaving the access region. Local recirculation occurs with inadequate access blood flow, i.e. if Q_b is larger than Q_a, and with close or reversed needle position. If a wrong placement of access needles and reversed placement of bloodlines can be excluded,

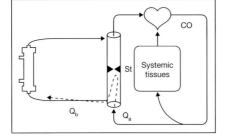

Fig. 2. Effect of mid-access stenosis. Access flow taking a functional bypass through the extracorporeal circulation during hemodialysis. Q_b = Extracorporeal blood flow; Q_a = access blood flow; St = intra-access stenosis; CO = cardiac output.

access recirculation is an indicator of an acute access problem. On the other hand, the absence of access recirculation does not necessarily exclude access problems since the presence of a significant stenosis between arterial and venous puncture sites is not detected by conventional recirculation measurements [9]. The explanation for the failure of access recirculation to detect a mid-access stenosis is as follows: with intra-access strictures which produce a significant resistance to access blood flow between arterial and venous needle puncture sites, the blood flow evades intra-access resistance during hemodialysis and takes a functional bypass through the extracorporeal circulation [10] (fig. 2). Even though the access is at risk for future thrombosis because of the intra-access stricture, there is sufficient blood supply to the inlet of the arterial bloodline and there is no recirculation.

Forced Recirculation

Inadvertent reversal of bloodlines is more frequent than anticipated [11]. Under these circumstances cleared blood is returned to the upstream section and pulled from the downstream section of the vascular access. Extracorporeal (Q_b) and access (Q_a) blood flows mix in the midsection between venous and arterial needles and the mixed blood is used to feed the extracorporeal circulation [12]. Forced recirculation is given as

$$R = \frac{Q_b}{Q_a + Q_b} \qquad\qquad \text{Eq. 2}$$

Forced recirculation induced by a wrong placement of bloodlines occurs even when access flow is sufficient or much larger than extracorporeal blood flow. To identify whether recirculation is caused by forced recirculation (a connection problem) or by access recirculation (an access problem), the lines have to be switched and the recirculation measurement has to be repeated at the same blood flow. The correct position of lines is characterized by the connection resulting in lower recirculation values.

Forced Recirculation in Central Venous Catheters

Reversal of bloodlines is common with central venous catheters in case the prescribed blood flow cannot be delivered. This procedure may do more

---

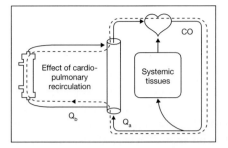

Fig. 3. Cardiopulmonary recirculation. Effects of cardiopulmonary recirculation (CPR = Q_a/CO) on extracorporeal circulation. Indicator entering the peripheral arteriovenous access through the venous line of the extracorporeal circulation mixes with systemic blood flow in the heart and returns to the arterial line without systemic equilibration. Q_b = Extracorporeal blood flow; Q_a = access blood flow; CO = cardiac output.

harm than good. Measured at the same blood flow recirculation in twin catheters (TwinCath, Medcomp) increased from 2.9 ± 5 to 12 ± 9% (mean difference 9.2%) when bloodlines were reversed [13]. Reversal of bloodlines may improve blood flow, but this may occur at the cost of recirculation, impairing the efficiency of hemodialysis.

Cardiopulmonary Recirculation

The cardiopulmonary component of recirculation is always present with a peripheral arteriovenous access [14]. Access blood flow bypasses systemic tissue compartments and returns to the arterial limb of the circulation feeding the access (fig. 3). The flow past systemic tissue compartments represents a significant amount of cardiac output (CO). The fraction Q_a/CO has been termed cardiopulmonary recirculation (CPR). Cardiopulmonary recirculation is in the range of 20–30% and may reach values up to 50% [15]. The effect of Q_a bypassing systemic tissue compartments and giving rise to recirculation is given as:

$$R = \frac{Q_b}{CO - Q_a + Q_b}$$

Eq. 3

Note that the magnitude of CPR is not necessarily identical to the degree of recirculation measured in the extracorporeal circuit. The recirculation in the extracorporeal circulation caused by access flow is usually much smaller than CPR, because Q_b is usually much smaller than Q_a. The recirculation in the extracorporeal circulation becomes equal to CPR when Q_b equals Q_a.

Methods

Even though the ultrasound Doppler technique has been used to detect retrograde blood flow between arterial and venous puncture sites with insufficient access blood flow [16], essentially all techniques to quantify and measure access recirculation are based on principles of indicator dilution. With perfect mixing of the indicator the concentration of the indicator measured downstream of the injection site is a measure for blood flow. Since recirculation refers to a ratio of flows (Eqs. 1–3) the determination of recirculation in general translates into the measurement of a ratio of concentrations.

Suitable indicators must be nontoxic, stable, and they must remain within the bloodstream. The classical indicators such as dyes or radiolabeled markers have been used to study access flow in hemodialysis; however, the treatment itself offers indicators much better suited for this purpose. The use of dialysate at different temperatures as an indicator is inherent to the technology of hemodialysis. Isotonic and hypertonic saline and glucose solutions are common in the clinical environment of hemodialysis, and these solutions have been studied or are currently in use to measure recirculation. An important variant of classical indicator dilution is offered by the controlled removal of indicators such as urea or ultrafiltrate by the process of hemodialysis and ultrafiltration so that urea concentration or measures of hemoconcentration can also be used to detect and quantify recirculation.

Because hemodialysis is associated with the controlled exchange of substances in the extracorporeal circulation, indicator dilution techniques have attracted most interest in the quantification of transport phenomena such as flow and recirculation.

Two points need to be considered for recirculation measurements:

Timing: As discussed above, recirculation consists of several components. Assessment of the vascular access using recirculation requires identification and separation of the local fistula component from the central, cardiopulmonary component of recirculation. The separation calls for exact timing of samples.

Variables: Since access recirculation depends on extracorporeal blood flow and access blood flow, studies on recirculation should include information on treatment variables such as extracorporeal blood flow and systemic blood pressures which determine access blood flow.

Bolus Techniques

The gold standard to measure access recirculation is based on the dilution of a bolus of indicator introduced into the venous line bloodstream by slug injection. This type of injection leads to a high and narrow pulse (a so-called Dirac pulse) at the injection site. As this high indicator pulse is carried downstream with the blood it first mixes with extracorporeal blood flow, then with access flow, finally with the venous return from all tissues which is equal to the cardiac output. After having passed the heart a fraction of the diluted indicator eventually returns to the access. On its way through the circulation the bolus is progressively more delayed and becomes wider and smaller the further downstream the concentration is measured. After a few circulations the dispersion of the indicator is complete as it is evenly distributed across the whole blood volume.

The principles of indicator dilution state that the blood flow mixing with the indicator can be determined from the first indicator transient measured downstream of the injection site [17]. More details on this technique are found in this contribution's companion chapter on the measurement of access blood flow [38].

Indicator added to the venous bloodstream is diluted by extracorporeal blood flow, enters the access, and in case of access recirculation reappears in the arterial bloodline with a delay of only a few seconds [18–20]. The transit of indicator recirculating through the access takes about 2–7 s. The exact transit times depend on blood flow, shunt volume between the needles, and the location of injection and sampling sites in the extracorporeal circulation. The transit of indicator recirculating through the veins, the cardiopulmonary loop and the arterial branch feeding the peripheral access takes about 6–25 s. Apart from blood flow and the location of injection and sampling sites, the exact times depend on access flow, cardiac output and central blood volume. Because of this time difference the two transients caused by access (short loop) and cardiopulmonary (long loop) recirculation are usually well separated when injection and sampling sites are close to the access and indicator is applied by slug injection.

The separation of the two transients is crucial for a high specificity to detect access recirculation. Failure to separate the transients will lead to false-positive results because cardiopulmonary recirculation is always found with a peripheral arteriovenous access. Minimizing the duration of the injection, injecting and measuring the indicator as close to the access as possible helps to separate and identify the possible access recirculation transient from the subsequent cardiopulmonary transient.

The magnitude of access recirculation is then determined by the amount of indicator retrieved in the arterial line (m_{art}) during its first transit relative to the amount of indicator delivered to the access using the venous line (m_{ven})

$$R = \frac{m_{art}}{m_{ven}} = \frac{AUC_{art}Q_{b,art}}{AUC_{ven}Q_{b,ven}} \qquad \text{Eq. 4}$$

where AUC is the area under the indicator concentration versus time curve. Typically, venous line blood flow ($Q_{b,ven}$) is not equal to arterial line blood flow ($Q_{b,art}$) because of ultrafiltration which has to be considered in the calculations [20].

The AUC measurement of the fast transients which only last a few seconds requires frequent sampling. For reasonable accuracy this can only be done by automatic sensors placed on or inserted in the extracorporeal bloodlines. Several techniques based on different indicators and different physical principles have been developed or adapted for this purpose.

Temperature
Temperature is one of the classic indicators to measure blood flow and it is not surprising that temperature was the prime choice for the first measurements of

access recirculation [18]. However, when temperature is used in the bolus approach temperature sensors must have short response times, which is difficult to realize in a noninvasive setting; therefore, the fistula assess monitors (FAM, Gambro AB, Lund, Sweden) which were based on the bolus-thermodilution technique remained at the prototype stage.

Isotonic Saline

Hemodialysis Monitor

The decrease in ultrasound velocity caused by the dilution of blood with isotonic saline is utilized by the Hemodialysis Monitor (HDM01, Transonic Systems, Inc., Ithaca, N.Y., USA) [19] to detect access recirculation. The magnitude of recirculation is displayed together with extracorporeal blood flow, which is also measured by ultrasonic means and which is an important variable in the development of access recirculation. The technique is often improperly referred to as 'ultrasound dilution'. Ultrasound is not diluted but used to detect dilution.

The manufacturer currently recommends to release saline from the saline bag (connected to the arterial line upstream of the dialyzer) for a duration of 4–5 s or to inject 10 ml of saline before or into the venous bubble trap. This type of administration simplifies handling, provides a smoother bolus, and causes less flow perturbation in the venous line, albeit requiring more sophisticated algorithms to separate true access recirculation from cardiopulmonary recirculation because of the dispersion of the bolus passing a significant section of the extracorporeal bloodline. In a study using 5 ml of saline as indicator volume the coefficient of variation of subsequent recirculation measurements was 9.3% [21]. The technique stands out for its ability to separate the components of recirculation such as access and cardiopulmonary recirculation and thus to measure true access recirculation [22, 23].

Crit-Line

The decrease in optical density caused by the dilution of blood with isotonic saline can also be used to detect and quantitate access recirculation [24]. The Crit-Line monitor (Crit-Line III, HemaMetrics, Kaysville, Utah, USA) measures optical density of blood passing a measuring cell inserted in the arterial limb of the extracorporeal circulation between the arterial line and the dialyzer [25]. Since only one measuring cell is used for the original purpose of this system to track ultrafiltration-induced hemoconcentration, the measurement of the venous transient entering the access (the denominator in Eq. 4) is substituted by an additional and identical injection of indicator into the arterial line before doing the actual recirculation test. This approach of performing a combination of arterial and venous injections when only one arterial sensor is available is also realized in other systems.

In a study injecting 10 ml of saline into the arterial line followed by 10 ml of saline into the venous line the coefficient of variation for the Crit-Line technique was 17.4% [21].

Hypertonic Saline
Hemodynamic Monitor
The change in blood conductivity (Λ) caused by the dilution with hypertonic saline can be measured noninvasively utilizing electromagnetic sensors. Such sensors are used by the Hemodynamic Monitor (HDM, Gambro Healthcare, Lakewood, Colo., USA). In this device a sensor measuring the difference between arterial and venous blood conductivities ($\Delta\Lambda = \Lambda ven - \Lambda art$) is clamped around both the venous and arterial lines. The sensor requires a modification of the bloodlines which have to contain closed loops (toroids) to be placed around the electromagnetic excitation and sensing cores of the measuring head.

A bolus of hypertonic saline (1 ml of 23.4% NaCl) is rapidly injected into the venous line as a conductivity tracer before the conductivity cell. The transient of hypertonic saline through the venous line produces a positive deflection whereas access recirculation into the arterial line leads to a subsequent negative deflection of the differential conductivity $\Delta\Lambda$. The venous and arterial signals are analyzed for plausibility with regard to timing and the fraction of access recirculation is calculated according to Eq. 4.

An in vitro analysis showed a coefficient of variation of $\approx 10\%$ for recirculation in the range between 5 and 20% [20]. The test is specific, i.e. it does not produce false positives in situations were access recirculation must be absent such as in situations were access needles are placed in different accesses. In vivo reproducibility determined as the coefficient of variation of subsequent measurements was 7.5% [21].

Even with the feature to accurately identify access recirculation (based on the ability to separate access recirculation from effects of CPR) the requirement to utilize dedicated disposable bloodlines probably explains why this technique remained at the prototype level.

Multimat
The transient of hypertonic saline can also be measured by conductivity cells originally designed for on-line measurement of blood urea concentration. The Multimat hemodialysis machine (Bellco-Sorin, Mirandola, Italy) is equipped with a sensor for a continuous measurement of urea in ultrafiltrate by the urease technique. In this machine ultrafiltrate undiluted by dialysate is obtained by the process of paired filtration and dialysis [26]. As with the Crit-Line device where only one measuring cell is available to measure arterial line concentrations, two subsequent injections of hypertonic saline (2.7 ml of 20% saline each) are required for measuring access recirculation. In a study done in 31 patients mean recirculation was between 5 ± 2 and $6 \pm 2\%$ when done early or late during hemodialysis and comparable to the blood side urea technique (6 ± 5 and $9 \pm 5\%$) [27]. However, blood side urea techniques are sensitive to effects caused by cardiopulmonary recirculation (see below) and it appears as if the paired filtration conductivity technique included effects of cardiopulmonary recirculation as well. This may

have to do with the dead space in the ultrafiltration filter and with the low ultrafil-tration flow causing an overlap with the cardiopulmonary transient. This will lead to false-positive results in the absence of access recirculation.

A comparison of three technologies showed that ultrasound (HDM01) and conductivity techniques (HDM) gave virtually identical results and showed good reproducibility. The optical technique (Crit-Line), however, appeared to underesti-mate access recirculation and provided less reproducible results [21].

Hypertonic Glucose

Bedside information on the plasma glucose concentration is of great clinical value and many devices offer an inexpensive and rapid measurement of this vari-able. Glucometers and glucose solutions are available in most dialysis wards. Thus, the measurement of recirculation by the dilution of hypertonic glucose injected into the venous bloodline is an interesting alternative to technically sophisticated and expensive approaches.

One of the protocols to measure recirculation is described as follows [28]. A base-line glucose concentration is measured in the arterial line (A) at the extracorporeal blood flow of 300 ml/min. Then, a 5-ml bolus of 20% glucose is injected into the venous drip chamber within 4 s while Q_b is 300 ml/min. Exactly 13 s later, 1 ml of blood is sampled from the arterial line for the duration of 4 s (sample B). The glucose concentrations in samples A and B are measured by the glucometer. The interpretation is straightforward: there is no recirculation if there is no rise in the glucose level (B ≤ A). When following the volumes, flows and times as specified above, recircula-tion can be calculated according to the following formula: R = 0.046(B − A) + 0.07. The glucose dilution test performed according to these specifications has a coefficient of variation of 8.6%. The test is easily done; however, strict adherence to the experi-mental conditions is mandatory.

Continuous Infusion Techniques

These techniques are based on constant infusion or removal of indicator to reach a more or less stable concentration in the mixed blood. In more detail, a sta-ble concentration is not reached because the indicator is added to or removed from a finite pool, but within a short period of time the change in indicator will be small so that the concentration of a single sample can be measured without additional technical equipment. However, for reasons of accuracy a continuous measurement of variables such as urea or temperature may be helpful.

Urea Technique

Urea has been the classic solute to identify and quantitate recirculation. Urea is one of the important solutes continuously cleared from the extracorporeal

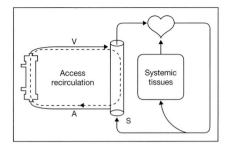

Fig. 4. Sampling sites. Location of samples to be taken for the measurement of urea recirculation are indicated (A, V, and S).

circulation during hemodialysis and it is easily measured. In terms of indicator dilution extracorporeal urea clearance can be viewed as a continuous infusion of blood with low urea concentration. Without access recirculation, the urea concentration in the arterial bloodline is equal to the urea concentration in the blood entering the access. However, with access recirculation, the concentration in arterial line blood is diluted by mixing with cleared blood.

The determination of urea recirculation requires three simultaneous samples: an arterial line sample (A), a venous line sample (V), and a sample representing the undiluted systemic concentration in the access inflow (S) (fig. 4).

$$R = \frac{S - A}{S - V} \qquad \text{Eq. 5}$$

There are no problems in getting the samples A and V; the difficulties reside with obtaining the proper sample S. S refers to the concentration of systemic arterial blood for an arteriovenous access and to mixed venous blood for a central venovenous access. If an arteriovenous access is used and if S is available from the arterial system such as from the femoral artery, the urea technique produces good results [29]. A peripheral venous sample from the contralateral access arm is not acceptable because venous urea concentration is systematically higher than arterial urea concentration so that the difference S − A becomes positive even without local recirculation [30].

An alternate approach for both arteriovenous and central venous accesses is to draw an arterial line sample 20 s after having stopped Q_b ('stop flow technique') or reduced Q_b to 70 ml/min ('low flow technique') and to assume that recirculation subsides with low Q_b [31]. However, the sample has to be drawn within 30 s as S starts to rebound shortly after having reduced or stopped extracorporeal clearance. The time window of 20–30 s to draw an undiluted sample S from the arterial bloodline after stopping or slowing Q_b is determined by the time necessary to clear the dead space between the needle tip and the sampling port, and by the transit time of uncleared access blood (because Q_b has been stopped or reduced) to recirculate through the heart and lungs and to reappear at the peripheral access and arterial sampling port because of cardiopulmonary recirculation. The problem with this approach is that there are many small albeit important variations to the same protocol [32].

Note that for stable venous concentrations (V) urea clearance and blood flow have to be stable for a period of a few minutes. Access complications leading to intermittent and low blood flows because of repeated machine alarms do not provide a good setting for reliable recirculation measurements. Urea recirculation can be measured any time during hemodialysis. Even though urea is an important marker and a familiar solute in hemodialysis, urea concentrations and test results are usually not available at the bedside. This is a major drawback as the immediate feedback offered by other techniques provides essential information to correct the problem on-site or to refer the patient for access revision.

Thermodilution

The fast response of temperature sensors required for the classic thermodilution approach is no longer required when temperature is used in a constant infusion approach. In case of access recirculation the temperatures of venous line blood and of access inlet blood mix to give the temperature measured in the arterial bloodline. Basically the same considerations apply as with the recirculation of urea, and Eq. 5 can be used to determine the amount of recirculation from the measurement of arterial and venous line temperatures. However, with thermodilution a different approach to solve the problem of measuring the sample S must be used. The temperature of venous blood returning to the access can easily be changed by changing the dialysate temperature without changing Q_b and without affecting the flow and recirculation conditions in the vascular access. If two sets of arterial and venous line temperatures (A_1, A_2, V_1, V_2) are measured as the result of changing the temperature of the dialysate Eq. 5 provides two sets of equations. S can then be eliminated to give the following relationship:

$$R = \frac{S-A_1}{S-V_1} = \frac{S-A_2}{S-V_2} = \frac{A_2-A_1}{V_2-V_1} = \frac{\Delta A}{\Delta V} \qquad \text{Eq. 6}$$

where ΔA and ΔV relate to the changes in arterial and venous line temperatures caused by the change in dialysate temperature. If changes in venous temperature are in the range of 2–3°C, the resolution in the measurement of arterial temperature changes needs to be better than 0.1°C.

Blood Temperature Monitor

The technique to measure arterial and venous line temperatures with the required accuracy without direct blood contact is realized in the Blood Temperature Monitor (BTM, Fresenius Medical Care, Bad Homburg, Germany). The BTM is designed to measure and control thermal balance in hemodialysis patients during their treatment. The BTM also performs automatic recirculation measurements by measuring the change in arterial and venous line temperatures caused by a change in dialysate temperature [33]. The technique is relatively slow since the infusion of cooled (or warmed) blood to produce a stable step change in arterial and venous line temperatures requires 2–3 min, long enough to overlap with effects caused by cardiopulmonary recirculation. The test result is available within minutes.

The standard deviation for BTM recirculation measurements is in the range of $\pm 1.2\%$ (full scale) and the coefficient of variation decreases with increasing recirculation ($\approx 5\%$ at 30% recirculation) [34].

Note that when measured in peripheral accesses BTM recirculation includes a component caused by cardiopulmonary recirculation. The exact value of this component depends on the magnitude of Q_b, Q_a, and CO (Eq. 3) but a threshold of 15% may help to detect 93% of accesses with access recirculation (sensitivity) and to reject 99% of accesses without access recirculation (specificity) [35]. The same threshold applied to detect fistulae for revision yields a sensitivity and specificity of 82 and 99%, respectively [36].

Clinical Implications

Access recirculation should be zero in a well-functioning access. It is indeed zero in the majority of patients [37]. While this condition can be attained in the peripheral arteriovenous access, access recirculation is more difficult to avoid with a central venous access.

If access recirculation is detected, the first question to be answered is whether needles and/or lines have been placed in the correct position. Switching the bloodlines and repeating the recirculation measurement may clarify the situation since the correct position of needles and lines relative to access blood flow yields smaller recirculation values (at the same or at a larger Q_b). If needles or lines are inadvertently reversed in an arteriovenous access (and this happens quite frequently, especially in loop grafts) the correct position will usually provide zero access recirculation.

If access recirculation is present with both positions of bloodlines, the next steps depend on the type of access used.

In the central venous access the situation is simplified with regard to the effect of cardiopulmonary recirculation, which is absent in this type of access, but the situation is more complicated with regard to access recirculation. In some cases there is no access recirculation even at high pump flows, and sometimes it is difficult to avoid access recirculation at small extracorporeal blood flows. In any case, it will be best to choose the connection producing the highest effective extracorporeal blood flow ($Q_{b,e}$)

$$Q_{b,e} = Q_b(1 - R) \qquad \text{Eq. 7}$$

and to use the access as long as the delivery of the dose of dialysis is not compromised.

Recirculation in the peripheral arteriovenous access indicates insufficient access blood flow so that this access is at a high risk of failing because of thrombosis. Access recirculation could also be due to a close position of access needles, in which case the space between puncture sites must be increased in subsequent treatments. A peripheral access with access recirculation requires careful further inspection, best by measurement of access flow as described in the following chapter of this book [38].

Conclusion

Even though the measurement of access flow has been proposed as the best test for fistula function [39, 40] daily measurements are not feasible and there remains an increased interest in practical alternatives [41–44].

Access recirculation has been regarded as a poor test for detecting access problems because it occurs after access flow has decreased to the point of impairing dialysis delivery and also because intra-access stenoses between the needles are not detected [40]. However, the interval between recirculation measurements in previous studies may have been too long to reflect the decline in access flow and the onset of access recirculation. Also, the correct clinical interpretation of recirculation data is difficult when using techniques that cannot distinguish between the different components of recirculation.

One of the most important features of recirculation measurements is that they can be done with every treatment and as often as required without interfering with the delivery of dialysis. The power of recirculation measurements increases with measuring frequency. Frequent recirculation measurements not only provide information on correct needle placement, but also yield instant bedside information on access function in routine dialysis. Therefore, access recirculation should not be dismissed as a gadget to monitor access function, especially when measurements can be easily performed on a daily basis.

References

1   Gotch FA: Models to predict recirculation and its effect on treatment time in single-needle dialysis; in Ringoir S, Vanholder R, Ivanovich P (eds): First International Symposium on Single-Needle Dialysis. Cleveland, ISAO Press, 1984, p 305.
2   Depner TA: Prescribing Hemodialysis: A Guide to Urea Modeling. Boston, Kluwer Academic Publishers, 1991.
3   Besarab A, Sherman R: The relationship of recirculation to access blood flow. Am J Kidney Dis 1997;29:223–229.
4   Schwab SJ, Raymond JR, Saled M, Newman GE, Dennis PA, Bollinger RR: Prevention of hemodialysis fistula thrombosis: Early detection of venous stenoses. Kidney Int 1989;36:707–711.
5   Sherman RA, Kapoian T: The role of recirculation in access monitoring. ASAIO J 1998;44:40–41.

6 Sherman RA, Kapoian T: Recirculation, urea disequilibrium, and dialysis efficiency: Peripheral arteriovenous versus central venovenous vascular access. Am J Kidney Dis 1997;29:479–489.

7 Schneditz D: Recirculation, a seemingly simple concept. Nephrol Dial Transplant 1998;13: 2191–2193.

8 Twardowski ZJ, Van Stone JC, Jones ME, Klusmeyer ME, Haynie JD: Blood recirculation in intravenous catheters for hemodialysis. J Am Soc Nephrol 1993;3:1978–1981.

9 Besarab A, Lubkowski T, Frinak S, Ramanathan S, Escobar F: Detection of access strictures and outlet stenoses in vascular accesses: Which test is best? ASAIO J 1997;43:M543–M547.

10 van Gemert MJ, Bruyninckx CM, Baggen MJ: Shunt haemodynamics and extracorporeal dialysis: An electrical resistance network analysis. Phys Med Biol 1984;29:219–235.

11 Shapiro W, Gurevich L: Inadvertent reversal of hemodialysis lines – A possible cause of decreased hemodialysis (HD) efficiency (abstract). J Am Soc Nephrol 1997;8:173A.

12 Krivitski NM: Novel method to measure access flow during hemodialysis by ultrasound velocity dilution technique. ASAIO J 1995;41:M741–M745.

13 Level C, Lasseur C, Chauveau P, Bonarek H, Perrault L, Combe C: Performance of twin central venous catheters: Influence of the inversion of inlet and outlet on recirculation. Blood Purif 2002;20:182–188.

14 Schneditz D, Kaufman AM, Polaschegg HD, Levin NW, Daugirdas JT: Cardiopulmonary recirculation during hemodialysis. Kidney Int 1992;42:1450–1456.

15 Schneditz D, Wang E, Levin NW: Validation of hemodialysis recirculation and access blood flow measured by thermodilution. Nephrol Dial Transplant 1999;14:376–383.

16 Weitzel WF, Rubin JM, Swartz RD, Woltmann DJ, Messana JM: Variable flow Doppler for hemodialysis access evaluation: Theory and clinical feasibility. ASAIO J 2000;46:65–69.

17 Lassen NA, Henriksen O, Sejrsen P: Indicator methods for measurement of organ and tissue blood flow; in Shepherd JT, Abboud FM (eds): Handbook of Physiology. Section 2. The Cardiovascular System. Bethesda, American Physiological Society, 1983, vol 3, pp 21–63.

18 Aldridge C, Greenwood RN, Cattell WR, Barrett RV: The assessment of arteriovenous fistulae created for haemodialysis from pressure and thermal dilution measurements. J Med Eng Technol 1984;8:118–124.

19 Depner TA, Krivitski NM, MacGibbon D: Hemodialysis access recirculation measured by ultrasound dilution. ASAIO J 1995;41:M749–M753.

20 Lindsay RM, Burbank J, Brugger J, Bradfield E, Kram R, Malek P, Blake PG: A device and a method for rapid and accurate measurement of access recirculation during hemodialysis. Kidney Int 1996;49:1152–1160.

21 Lindsay RM, Bradfield E, Rothera C, Kianfar C, Malek P, Blake PG: A comparison of methods for the measurement of hemodialysis access recirculation and access blood flow rate. ASAIO J 1998;44:62–67.

22 Alloatti S, Molino A, Bonfant G, Ratibondi S, Bosticardo GM: Measurement of vascular access recirculation unaffected by cardiopulmonary recirculation: Evaluation of an ultrasound method. Nephron 1999;81:25–30.

23 Krivitski NM, MacGibbon D, Gleed RD, Dobson A: Accuracy of dilution techniques for access flow measurement during hemodialysis. Am J Kidney Dis 1998;31:502–508.

24 Hester RL, Ashcraft D, Curry E, Bower J: Non-invasive determination of recirculation in the patient on dialysis. ASAIO J 1992;38:M190–M193.

25 Steuer RR, Harris DH, Conis JM: A new optical technique for monitoring hematocrit and circulating blood volume: Its application in renal dialysis. Dial Transplant 1993;22:260–265.

26 Ghezzi PM, Frigato G, Fantini GF, Dutto A, Meinero S, Cento G, Marazzi F, D' Andria V, Grivet V: Theoretical model and first clinical results of the paired filtration-dialysis (PFD). Life Support Syst 1983;1(suppl 1):271–274.

27 Bosc JY, Leblanc M, Garred LJ, Marc JM, Foret M, Babinet F, Tetta C, Canaud B: Direct determination of blood recirculation rate in hemodialysis by a conductivity method. ASAIO J 1998;44:68–73.

28 Magnasco A, Alloatti S, Bonfant G, Copello F, Solari P: Glucose infusion test: A new screening test for vascular access recirculation. Kidney Int 2000;57:2123–2128.

29 Buur T, Will EJ: Haemodialysis recirculation measured using a femoral artery sample. Nephrol Dial Transplant 1994;9:395–398.
30 Tattersall JE, Chamney P, Aldridge C, Greenwood RN: Recirculation and the post-dialysis rebound. Nephrol Dial Transplant 1996;11:75–80.
31 Tattersall JE, Farrington K, Raniga PD, Thompson H, Tomlinson C, Greenwood RN: Haemodialysis recirculation detected by the three-sample method is an artefact. Nephrol Dial Transplant 1993;8:60–63.
32 Kapoian T, Steward CA, Sherman RA: Validation of a revised slow-stop flow recirculation method. Kidney Int 1997;52:839–842.
33 Kaufman AM, Krämer M, Godmere RO, Morris AT, Amerling R, Polaschegg HD, Levin NW: Hemodialysis access recirculation (R) measurement by blood temperature monitoring (BTM) – A new technique (abstract). J Am Soc Nephrol 1991;2:324.
34 Schneditz D, Fan Z, Kaufman AM, Levin NW: Measurement of access flow during hemodialysis using the constant infusion approach. ASAIO J 1998;44:74–81.
35 Wang E, Schneditz D, Kaufman AM, Levin NW: Sensitivity and specificity of the thermodilution technique in detection of access recirculation. Nephron 2000;84:134–141.
36 Wang E, Schneditz D, Ronco C, Levin NW: Surveillance of fistula function by frequent recirculation measurements during high-efficiency dialysis. ASAIO J 2002;48:394–397.
37 MacDonald S, Sosa M, Krivitski NM, Glidden D, Sands JJ: Identifying a new reality: Zero vascular access recirculation using ultrasound dilution. ANNA J 1996;23:603–608.
38 Krivitski NM, Schneditz D: Arteriovenous vascular access flow measurement: accuracy and clinical implications; in Ronco C, Levin NW (eds): Hemodialysis Vascular Access and Peritoneal Dialysis Access. Contrib Nephrol. Basel, Karger, 2004, vol 142, pp 269–284.
39 NKF-DOQI Clinical Practice Guidelines for Vascular Access. National Kidney Foundation-Dialysis Outcomes Quality Initiative. Am J Kidney Dis 1997;30:S150–S191.
40 Besarab A, Lubkowski T, Frinak S, Ramanathan S, Escobar F: Detecting vascular access dysfunction. ASAIO J 1997;43:M539–M543.
41 Skladany M, Vilkomerson D, Lyons D, Chilipka T, Delamere M, Hollier LH: New, angle-independent, low cost Doppler system to measure blood flow. Am J Surg 1998;176:179–182.
42 Steuer RR, Miller DR, Zhang S, Bell DA, Leypoldt JK: Noninvasive transcutaneous determination of access blood flow rate. Kidney Int 2001;60:284–291.
43 Ezzahiri R, Lemson MS, Kitslaar PJ, Leunissen KM, Tordoir JH: Haemodialysis vascular access and fistula surveillance methods in The Netherlands. Nephrol Dial Transplant 1999;14:2110–2115.
44 Bonucchi D, D'Amelio A, Capelli G, Albertazzi A: Management of vascular access for dialysis: An Italian survey. Nephrol Dial Transplant 1999;14:2116–2118.

Daniel Schneditz, PhD,
Harrachgasse 21/5,
AT–8010 Graz (Austria)
Tel. +43 316 380 4269, Fax +43 316 380 9630, E-Mail daniel.schneditz@uni-graz.at

Ronco C, Levin NW (eds): Hemodialysis Vascular Access and Peritoneal Dialysis Access.
Contrib Nephrol. Basel, Karger, 2004, vol 142, pp 269–284

....

Arteriovenous Vascular Access Flow Measurement: Accuracy and Clinical Implications

Nikolai Krivitski, Daniel Schneditz

Transonic Systems, Inc., Ithaca, N.Y., USA; Department of Physiology,
University of Graz, Graz, Austria

'Prospective surveillance of AV grafts for hemodynamically significant stenosis, when combined with correction, improves patency and decreases the incidence of thrombosis'

'Sequential timely repetitive measurement of access flow is the preferred method for surveillance of AV grafts'

K/DOQI guidelines [1]

Introduction

Since the introduction of native AV fistulas for use in hemodialysis, multiple approaches have been developed to estimate access blood flow. The first method used dye dilution [2], which was followed by use of isotopes [3], and then videodensitometry [4]. Color Doppler was first used to estimate flow and structure by Forseberg et al. [5] in 1980. More sophisticated technologies such as magnetic resonance imaging were introduced by Oudenhoven et al. [6] in 1993. Of the many approaches developed, none found routine use in the clinics on account that they were expensive, difficult to use (requiring specially trained personnel), had interobserver variations, and were not available for every hemodialysis unit.

In 1995, a reversed-line dilution method for measuring vascular access blood flow during hemodialysis was introduced [7]. This method allowed for routine, operator-independent measurements to be made by a nurse and required only 3–5 min to perform. This development initiated widespread use of access flow measurements in hemodialysis clinics. Since 1995, more than 100 papers

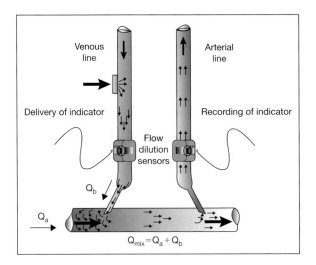

Fig. 1. Scheme of reversed placement of extracorporeal blood lines. Q_a = Blood flow entering the access; Q_b = pump flow; Q_{mix} = sum of mixed access flow and pump flow.

have been published addressing the accuracy, prognostic value, and economic impact of ultrasound velocity dilution technology [8].

Following the use of blood ultrasound velocity to perform dilution measurements (Transonic Systems, Inc.) [9], multiple technologies have been developed to perform access flow measurements with line reversal: conductivity dilution by Gambro [10], thermodilution by Fresenius [11], the Delta H method by HemaMetrics [12], dialysance by Fresenius [13] and Hospal [14], and urea sampling [15]. Three technologies that do not require line reversal have been recently introduced: variable flow Doppler [16], transcutaneous access flow monitor (TQA; HemaMetrics) [17] and the glucose pump test (GPT) [18].

The purpose of this paper is to review and analyze the major factors that can influence accuracy of access flow measurement technologies to ensure successful clinical outcomes of flow surveillance programs.

Methodologies

Reversed-Line Position Methodologies
The purpose of line reversal is to enable delivery of indicator into the venous dialyzer outflow line upstream of the access, and then be able to sample downstream of the access (after the indicator has mixed) in the withdrawal/arterial line (fig. 1).

The most often used formula to calculate access flow utilizes the relationship between access flow (Q_a) and the access recirculation (R) introduced by line reversal [7]:

$$Q_a = Q_b \left(\frac{1}{R-1} \right)$$

Eq. 1

where Q_b represents pump flow. Use of this formula assumes that delivery of pump flow upstream of the access does not change the initial access inflow.

Any technology that measures recirculation can be used to measure access flow with the reversed-line position [7]. All such technologies use formulas that are mathematically equivalent to Eq. 1. Thus, all the methods share the same methodological pitfalls related to line reversal and have additional ones related to the specific indicator used.

Blood Ultrasound Velocity

Measurement of the changes in the blood ultrasound velocity are used in Transonic System's HD01/HD02 monitor to measure access flow. Two ultrasound flow dilution sensors are clamped onto the bloodlines, one on the arterial and the other on the venous one [7, 9]. The sensors simultaneously measure blood flow in the tubing line and changes in ultrasound velocity caused by the introduction of the indicator isotonic saline. Saline may be administrated in two ways: as a 10-ml bolus injected before/into the venous bubble trap, or it may be released over a 4- to 5-second count from the infusion bag connected to the arterial side of the dialyzer (routinely used to flush the dialyzer and bloodlines). The dilution of blood in the venous line caused from the introduction of saline is recorded as it passes the venous line sensor (S_v). After entering the access, the indicator mixes with the access flow. Some portion of this diluted blood reenters the extracorporeal circuit via the arterial line where the dilution is now recorded by the arterial sensor (S_a). Access flow is calculated with Eq. 2:

$$Q_a = Q_b \left(\frac{S_v}{S_a} - 1 \right)$$

Eq. 2

where Q_b represents pump flow in the venous line, and S_v and S_a represent the areas under the venous and arterial dilution curves, respectively. The performance of the measurement takes 2–3 min.

This technology was validated on the bench [7, 9], was independently validated in direct animal experiments [19], and was successfully compared with the magnetic resonance imaging technique [20] and in multiple comparisons with color Doppler [21–23]. At this time, it is the most widely used technology for access flow measurement. Practically the major part of the new knowledge about blood flow phenomena in a variety of artificial AV grafts and native fistulas, including major guidelines, was developed based on scientific publications that used this technology.

Differential Conductivity Monitor

This method was initially developed by Cobe-Gambro to measure access recirculation and then was used to measure access flow [10]. One sensor with magnetic coils is clamped around specially designed tubing loops in the arterial and venous bloodlines. Bolus injection of 24% hypertonic saline into the venous line changes the electrical impedance of blood. In the reversed-line position, the saline bolus passes the sensor and enters the vascular access. Analogous to the ultrasound method, the saline bolus mixes with access flow and is recorded by the sensor when it appears in the arterial line. Access flow is calculated with an equation analogous to Eq. 1. At this time, this technology is unavailable for commercial use.

Thermodilution

The Fresenius Blood Temperature Monitor (BTM) uses two temperature sensors attached to the bloodlines, one on the arterial and one on the venous line [11]. Changes in dialysate temperature alter the temperature of the blood flowing through the dialyzer. In the reversed-line position, the cooled/warmed bolus of blood passes the venous line sensor and enters the vascular access without adding any indicator volume. In the same manner as described for the saline dilution method, the temperature bolus mixes with access flow and then is recorded by the arterial temperature sensor. Access flow is calculated with an equation analogous to Eq. 1. Because the time duration of the temperature bolus is minutes, the artificially induced recirculation overlaps with cardiopulmonary recirculation (CPR), which introduces an error into the access flow measurements. To compensate for CPR, a second measurement is performed with the normal line position, and this result is used for compensation [11].

$$Q_a = \frac{(1-R_x)(Q_n) \cdot (1-R_n)(Q_x - UFR)}{(1-R_n)(Q_n) - (1-R_x)(Q_x - UFR)}$$

Eq. 3

where R_n and R_x represent recirculation at normal and reversed-line positions, respectively; Q_n and Q_x represent pump flow at normal and reversed-line positions, respectively, and UFR represents the ultrafiltration rate.

There is one independent study of BTM use for access flow measurements (using the double recirculation approach described above) in 56 patients [24]. The thermodilution technique gave a 95% confidence limit of ± 70 ml/min at access flows of 500 ml/min, and the confidence limits widened as access flow increased. The authors concluded that the technology's limited sensitivity at a higher flow range would not allow for accurate recording of the 20–25% flow drop recommended by the K/DOQI guidelines.

Dialysance

This technology is used to measure access flow in the On-Line Clearance Monitor (OLC, Fresenius Medical Care, Germany) [13] and in the Diascan clearance monitor (Hospal Dasco SpA, Medolla, Italy) [14]. Two electrical impedance sensors (Fresenius) are attached to the dialysate lines: one on the outflow and the other on the inflow to measure dialysate conductivity. A change in dialysate sodium concentration (and conductivity) causes a corresponding change in the sodium concentration of the blood flowing through the dialyzer without addition of indicator volume. The blood with altered sodium concentration is delivered through the venous line to the vascular access. Dialysance measurements are performed at the normal and reversed-line positions. With the reversed-line position, analogous to the saline dilution method, the high sodium venous line blood mixes with access flow and a portion of the mixed blood enters the arterial line. These changes in sodium concentration are recorded by electrical impedance sensors in the dialysate. Access flow can be calculated using dialysance measurements at the normal and reversed-line position with a formula that is theoretically identical to Eq. 1:

$$Q_a = D_x \frac{(D_n - UFR)}{(D_n - D_x)} \qquad\qquad \text{Eq. 4}$$

where D_n and D_x represent dialysance at normal and reversed-line positions, respectively.

There are no independent studies of accuracy and reproducibility of the Fresenius monitor at this time. An independent comparison of access flow determined by Diascan versus Transonic produced a difference of 44 ± 661 ml/min $(9 \pm 70\%)$ between methods in 19 hemodialysis patients [25].

Ultrafiltration Step Change Method

This method uses the HemaMetrics monitor. Ultrafiltration is increased as a step change to produce a 4-min bolus of blood with a higher hematocrit [12]. In the reversed-line position, analogous to the saline dilution method, the concentrated blood mixes with the access flow and some of it enters the arterial line. These changes in hematocrit are recorded by an optical sensor on the arterial line. Because the hematocrit bolus is minutes long, the artificially induced recirculation overlaps with CPR introducing an error into the access flow measurements. To compensate for the CPR influence, the result of the ultrafiltration step change is first measured in the normal line position and then used for compensation:

$$Q_a = UFR \cdot \frac{H_o}{(\Delta H_x - \Delta H_n)}$$

Eq. 5

where H_o represents the initial hematocrit, and ΔH_n and ΔH_x represent the hematocrit change due to the ultrafiltration step at normal and reversed-line positions, respectively. In this case volume is not added but removed from the blood by ultrafiltration.

The technique points to a potential problem of excessive hemoconcentration in the extracorporeal system for all reversed bloodline techniques when ultrafiltration is on and forced access recirculation is high.

It does not appear that there are any independent studies on the accuracy and reproducibility of the Delta H method.

BUN Dilution Technique

Different groups of authors [15, 26, 27] have tried to use the three-BUN sample low-flow method for access recirculation measurement in the reversed-line position to measure access flow. The formula they used is based on Eq. 1. Lindsay et al. [27] concluded that the urea method is a poor predictor of access outcome.

Standard Line Position Methodologies
Variable Flow Doppler

This nondilution method is based on the idea of using Doppler to measure changes in linear velocity in blood between the needles and during pump flow changes. Access flow is calculated based on known changes in pump flow and measured changes in blood flow velocity [16]. At this time, this technology is not available commercially.

Transcutaneous Access Flow Monitor (TQA)

The TQA technology employs optical detection of hematocrit decreases induced by injection of 30 ml of saline directly into the venous line during hemodialysis using a special adaptor [17]. A pad with optical sensors is placed on the skin above the outflow section of the AV access to record dilution curves. The sensors use differential readings to compensate for individual differences in tissue illumination. A recent modification to the technique uses a rapid (3–4 s) injection of 20 ml of saline directly into the access through the arterial hemodialysis needle instead of into the venous line of a working dialysis system. The access flow is calculated with the assumption that the injection flow does not influence the initial access flow [17]. The first independent studies of the TQA technology [28–30] presented unfavorable and sometimes confusing results.

Glucose Pump Test

The GPT is implemented by pump infusion of hypertonic glucose at a constant rate of 25 ml/min into the arterial needle. Blood samples taken before and during the infusion (the latter is obtained with rapid blood withdrawal) are analyzed for glucose content [18]. Access flow is calculated with the assumption that both the glucose infusion and the rapid blood withdrawal do not change the initial access flow. There is no independent study at this time.

Factors Affecting Access Flow Measurement Accuracy

Over the process of developing these dilution techniques, it has become clear that there are many factors that affect the accuracy of access flow measurement and may have clinical implications:
(1) the quality of mixing of indicator with access flow between the introduction and recording sites, (2) second pass of the indicator through the cardiopulmonary system, (3) distortion of initial access flow by line reversal, indicator introduction, or indicator withdrawal, and (4) indicator loss.

Indicator Mixing with Access Flow between the Introduction and Recording Sites

The major difference between using dilution techniques for assessing central hemodynamics and for assessing access flow is the absence in the latter of a mixing chamber like the heart. The specific issue of mixing conditions in AV accesses has previously been addressed for reversed-line methods [7, 31]. Mixing is aided in artificial grafts by their relatively small inner diameter (4–6 mm), the relatively large distance between the needles (usually more than 4–5 cm) and turbulent flow. Thus, adequate mixing can be achieved regardless of needle position, as long as the pump flow for the reversed-line position is set at 200–300 ml/min.

In native fistulas, two major factors pose problems for indicator mixing. The first is their inner diameter which may be large and may also include aneurysms. The second is that upper arm fistulas that have been observed to reach high flows of 4–5 liters/min or more. To overcome these factors, it has been suggested that the arterial needle be placed facing the flow (just for the day of the measurement); this produces the best conditions for mixing when the lines are reversed [7].

For the TQA method, mixing should not be a problem since the injection flow is relatively large: $Q_i = 20$ ml/min/(3–4 s) = 300–400 ml/min.

For the GPT, the slow infusion of hypertonic glucose (25 ml/min) may not produce adequate mixing, especially in native fistulas with small distances

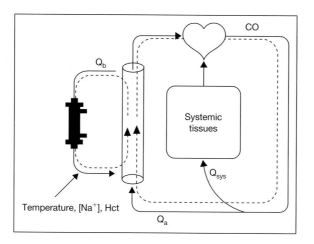

Fig. 2. Scheme of reversed placement of extracorporeal bloodlines. The characteristics of blood entering the extracorporeal circulation under conditions of forced recirculation (short dashed loop) are also influenced by CPR (long dashed loop). Q_b = Extracorporeal blood flow with reversed placement of bloodlines; Q_a = access blood flow; Q_{sys} = systemic blood flow; CO = cardiac output; Hct = hematocrit of blood leaving the dialyzer.

between needles. The recommendation of rapid sample withdrawal [18] possibly is an attempt to produce turbulence to enhance mixing at the tip of the withdrawal needle.

Influence of the Second Pass of the Indicator through
the Cardiopulmonary System

Adequate time separation between the first and second passes of indicator can be achieved with the relatively rapid indicator introduction by saline injection or saline release used for the Transonic HD01/02 system [32].

The difficulties with constant infusion techniques in the presence of CPR have previously been described [11, 32]. Regardless of whether the lines of the extracorporeal circulation are connected to the patient in the normal or reversed positions, CPR will be present when a peripheral AV access is used. CPR will affect recirculation, clearance, and hemoconcentration whether measured with normal or reversed position of extracorporeal bloodlines (fig. 2).

If the effects of CPR cannot be separated from recirculation, as is done in HD01/02, recirculation measured with reversed placement of blood lines will be erroneously high and accordingly access flow (Q_a) calculated from the original formula (Eq. 1) will be erroneously low. This is because recirculation is inflated

---

by the combined effects of forced access recirculation and CPR which cannot be separated from each other by the constant infusion approach [32]. The resulting underestimation of access flow was shown to be proportional to the term (1 − cardiac output/access flow) [33].

To solve this problem, measurements are made with both the normal and reversed-line positions, with the assumption that the influence of CPR does not change when bloodlines are switched. This approach has been termed the 'double recirculation technique', and it is the basis for measuring access flow with the thermodilution [11], on-line clearance [13, 14], and ultrafiltration techniques [12].

There are multiple assumptions to make this double recirculation approach reliable: (1) The influence of CPR on the measurements at normal and at reversed-line positions should be the same. (2) Hemodynamic status during the measurement time, which in some methods exceeds 20 min, should be unchanged. (3) The indicator baseline level should remain unchanged over the same measurement time. (4) The concentration level of the indicator (sodium for dialysance and hematocrit for Delta H methods) should reach a stable plateau during the time allotted for measurement (4 min).

A review of Eqs. 3–5 suggests that if the difference in the denominator becomes small, the equations require extremely high accuracy of the measured parameters; otherwise the results become unreliable. It is practically difficult to expect that all four of the above conditions will always take place to guarantee high accuracy of measured parameters. The situation of small values in the denominator takes place with increases of the access blood flow. Values R_x (Eq. 3) and ΔH_x (Eq. 5) will decrease and value D_x (Eq. 4) will increase. Measurement results may become less repeatable as access flow exceeds the level of 500 ml/min [24].

Small flows can be more reliably measured by the double recirculation techniques, as the values in the denominator (level of reversed recirculation) will be relatively high. One can expect that K/DOQI recommendations on low flow (500–600 ml/min) may be detectable with constant infusion techniques. The ability to identify a flow decrease of 25% over the flow range of 1,300–600 ml/min according to K/DOQI guidelines is doubtful at this time and should be proven in clinical studies.

*The Effect of Line Reversal and Indicator Introduction on
Initial Access Flow (Do We Influence What We Measure?)*

The necessity for complete indicator mixing within the small distance of the vascular access requires the introduction of a significant flow to artificially create turbulence. At the same time, the influence of this introduced flow on the initial access flow must be compensated for or minimized.

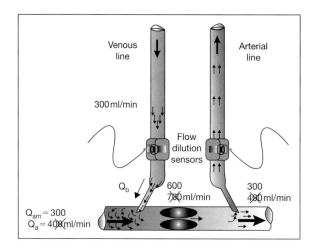

Venous
line

Arterial
line

300 ml/min

Flow
dilution
sensors

Q_b

600
780 ml/min

300
480 ml/min

$Q_{am} = 300$
$Q_a = 408$ ml/min

Fig. 3. Influence of line reversal on initial access flow in the case of significant stenosis between the needles. Q_a = Initial access flow; Q_{am} = measured access flow.

Reversed-Line Methods

The initial access flow Q_a can be considered to be the access flow that could theoretically be measured with the pump stopped. Once the lines are reversed creating local recirculation, the initial access flow may be altered. The mechanism of these changes is described below.

Eq. 1 calculates blood flow with the reversed-line position. The major assumption of Eq. 1 is that the initial flow Q_a is not changed when pump flow Q_b is added upstream. Under these conditions, the flow between the needles (Q_{mix}) is simply the sum of the access and pump flows: $Q_{mix} = Q_a + Q_b$. Q_{mix} is the flow actually measured by the dilution method, so Q_a can be calculated by subtracting Q_b from Q_{mix}. Errors may appear if in reality the inflow is altered (generally becoming smaller) because of Q_b. This leads to underestimation of Q_a that affects all reversed-line methods as their formulas are all mathematically equivalent to Eq. 1 (fig. 3).

The above discussion shows that a trade-off must be made between achieving adequate mixing and minimizing initial flow disturbance. To ensure complete mixing, pump flow (Q_b) must be in the range of 200–300 ml/min [7]. The major question becomes whether the resulting underestimation of initial flow measurement is clinically significant. This issue was addressed by mathematical modeling, bench studies, animal experiments, and clinical studies [31, 34]. The commonly reached conclusion was that the underestimation of the flow was in the order of 40–60 ml/min. The only case in which the magnitude of this discrepancy may increase up to the range of the extracorporeal blood flow is with the development of significant stenosis between the needles. The results of these investigations also suggest that whenever a significant discrepancy is observed between measured and initial access flow this vascular access is already severely compromised.

In the reversed-line approach with an HD01/02 monitor, a 10-ml saline injection is introduced into the venous bubble trap. By the time the saline enters the access, all pressure changes related to the injection have dissipated, and the access flow has already returned to its initial level [31, 32].

Reversal of bloodlines to produce forced access recirculation reduces dialysis efficiency. Therefore, the duration during which bloodlines are kept in reversed position should be minimized. Bolus techniques have the advantage that this time is kept at a minimum. The loss of efficient dialysis time can be further reduced and the handling can be simplified by utilizing special line extensions inserted between the access needles and the extracorporeal circulation [14, 35]. Such line extensions allow to reverse the extracorporeal blood flow at the access without manual disconnection and reconnection of bloodlines, which also reduces the risk for contamination.

Methods with Direct Injection/Withdrawal of Indicator
into the AV Access

Three factors determine how much injection flow affects the measurement result [32, 36]: (1) time duration of indicator injection/withdrawal, (2) indicator transit time from injection site to recording site, and (3) distribution of hemodynamic resistances in the AV access. As soon as the indicator is injected with a significant volume, an injection flow is created, and there are transient changes to the pressure and flow in the access. Depending on the distance between the needles and the indicator transit time in the access, the pressure and flow disturbances may or may not have dissipated by the time the dilution curve reaches the recording sensor.

The effect of the injection of indicator volume on flow in the access is a function of the distribution of hemodynamic resistances in the AV access. For example, if the outflow resistance is much larger than the inflow resistance (outflow stenosis), blood flow will not change much at the outflow location, because the introduced injection flow into the access will slow down incoming flow from the artery (fig. 4a). In the case where the major resistance is at the inflow (as with a new fistula) injection flow will add to initial flow increasing the value of outflow (fig. 4b).

For the TQA method, the manufacturer recommends rapid injection (within 3–4 s) of 20 ml of saline into the AV access. This creates an injection flow Q_i on the order of 300–400 ml/min that will add to initial flow in case

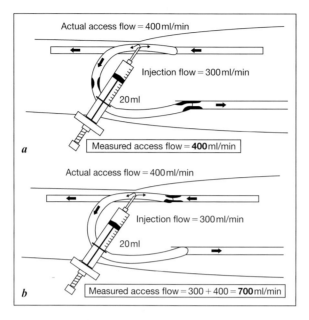

Fig. 4. Influence of injection flow on measured flow in the case of dominant outflow resistance (*a*) and in the case of dominant inflow resistance (*b*).

of a dominant inflow resistance. The access flow calculation is based on the assumption that the injection flow does not influence the initial blood flow [17]; in other words, it is assumed that all resistance in the access is located at the outflow site. As this it obviously not always correct TQA technology will tend to overestimate the blood flow in the access with inflow resistance. The above consideration may help to explain why the first independent studies of the TQA technology [28–30] presented unfavorable and sometimes confusing results.

Indicator Loss

All dilution methods will have problems with indicator loss in native fistulas constructed with a side-to-side anastomosis that created two branches when needles are in different branches (fig. 5a). When dialysis lines are reversed, there will be no recirculation for access flows greater than pump flow. This means that the indicator does not get pulled into the arterial line after it has been introduced into the access flow. The indicator will only appear in the arterial line after it has passed through the cardiopulmonary system. The Transonic HD01/02 monitor will automatically detect this situation and will ask the operator to check the needle position and check for line reversal. If this situation is confirmed, the operator should apply pressure with a finger

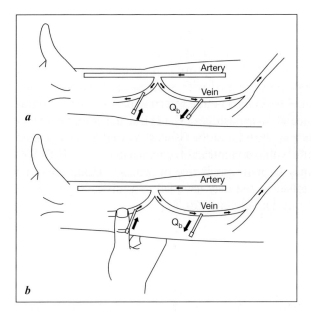

Fig. 5. *a, b* Methodology of performing flow measurements for needles located in two separate branches of native fistula (side-to-side AV anastomosis).

(stopping the flow) proximal to the outflow needle of one of the veins (preferably a distal, more superficial vein) for 1 min to perform the measurement (fig. 5b). A more complicated approach is to place both needles in the same branch and to repeat the measurements in both branches over two consecutive sessions.

With the TQA methodology, indicator may additionally be lost into arterial branches. The tip of the arterial needle where the injection is performed is often located within 2–3 ml of the priming blood volume from the arterial anastomosis. When 20 ml of saline are injected at the peak flow rate exceeding shunt flow rate, part of the indicator may flow retrograde into arterial branches. The loss of indictor prior to mixing with access flow decreases the area under dilution curve. This will produce erroneously high flow values, as has been observed experimentally [28].

Summary and Suggestions

The wide use of access flow surveillance has produced multiple papers supporting the concept that the high predictive power of access flow surveillance in identifying hemodynamically significant stenosis and predicting thrombosis may be used to decrease the thrombosis rate in grafts and native fistulas through timely interventions [37–49]. Blood flow measurement is only a tool for surveillance of AV grafts and fistulas. To apply it effectively the following two recommendations may be useful to improve clinical outcomes: (1) Use a reliable access flow technology combined with analysis of all hemodynamic data (including mean arterial pressures) before referring patients for angiography to decrease surveillance of false positives [8]. (2) Use the absolute threshold (600 ml/min for grafts and 500 ml/min for fistulas) as well as the dynamic threshold of a 25% decrease within 4 months as recommended by the K/DOQI. The dynamic threshold may be more predictive of stenosis. Using only one threshold may not be as effective and may have led to a misleading message about the effectiveness of flow surveillance [50, 51].

References

1   National Kidney Foundation-K/DOQI Clinical Practice Guidelines for Vascular Access: Update 2000. Am J Kidney Dis 2001;37(suppl 1):S137–S181.
2   Lindstedt E: Use of arterio-venous shunts (external and internal) for haemodialysis. Proceedings of the 4th International Congress on Nephrology, Stockholm, 1969. Basel, Karger, 1970, pp 188–197.
3   Kaye M, Lemaitre P, O'Regan S: A new technique for measuring blood flow in polytetrafluoroethylene grafts for hemodialysis. Clin Nephrol 1977;8:533–534.
4   Lantz BM, Holcroft JW, Foerster JM, Link DP, Reid MH: Determination of blood flow through arteriovenous fistulae and shunts. Acta Radiol 1979;20:727–736.
5   Forsberg L, Tylen U, Olin T, Lindstedt E: Quantitative flow estimations of arteriovenous fistulas with Doppler and dye-dilution techniques. Acta Radiol Diagn (Stockh) 1980;21:465–468.
6   Oudenhoven L, Pattynama P, De Roos A, Seeverens H, Rebergen SA, Chang PC: Magnetic resonance, a new method for measuring blood flow in hemodialysis fistulae. Kidney Int 1993; 45:884–889.
7   Krivitski NM: Theory and validation of access flow measurement by dilution technique during hemodialysis. Kidney Int 1995;48:244–250.
8   Krivitski NM: Access flow measurement during surveillance and percutaneous transluminal angioplasty intervention. Semin Dial 2003;16:304–308.
9   Krivitski NM: Novel method to measure access flow during hemodialysis by ultrasound velocity dilution technique. ASAIO J 1995;41:M741–M745.
10 Lindsay RM, Bradfield E, Rothera C, Kianfar C, Malek P, Blake PG: A comparison of methods for the measurement of hemodialysis access recirculation and access blood flow rate. ASAIO J 1998;44:62–67.
11 Schneditz D, Fan Z, Kaufman AM, Levin NW: Measurement of access flow during hemodialysis using the constant infusion approach. ASAIO J 1998;44:74–81.
12 Yarar D, Cheung AK, Sakiewicz P, Lindsay RM, Paganini EP, Steuer RR, Leypoldt JK: Ultrafiltration method for measuring vascular access flow rates during hemodialysis. Kidney Int 1999;56:1129–1135.
13 Gotch FA, Buyaki R, Panlilio F, Folden T: Measurement of blood access flow rate during hemodialysis from conductivity dialysance. ASAIO J 1999;45:139–146.
14 Mercadal L, Hamani A, Béné B, Petitclerc T: Determination of access blood flow from ionic dialysance: Theory and validation. Kidney Int 1999;56:1560–1565.
15 Depner T, Krivitski N: Access flow measured from recirculation of urea during hemodialysis with reversed blood lines. J Am Soc Nephrol 1995;6:486.

16   Weitzel WF, Rubin JM, Leavey SF, Swartz RD, Dhingra RK, Messana JM: Analysis of variable flow Doppler hemodialysis access flow measurements and comparison with ultrasound dilution. Am J Kidney Dis 2001;38:935–940.

17   Steuer RR, Miller DR, Zhang S, Bell DA, Leypoldt JK: Noninvasive transcutaneous determination of access blood flow rate. Kidney Int 2001;60:284–291.

18   Magnasco A, Alloatti S, Martinoli C, Solari P: Glucose pump test: A new method for blood flow measurements. Nephrol Dial Transplant 2002;17:2244–2248.

19   Gleed RD, Harvey HJ, Dobson A: Validation in the sheep of an ultrasound dilution technique for haemodialysis graft flow. Nephrol Dial Transplant 1997;12:1464–1467.

20   Bosman PJ, Boereboom FTJ, Bakker CJ, Mali WPT, Eikelboom BC, Blankestijn PJ, Koomans HA: Access flow measurements in hemodialysis patients: In vivo validation of an ultrasound dilution technique. J Am Soc Nephrol 1996;7:966–969.

21   May RE, Himmelfarb J, Yenicesu M, Knights S, Ikizler TA, Schulman G, Heranz-Schulman M, Shyr Y, Hakim RM: Predictive measures of vascular access thrombosis: A prospective study. Kidney Int 1997;52:1656–1662.

22   Sands JJ, Glidden D, Miranda C: Hemodialysis access flow measurement – Comparison of ultrasound dilution and duplex ultrasonography. ASAIO J 1996;42:M899–M901.

23   Zanen AL, Toonder IM, Korten E, Wittens CH, Diderich PN: Flow measurements in dialysis shunts: Lack of agreement between conventional Doppler, CVI-Q, and ultrasound dilution. Nephrol Dial Transplant 2001;16:395–399.

24   Ragg JL, Treacy JP, Snelling P, Flack M, Anderton S: Confidence limits of arteriovenous fistula flow rate measured by the 'on-line' thermodilution technique. Nephrol Dial Transplant 2003; 18:955–960.

25   Colzani S, La Milia V, Andrulli S, Bacchini G, De Filippo S, Locatelli F: Graft access blood flow (Qa) estimated by different methods (abstract). J Am Soc Nephrol 2001;12:285A.

26   Raja R, Velasques M: Access flow rate (Qa) with reverse urea recirculation: Better than outlet pressure to predict graft thrombosis (abstract). J Am Soc Nephrol 1998;9:180A.

27   Lindsay RM, Blake RG, Bradfield E: Estimation of hemodialysis access blood flow rates by a urea method is a poor predictor of access outcome. ASAIO J 1998;44:818–822.

28   Spergel L, Tucker T, Nadolski S, Hamilton T, Lasseter P: Access flow measurements by new TQA technology (abstract). J Am Soc Nephrol 2002;13:233A.

29   Roca-Tey R, Ibrik O, Samon R, Viladoms J: Study of vascular access blood flow rate prior to HD in 32 patients with native arteriovenous fistula by the optical transcutaneous method (abstract). Nephrol Dial Transplant 2002;17(suppl 1):286.

30   Ronco C, Brendolan A, Crepaldi C, D'Intini V, Sergeyeva O, Levin NW: Noninvasive transcutaneous access flow measurement before and after hemodialysis: Impact of hematocrit and blood pressure. Blood Purif 2002;20:376–379.

31   Krivitski NM, Depner TA: Development of a method for measuring hemodialysis access flow: From idea to robust technology. Semin Dial 1998;11:124–130.

32   Krivitski NM, MacGibbon D, Gleed RD, Dobson A: Accuracy of dilution techniques for access flow measurement during hemodialysis. Am J Kidney Dis 1998;31:502–508.

33   Schneditz D, Wang E, Levin NW: Validation of haemodialysis recirculation and access blood flow measured by thermodilution. Nephrol Dial Transplant 1999;14:376–383.

34   Bos C, Smits JH, Zijistra JJ, Blankestijn PJ, Bakker CJ, Viergever MA: Underestimation of access flow by ultrasound dilution flow measurements. Phys Med Biol 2002;47:481–489.

35   Sakiewicz PG, Paganini EP, Wright E: Introduction of a switch that can reverse blood flow direction on-line during hemodialysis. ASAIO J 2000;46:464–468.

36   Krivitski N: Errors of access flow dilution methods resulting from procedural technique, EDTA (abstract). Nephrol Dial Transplant 2003;18(suppl 1):296.

37   Lindsay RM, Blake PG, Malek P, Posen G, Martin B, Bradfield E: Hemodialysis access blood flow rates can be measured by a differential conductivity technique and are predictive of access clotting. Am J Kidney Dis 1997;30:475–482.

38   Tonelli M, Jindal K, Hirsh D, Taylor S, Kane C, Henbrey S: Screening for subclinical stenosis in native vessel arteriovenous fistulae. J Am Soc Nephrol 2001;12:1729–1733.

39   Tessitore N, Mansueto G, Bedogna V, Poli A, Gammaro L, Baggio E, Morana G, Loschiavo C, Laudon A, Oldrizzi L, Maschio G: A prospective control trail of affect of percutaneous transluminal angioplasty on functional arteriovenous fistulae survival. J Am Soc Nephrol 2003;14: 1623–1627.

40   Bosman PJ, Boereboom FTJ, Eikelboom BC, Koomans HA, Blankenstijn PJ: Graft flow as predictor of thrombosis in hemodialysis grafts. Kidney Int 1998;54:1726–1730.

41   May RE, Himmelfarb J, Yenicesu M, Knights S, Ikizler TA, Schulman G, Heranz-Schulman M, Shyr Y, Hakim RM: Predictive measures of vascular access thrombosis: A prospective study. Kidney Int 1997;52:1656–1662.

42   Neyra NR, Ikizler TA, May RE, Himmelfarb J, Schulman G, Shyr Y, Hakim RM: Change in access blood flow over time predicts vascular access thrombosis. Kidney Int 1998;54:1714–1719.

43   Sands JJ, Jabyac PA, Miranda CL, Kapsick BJ: Intervention based on monthly monitoring decreases hemodialysis access thrombosis. ASAIO J 1999;45:147–150.

44   Schon D, Mishler R: Salvage of occluded autologous arteriovenous fistulae. Am J Kidney Dis 2000;36:804–810.

45   Schwab SJ, Oliver MJ, Suhocki P, McCann R: Hemodialysis arteriovenous access: Detection of stenosis and response to treatment by vascular access blood flow. Kidney Int 2001;59:358–362.

46   Wang E, Schneditz D, Nepomuceno C, Lavarias V, Martin K, Morris AT, Levin NW: Predictive value of access blood flow in detecting access thrombosis. ASAIO J 1998;44:M555–M558.

47   McCarley P, Wingard RL, Shur Y, Pettus W, Hakim RM, Ikizler TA: Vascular access blood flow monitoring reduces access morbidity and costs. Kidney Int 2001;60:1164–1172.

48   Van Der Linden J, Smits JHM, Assink JH, Wolterbeek DW, Zijlstra JJ, De Jong GHT, Van Den Dorpel MA, Blankestign PJ: Short- and long-term functional effects of percutaneous transluminal angioplasty in hemodialysis vascular access. J Am Soc Nephrol 2002;33:708–714.

49   Tonelli M, Hirsh D, Clark T, Wile C, Mossop P, Marryatt J, Jindal K: Access flow monitoring with native vessel arteriovenous fistulae and previous angioplasty. J Am Soc Nephrol 2002;13: 2969–2973.

50   McDougal G, Agarwal R: Clinical performance characteristics of hemodialysis graft monitoring. Kidney Int 2001;60:762–766.

51   Ram SJ, Work J, Caldito GC, Eason JM, Pervez A, Paulson WD: A randomized controlled trial of blood flow and stenosis surveillance of hemodialysis grafts. Kidney Int 2003;64:272–280.

Nikolai M. Krivitski, PhD, DSc,
Transonic Systems, Inc.,
34 Dutch Mill Road, Ithaca, NY 14850 (USA)
Tel. +1 607 257 5300, Fax +1 607 257 7256, E-Mail nikolai.krivitski@transonic.com

Ronco C, Levin NW (eds): Hemodialysis Vascular Access and Peritoneal Dialysis Access.
Contrib Nephrol. Basel, Karger, 2004, vol 142, pp 285–322

....

Interventional Techniques for Malfunctioning Accesses

Joseph Shams

Albert Einstein College of Medicine, Division of Vascular and Interventional
Radiology, Beth Israel Medical Center, New York, N.Y.

Vascular access failure is a major source of morbidity, mortality, and
expense for patients undergoing hemodialysis. Vascular access complications
account for up to USD 1 billion in expenditure, 15% of hospitalizations and
many of the longest hospital stays for patients on hemodialysis in the United
States [1, 2]. Percutaneous endovascular techniques have revolutionized maintenance of hemodialysis access by prolonging the life span of failing grafts and
fistulae and allowing rapid recanalization of occluded accesses [3, 4]. This
chapter will discuss the various techniques available to the interventionalist for
treatment of the failing or failed dialysis access at the present time.

Vascular access is defined as a conduit to draw blood from and return
blood to a patient's circulation for hemodialysis. Access may include a native
arteriovenous (AV) fistula, a prosthetic bridge graft interposed between an
artery and a vein, or a double lumen central venous catheter. According to the
National Kidney Foundation/Kidney Disease Dialysis Outcomes Quality
Initiative (DOQI), a native AV fistula is the access of choice for patient's requiring long-term hemodialysis [5]. Native fistulae include radiocephalic, brachiocephalic and transposed brachiobasilic vein fistulae. The radiocephalic fistula
is the preferred and most common native hemodialysis fistula. This fistula is
created via surgical end-to-side anastomosis of the cephalic vein to the radial
artery near the wrist. The brachiocephalic fistula, with a higher incidence of
development of high-flow steal syndrome as compared to the wrist fistula, is
created via surgical anastomosis of the brachial artery to the cephalic vein in
the region of the antecubital fossa. Transposed brachiobasilic vein fistulae are
created via surgical mobilization of the basilic vein in the upper arm, which is
tunneled through a superficial subcutaneous tract to allow percutaneous access

for hemodialysis. Native fistulae have the distinct advantage of improved long-term patency as compared to grafts, as well as decreased infectious and thrombotic complications. Disadvantages include a 4- to 16-week requirement of fistula maturation prior to initial use as well as a 4–30% maturation failure rate [5, guideline 9].

Interposition bridge grafts are typically constructed using tubular 6-mm polytetrafluoroethylene (PTFE) graft material that is tunneled subcutaneously and anastomosed to an inflow artery and an outflow vein. Upper extremity grafts include a forearm U-loop graft from the brachial artery to the basilic or cephalic vein at or near the antecubital fossa, a straight graft from the radial artery at the wrist to the basilic or cephalic vein at the elbow, and a C-loop graft from the brachial artery to the basilic, brachial or axillary veins in the mid to upper portion of the upper arm. Composite grafts, with a synthetic graft anastomosed to a venous remnant of a native fistula, may be used to salvage a failed or failing fistula. Subclavian artery to ipsilateral subclavian venous shunts may be created but are associated with poor long-term patency. If no access site within the upper extremities is available, a lower extremity loop graft from the superficial femoral artery to the saphenous vein is constructed.

Central venous catheters are large bore (13–15 french) double-lumen catheters which allow rapid blood flow exchange required for hemodialysis. Complications of these devices have been discussed in previous chapters.

Treatment of Failing Dialysis Bypass Grafts

The bane of the dialysis graft and fistula is the development of stenoses at predictable sites, which eventually result in access failure (fig. 1). According to DOQI, 85–90% of dialysis graft thromboses are associated with venous outflow stenotic lesions caused by endothelial and fibromuscular hyperplasia [5, guideline 19]. Stenoses may also occur at the arterial anastomosis within the graft or within the central veins. Native fistulae develop stenoses at or just beyond the AV anastomosis and within the venous outflow. Treatment of these lesions prior to access failure has been shown to lengthen the life of the access.

Surveillance is a major component of dialysis access maintenance. Schwab et al. [6] were among the first investigators to publish data supporting prophylactic balloon angioplasty of venous stenoses to prevent graft thrombosis. Venous pressures were measured in a series of 168 patients on a monthly basis. Patients with venous pressure elevation >150 mm Hg were referred for angiography and balloon angioplasty. 86% of patients with significant pressure elevations were shown to have venous stenoses by angiography. Patients with venous pressure elevation >150 mm Hg who underwent angiography and

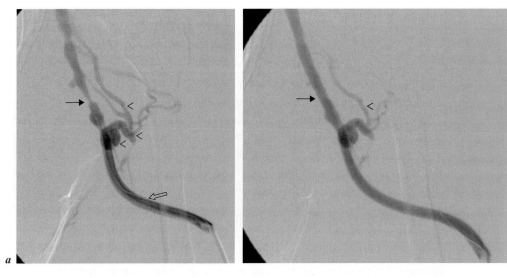

Fig. 1. Digital subtraction images from angiographic study of left upper arm loop graft in a patient who presented with low access blood flow. *a* Venous graft limb (open arrow) is widely patent. Focal narrowing (arrow) is identified within the outflow basilic vein beyond the graft/venous anastomosis. Note prominent collateral (arrowheads) proximal to the stenosis. *b* Following angioplasty with an 8 mm × 4 cm balloon, wide vessel patency is noted (arrow). Note decreased opacification of collaterals consistent with improved blood flow through the basilic vein.

percutaneous angioplasty of an underlying stenosis had 0.15 episodes of graft thrombosis per patient-year while patients with elevated pressures who underwent no treatment had 1.4 episodes of graft thrombosis per patient-year. Sands et al. [7] confirmed these findings using access blood flow measurement with the Transonics device (Transonic HD01 hemodialysis monitor; Transonic Systems, Ithaca, N.Y., USA). Several other studies have confirmed the utility of surveillance programs utilizing various parameters [8–11].

Several indicators have been identified which correlate with developing access stenoses. These include poor palpable thrill or conversion of a normal thrill to pulse, increasing Kt/V, blood flow <600 ml/min by Transonic blood flow measurement or 25% decrease in baseline blood flow, increased recirculation within the graft, elevated venous pressures, difficult placement of dialysis needles, extremity edema, and increased time to hemostasis following dialysis. When indicators are suggestive of potential graft failure, the patient should be referred for angiographic evaluation of the access.

Angiographic evaluation of the access (fistulagram) may be performed on an outpatient basis and should include evaluation of the arterial inflow, anastomoses of the graft with the inflow artery and the outflow vein, the graft itself and the outflow vein to the level of the right atrium.

Patient Evaluation

Preoperative evaluation of the patient should include a directed history and physical examination. A history of coronary artery disease, pulmonary disease, diabetes mellitus, and hypertension should be noted. Time of the patient's last hemodialysis session should be documented. If an allergy to iodinated contrast is noted, premedication with steroids (prednisone 50 mg p.o. q.d. ×3 days or 50 mg prednisone 24 h and Solucortef 100 mg i.v. 2 h before the procedure) should be considered. (Alternatively, a contrast study may be performed with gadolinium or CO_2 contrast, which will be discussed later.) Some interventionalists recommend the routine use of prophylactic antibiotics. However, most reserve them for selected, high-risk cases. If the patient is on anticoagulant medication, elective studies may be deferred until the coagulation profile is normalized. Diabetic patients should not receive NPH insulin on the morning of their study and should only receive half their normal regular insulin dose.

Physical examination should include evaluation of the heart and lungs. If wet rales are present at the lung bases, elective studies should be deferred as the patient may develop fluid redistribution and respiratory insufficiency when placed in the supine position on the procedure table. Arterial pulses proximal and distal to the access should be recorded.

The vascular access should be carefully examined. If there is evidence of erythema, swelling or tenderness to palpation overlying the access, particularly a prosthetic graft, graft infection should be suspected and the patient referred to an access surgeon for evaluation. The location, course and orientation of the arterial and venous limbs of a bridge graft should be determined. Any extension (jump) grafts should be noted as well as scars or sutures from previous surgical revision. Old grafts and fistula sites should also be examined as they may give clues to the cause of present access dysfunction.

If a graft is patent, the arterial limb may be identified via graft compression. The venous limb will collapse and pulsation will be lost beyond the site of compression while the arterial limb will remain pulsatile. Dampening of palpable thrill or ausculatory bruit with development of increasing pulsatility is consistent with a venous outflow lesion. Graft pulsatility, which does not increase in intensity with compression of the venous anastomosis, is also indicative of an outflow lesion. A faintly palpable pulse within the graft may be the result of an inflow lesion or may indicate imminent graft thrombosis. Absence of palpable thrill with absence of an auculatory bruit using a stethoscope is consistent with graft thrombosis.

Shams

Contraindications

Absolute contraindications to balloon dilatation include graft infection as noted previously. A patient with symptoms of vascular steal syndrome, such a cool, cyanotic hand with poor or absent radial pulse which improves during graft compression, should not undergo percutaneous angioplasty of a venous outflow lesion as this will exacerbate steal symptoms. Percutaneous angioplasty of a newly constructed surgical anastomosis should not be performed until several weeks have passed from the date of construction.

Technique

The patient is placed supine on the angiographic table and the extremity prepped in a sterile fashion. We routinely administer sedative medication (Versed 1 mg and fentanyl 50 μg) intravenously prior to the procedure. The graft is accessed via single wall puncture with an 18-gauge wing-tipped needle (Cook, Bloomington, Ind., USA) or a 21-gauge micropuncture needle (Cook). For right-handed operators, holding the graft in place with the thumb and forefinger of the left hand may facilitate puncture. A shallow needle angle (no greater than 30–45°) should be used to allow easy passage of the wire through the graft limb. If a venous anastomotic lesion is suspected, antegrade puncture of the outflow limb of the loop graft is performed. After exchanging for a 0.035-inch guidewire, a 5- or 6-french vascular sheath is placed. A preliminary fistula gram is performed to delineate venous outflow lesions. Examination should include evaluation of the central outflow veins to the level of the right atrium. Contrast injection through the sheath while obstructing graft outflow via manual compression or by inflating a balloon within the venous (outflow) graft limb will provide retrograde opacification of the arterial (inflow) graft limb and the arterial anastomosis.

If an inflow lesion is identified, a second puncture aiming towards the arterial anastomosis will be required. If more than one lesion is suspected prior to initial puncture, apical puncture of the graft may be considered. For this technique, described by Hathaway and Vesely [12], an initial puncture is made at the apex (tip of loop) of the graft through a 1- to 2-cm subcutaneous tunnel. The side of the graft is punctured. A sheath is placed aiming towards the venous outflow. When venous manipulations have been completed, the sheath may be redirected towards the arterial graft limb using a reversed curve catheter without requiring additional graft puncture.

If a venous lesion is identified, 3,000–5,000 units of heparin are administered intravenously and the lesion crossed with a floppy or hydrophilic guidewire. (Some operators do not routinely administer heparin.) An appropriately sized balloon catheter should be selected, determined by the diameter of the PTFE graft and the outflow vein. In general, a balloon size 10–20%

greater than the vessel diameter is selected. In our practice, we typically use 7-mm balloons for venous lesions at or distal to the antecubital fossa and 8-mm balloons for lesions within upper arm veins. As these lesions represent areas of neointimal hyperplasia, they may be highly resistant to balloon dilatation. We routinely use high-pressure balloons (Conquest, Bard) with rated inflation pressures up to 30 mm Hg. If a lesion is resistant to dilatation, repeated inflations with prolonged inflation times (1–5 min) should be attempted initially. If the lesion is still unresponsive, an atherectomy device may be used to create a small tear within the lesion, making it more amenable to dilatation with a balloon [13]. However, atherectomy devices are expensive and are not widely accepted for this indication in the US. Cutting balloons or balloons with small, sharp metallic strips embedded in the balloon wall have been used successfully for this indication [14, 15] but are currently only available, on a limited basis in the US, in small-diameter (4 mm) sizes. The use of larger diameter cutting balloons is presently under investigation in clinical trials. We have successfully used a 'buddy wire' technique whereby a stiff, 0.035 Amplatz guidewire is advanced across the lesion adjacent to the balloon. (This will require placement of a larger sheath.) The balloon is then inflated and the wire 'embedded' into the lesion mimicking a cutting balloon. The wire is then removed and the lesion redilated with a high-pressure balloon. If all attempts fail, the patient should be referred for surgical revision. Stents should *not* be deployed across these lesions as the radial force of the presently available stents will not overcome the stenosis.

Following successful angioplasty, fistulography is repeated. If greater than 30% residual stenosis is present, the graft remains highly pulsatile with minimal thrill, or if pressure measurements are suggestive of persistent stenosis, repeated inflation with a larger balloon (1 mm diameter larger) should be considered. If still unresponsive, a stent may be deployed across the lesion or the patient referred for surgical revision (fig. 2).

Intimal hyperplastic lesions may be associated with significant elastic recoil. Some interventionalists recommend waiting 15 min after successful angioplasty to perform final fistulography to determine if a recoiling lesion is present. This technique should be considered in patients with rapidly recurring stenoses.

Central vein stenoses are a rare cause of graft failure. Symptomatic lesions occur in 5–17% in the dialysis population [13]. Most patients present with worsening arm swelling resulting from unilateral subclavian or brachiocephalic lesions. Bilateral upper extremity or facial swelling may result from superior vena cava or bilateral central venous lesions. Most lesions are related to previously placed central venous catheters that initially cause trauma to the vessel wall, exacerbated by high, turbulent flow within the vessel, leading to the

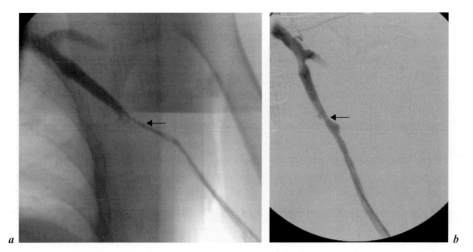

Fig. 2. Images from angiographic study of a dialysis patient who presented with recurrent episodes of thrombosis of his left upper arm C-loop graft. *a* Following graft thrombectomy and angioplasty of a venous anastomotic stenosis the previous day, the patient returned with a pulsatile graft and elevated venous pressures during dialysis. Note recoiling of the stenosis at the angioplasty site (arrow). *b* A 10 × 48 mm wallstent was deployed across the lesion and dilated with a 8 mm × 4 cm angioplasty balloon with an excellent cosmetic result. Good thrill was palpated within the graft at termination of the procedure.

formation of intimal hyperplasia and fibrosis within the vessel [16]. Subclavian venous stenoses are most commonly seen, followed by brachiocephalic and superior vena cava lesions. These stenoses can be treated via dilatation with 10–16 mm angioplasty balloons depending on vessel size (fig. 3). Most studies report technical success between 70 and 100% and 6-month patency of 13–38%. In view of these findings, some interventionalists have advocated the routine use of stents for central venous stenoses. In a series of 50 patients, Haage et al. [17] treated 57 central venous lesions with primary wallstent placement with 100% technical success and 1 episode of early rethrombosis. Primary patency at 3, 6, 12 and 24 months was 92, 84, 56 and 28%, respectively. Secondary patency at 6, 12, 24 and 48 months was 97, 97, 89 and 81%, respectively. DOQI [5, guideline 20] guidelines recommend central vein stent placement for angioplasty failure secondary to elastic recoil or for early recurrence (<3 months) following an initially successful PTA.

In our practice, we advocate a conservative approach which limits central venous stenting to lesions that have recurred twice within a 6-month period, recoiling lesions (lesions with >50% residual stenosis following PTA), venous ruptures resulting from balloon angioplasty and occlusions. Stent placement has been

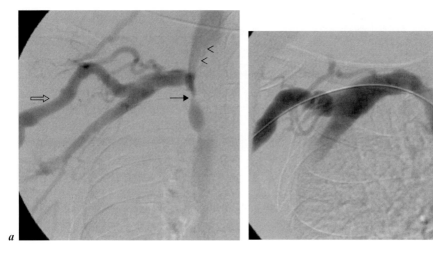

Fig. 3. Digital subtraction and fluoroscopic images from angiographic study of a patient with a right upper arm brachiocephalic fistula who presents with arm swelling. The patient was dialyzed through a right internal jugular permcath for several months prior to maturation of his fistula. *a* The cephalic outflow vein (open arrow) is widely patent. Severe focal narrowing of the proximal and distal segments of the brachiocephalic vein is seen (arrow). Note contrast reflux into the right internal jugular vein (arrowheads). The lesions were dilated with a 14 × 4 cm balloon (not shown). *b* Postangioplasty fistulagram demonstrates wide patency of the brachiocephalic vein.

shown to at least double the long-term patency rate [13]. However, supplementary collateral channels covered by the stent are compromised leading to worsening extremity edema when stent occlusion invariably occurs. Also, central branch veins (internal and external jugular and contralateral innominate) may be covered and therefore compromise future dialysis catheter access (fig. 4). If treatment with angioplasty is chosen, repeat fistulagrams should be performed every 2–3 months and recurrent lesions aggressively retreated to prevent vessel occlusion.

We reserve peripheral stent placement for stenoses that are surgically inaccessible or for acute venous ruptures. We believe that surgical revision should remain the first line therapy for stenoses that are suboptimally treated with balloon angioplasty.

In patients with residual renal function that the nephrologist does not wish to jeopardize or in patients with severe iodine contrast allergies, angiographic evaluation may be performed with carbon dioxide (CO_2) or gadolinium.

Complications

Complications occur in <2–3% of cases and most are easily treated. Complications include allergic reaction to contrast, vessel rupture during

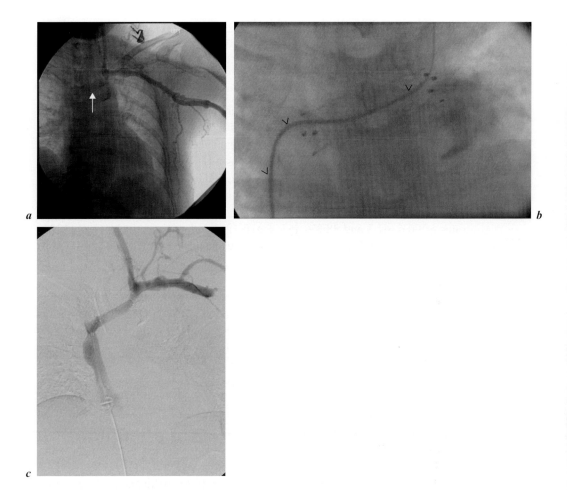

Fig. 4. 55-year-old woman presents with a failing left radiocephalic fistula and chronic left arm swelling. Fistulagram (not shown) demonstrated patency of the radial artery with a high-grade juxta-anastomotic stenosis that was successfully treated via angioplasty with a 6-mm balloon. ***a*** Evaluation of central veins demonstrates occlusion of the left braciocephalic venous stent (arrow). Contrast drainage (not shown) was across the neck and into the right internal jugular venous system. Attempts to cross the braciocephalic vein occlusion were unsuccessful. ***b*** The patient was brought back 3 weeks later for attempted recanalization of braciocephalic vein via retrograde femoral approach. Note catheter (arrowheads) extending through the stent. ***c*** Following dilatation with 12- and 14-mm balloons, the stent is widely patent.

angioplasty, vessel perforation or dissection, graft thrombosis and angioplasty balloon rupture. Most vessel perforations may be treated conservatively with prolonged balloon inflation or stent placement. Although uncovered stents have been utilized successfully for the treatment of perforations, the use of newly available covered stents may provide durable treatment of these lesions. For a more extensive discussion of complications, the reader is referred to the Complications section of Treatment of the Thrombosed Dialysis Graft.

Results

Glanz et al. [18] reported one of the earliest series of percutaneous balloon dilatation for the salvage of hemodialysis access in 1984. In a series of 56 balloon dilatations, they reported a technical success rate of 70% with a complication rate of 5%. Primary patency rates reported were 80, 70, 55, 50, and 33% at 3 months, 6 months, 1 year, 2 years, and 3 years, respectively. Beathard [19] reported a series of 536 percutaneous angioplasty procedures for graft salvage in 1992. He reported a technical success of 94% with primary patency rates of 90.6, 61.3 and 38.2% at 3, 6 and 12 months, respectively. Gray [13] in a review of multiple studies reported primary patency rates of 38–64 and 10–40% at 6 and 12 months, respectively. Secondary patency rates were reported as 85 and 79% at 6 and 12 months, respectively.

SIR guidelines determine anatomic success as less than 30% residual stenosis at the venous angioplasty site following PTA and clinical success as resolution or normalization of the clinical parameter which initiated the study [20]. Anatomic success may not result in clinical success and vice versa. Schwab et al. [21] noted that in a study of vascular access blood flow following angioplasty, 21% of patients did not improve their baseline blood flow measurement by more than 20%. van der Linden et al. [22] also measuring access flow following PTA noted a 34% incidence of <600 ml/min blood flow in treated grafts and a 50% incidence in treated native fistulae. Funaki et al. [23], in a study of venous stenoses following angioplasty using pullback pressure measurements, found that 18% of lesions had significant pressure gradients across them following PTA requiring further treatment with larger balloons. In our practice, each patient who undergoes an angioplasty or recanalization procedure has access blood flow measured at the dialysis unit within 24–72 h following the procedure. If the results are abnormal, the patient is returned to the angiography suite for redilatation with a larger angioplasty balloon or stent placement.

Treatment of the Thrombosed Dialysis Byass Graft

Dialysis graft thrombosis remains a major source of morbidity for dialysis patients. In the past, patients frequently required hospital admission for graft recanalization and would miss dialysis treatments. Percutaneous recanalization techniques have revolutionized the rapid outpatient treatment of this clinical problem with substantial benefit for dialysis patients.

Prior to the development of percutaneous techniques, surgical thrombec-tomy with or without revision of the venous anastomosis was the primary method of treatment for hemodialysis graft thrombosis. Surgical thrombectomy is performed via access to the graft through a short incision overlying the venous graft limb. Thrombectomy is performed via passage of a compliant Fogarty balloon catheter in both the arterial and venous directions. Vascular dilators are then passed through the venous anastomosis and outflow veins in an attempt to uncover any underlying venous stenoses. If difficulty in passage of the dilators is noted, surgical revision (patch angioplasty) of the venous anas-tomosis, jump graft placement to a more central vein or new graft placement is performed. Alternatively, the patient is referred for percutaneous angioplasty of the venous outflow lesion.

With the advent of minimally invasive techniques, percutaneous therapy has quickly become the gold standard for recanalization of thrombosed grafts. The dialysis graft is uniquely suited to percutaneous recanalization. In vivo measurement has determined that only about $3\,cm^3$ of thrombus is typically present within a nonaneurysmal, thrombosed hemodialysis graft. Acute throm-bus tends to be soft or poorly adherent to the graft wall. The graft is generally easily palpable, may be accessed percutaneously with minimal effort, and is a closed system with single inflow and outflow vessels, allowing controlled thrombolysis or thrombectomy.

Percutaneous therapy has several advantages over surgical thrombectomy. The procedure can be performed in a single session on an outpatient basis and the patient can return home or to the dialysis unit immediately following the procedure. The graft may be evaluated angiographically and all underlying lesions contributing to graft failure may be identified and treated. Postoperative discom-fort and edema are minimized as no surgical incisions are made. As opposed to surgical thrombectomy with revision, where the graft may not be able to be used for 24–72 h following the procedure, the graft may be used immediately and sheaths used during the procedure may be utilized for hemodialysis. No tempo-rary dialysis catheter need be placed. This decreases expenses as well as the thrombotic and infectious complication risk of hemodialysis catheters. Several studies have shown comparable patency rates, procedure time and complications associated with both therapies although procedure-related costs may vary [24, 25].

Patient Selection
Preoperative evaluation of the patient with a thrombosed dialysis graft should be performed in similar fashion to that of the patient with a patent graft (please refer to the preceding section on the Treatment of Failing Dialysis Bypass Grafts). In addition, several contraindications to graft recanalization should be noted.

Graft infection is an absolute contraindication to graft thrombolysis. Attempted thrombolysis of an access with an infected clot may precipitate bacteremia, septic emboli or frank sepsis. Typical signs of graft infection include erythema surrounding the graft, overlying skin which is warm and tender to palpation, and fluctuance of the overlying soft tissues secondary to edema or frank abscess formation. Late signs include purulent discharge from the graft or skin breakdown. Signs should be distinguished from a localized allergic reaction, such as a reaction to tape, in which case the reaction is localized to the borders of the inciting agents. If the diagnosis is in doubt, aspiration of graft thrombus or purulent fluid may be performed. If graft infection is suspected, the patient should be immediately referred to an access surgeon for evaluation and possible graft removal.

Patients with severe cardiopulmonary disease should be considered for surgical thrombectomy. Thrombus fragments invariably escape from the graft during percutaneous recanalization procedures and embolize to the lungs. These small emboli are generally well tolerated by most patients but may lead to acute respiratory decompensation in patients with compromised cardiopulmonary status. Patients with pulmonary hypertension, baseline room air oxygen saturation of <90%, right-sided heart failure or right to left shunts should be referred for surgical thrombectomy, as this will allow controlled clamp occlusion of the outflow vein preventing central embolization. (Mortality was recently reported secondary to paradoxical embolus through a right to left shunt with the development of massive stroke and death.)

If occlusion occurs less than 2–4 weeks following surgical creation of a graft, it is most likely the result of a surgical technical problem. As graft incorporation into the subcutaneous tissues may not have occurred yet in these newly placed grafts, bleeding into the adjacent soft tissue may develop rapidly and may be poorly controlled. In our practice, we avoid use of thrombolytic agents in these patients but we will recanalize these grafts using mechanical thrombectomy and aspiration devices beginning 4–5 days following graft creation. Although a high incidence of rapid reocclusion is noted in these patients, percutaneous recanalization may uncover an underlying lesion that may be corrected surgically. Percutaneous angioplasty of a recent surgical anastomosis should be avoided or approached with gentle, submaximal angioplasty balloon inflation to avoid rupture of the anastomosis.

Absolute contraindications to the administration of thrombolytic agents include recent stroke (<3 months), recent head trauma, uncontrolled hypertension and active bleeding. Recent abdominal surgery is a relative contraindication. Hemodialysis patients, particularly elderly ones, may be prone to falling episodes and any recent head trauma should be carefully investigated prior to administration of thrombolytic agents.

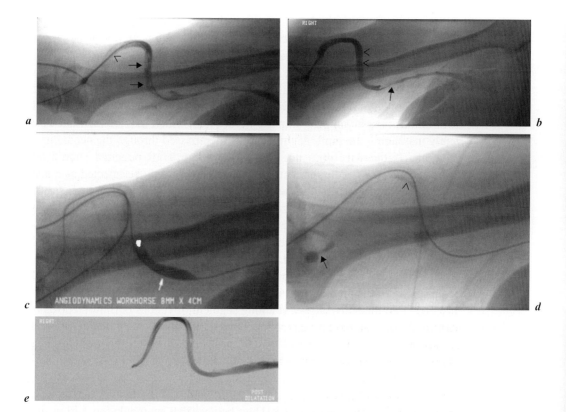

Fig. 5. 49-year-old female who presents with thrombosis of her right upper arm C-loop dialysis graft. *a* The graft was accessed in its arterial limb aiming cephalad and a sheath placed (arrowhead). Contrast injection demonstrates thrombus (arrows) throughout the graft. *b* Clot removed via aspiration thrombectomy. No significant residual thrombus noted within the graft (arrowhead). Note venous anastomotic stenosis (arrow) with minimal adjacent thrombus. *c* Venous anastomotic stenosis is dilated with an 8-mm angioplasty balloon. *d* Arterial plug is dislodged using a Fogarty balloon (arrow) introduced through a crossing sheath (arrowhead). Note how this noncompliant balloon conforms to the contour of the anastomotic site. The balloon catheter is gently withdrawn into the graft. *e* Final angiogram demonstrates wide graft patency with excellent antegrade contrast flow.

Technique

Three basic steps are required for percutaneous recanalization of a dialysis bypass graft: (1) clot removal or lysis, (2) percutaneous angioplasty of underlying arterial inflow, intragraft or venous outflow stenoses and (3) dislodgment and/or maceration of the arterial plug (fig. 5).

The graft is initially punctured in its arterial limb (segment of graft closest to the AV anastomosis) aiming towards the venous outflow. Puncture should be performed approximately 2–3 cm beyond the AV anastomosis as grafts may taper from 6 to 4 mm in diameter proximal to this region. In our practice, we prefer to access the graft with an 18-gauge wing-tipped needle (Cook) or a 21-gauge micropuncture needle (Cook). With the 18-gauge needle, a faint 'popping' or 'give' will be felt as the graft wall is traversed. In a thrombosed graft, no frank blood return will be noted from the needle. However, dark blood or thrombus may be noted within the needle hub, which may be facilitated by gently massaging the graft. A guidewire is then passed through the needle into the graft. If the wire does not pass easily, extra graft puncture should be suspected and the needle redirected. Contrast should only be injected as a last resort as extraluminal contrast will obscure the graft during the remainder of the procedure. Once an intragraft position is confirmed, a 4- to 5-french Berenstein (AngioDynamics) is advanced into the venous outflow and an upper extremity venogram is performed. The entire venous outflow including the central veins should be evaluated. Of note, if contrast is injected into the throm-bosed graft itself prior to clot removal, contrast should be injected gently and compression of the arterial graft limb should be performed to prevent reflux of thrombus into the native artery. If a long segment of venous outflow stenosis is identified, some authors have recommended terminating the procedure prior to graft recanalization while others have described success treating these lesions. In most cases, a single venous anastomotic lesion amenable to balloon dilata-tion is uncovered.

Cynamon and Pierpont [26] advocate dilatation of the venous anastomotic lesion prior to thrombus removal. They believe that manipulation within the graft during thrombus removal or lysis will predispose to arterial embolization unless an exit pathway is provided. In our practice, the venous anastomotic lesion is dilated following thrombus removal. Prior to venous dilatation, a close system is present which allows easy thrombus removal or lysis. This method also prevents significant embolization of the thrombus to the lungs. We have not found an increased incidence of arterial embolization with this method.

Clot Removal

As long-term graft patency is related to the treatment of underlying stenoses and not thrombus removal, any method that adequately removes the thrombus may be utilized. Several methods have been described for percuta-neous dissolution of thrombus. Thrombolysis of occluded dialysis grafts was initially described approximately 20 years ago utilizing streptokinase [27] and later with continuous infusion of urokinase [28]. In these initial studies, continuous infusion of urokinase through an end-hole catheter lodged within the thrombus was performed over a 2- to 20-hour period. Technical success rates ranged from 49 to 79% as significant residual thrombus remained within the graft following infusion and bleeding complications were exceedingly high. With the advent of pulse spray infusion technique, pharmacomechanical thrombolysis became the preferred method of clot lysis for dialysis grafts. With this technique, the graft is accessed in each limb in a crisscrossing fashion. 4- to 5-french multi-side-hole infusion catheters are placed into the graft. 250,000 units of urokinase or 3–5 mg of alteplase are reconstituted with saline or sterile water in a defined volume (5–50 ml). The thrombolytic agent is then injected through the infusion catheters in short, 0.2- to 1-ml pulses, adding a 'jet-spray' effect to the administration of the agent. The thrombolytic agent is administered over a 5- to 60-min interval. In an initial series [29], technical success was achieved in 97.9% of cases with a mean infusion time of 49 min. In a 1995 series, Valji et al. [30] compared pulse spray infusion with continuous thrombolytic infusion for the treatment of thrombosed grafts. Infusion time decreased from 44 to 23 min and initial success increased from 86 to 96% with a 92% patency at 24 h. Beathard [31] described pulse spray infusion of heparinized saline solution with a similar technical success and patency rates.

'Lyse and Wait'

The 'lyse and wait' technique has been widely accepted in United States since first described by Cynamon et al. [32] in 1999. It has since been described using alteplase [33], retaplase [34] and low-dose (5,000 to 10,000 units) urokinase [35]. The patient is brought into the radiology recovery or holding area and the skin overlying the access is prepped in a sterile fashion. An 18- to 22-gauge Angiocath (using an 18-gauge Angiocath allows placement of a 0.035-inch guidewire through it but leaves a larger hole if the graft is not accessed properly) or a 21-gauge micropuncture needle is placed into the arterial graft limb aiming towards the venous outflow. The thrombolytic agent (2–5 mg TPA or 250,000 units of urokinase) is injected into the graft while the arterial and venous graft limbs are compressed. The catheter is capped and the patient observed in the holding area. Heparin may also be injected into the graft but should not be mixed with the thrombolytic agent to avoid precipitation. After waiting 30–90 min, the patient is brought into the angiographic suite and the access site is reprepped. A venogram is then performed frequently demonstrating minimal to no residual clot within the graft. Treatment of the venous outflow lesion and the arterial plug is then performed. The advantage of this technique is that it allows thrombolysis to occur before the patient enters the angiographic suite decreasing patient time on the angiographic table. As less time is expended on thrombus removal, attention may be focused on evaluating and treating the lesion that led to graft failure. Disadvantages of this technique include bleeding from previous dialysis puncture or attempted puncture sites. (Dialysis nurses should be educated to avoid punctures of thrombosed grafts to confirm graft occlusion.) If a patient bleeds from one of these sites and bleeding is poorly controlled with manual compression, a 4-french dilator may be placed through the puncture wound to occlude it or a small purse-string suture may be placed across the site. Other disadvantages of this technique include injection of a thrombolytic agent prior to evaluation of the venous outflow (vein may not be amenable to percutaneous treatment), poor lysis of thrombus within pseudoaneurysms and a possible increased risk of arterial embolization with overaggressive thrombolytic injection.

Mechanical Thrombectomy

Thrombus may also be removed or macerated into small fragments with mechanical thrombectomy devices [36, 37]. The following devices have been approved by the US Food and Drug Administration for use in hemodialysis access grafts: Amplatz thrombectomy device (Microvena, White Bear Lake, Minn., USA), Arrow-Trerotola percutaneous thrombolytic device (Arrow, Reading, Pa., USA), Cragg-Castaneda thrombolytic brush (Microtherapeutics, Aliso Viejo, Calif., USA), AngioJet (Possis, Minneapolis, Minn., USA), Oasis Thrombectomy System (Boston Scientific/Medi-tech, Natick, Mass., USA), Hydrolyser (Cordis, Miami, Fla., USA), Gelbfish-Endovasc device (NeoVascular Technologies, Brooklyn, N.Y., USA), and the PMT device (Baxter, Irvine, Calif., USA).

Thrombectomy devices may be classified as 'wall contact' or as hydrodynamic/vortex aspiration devices. Wall contact devices include the Arrow-Trerotola device (rotating modified stone basket) and Castaneda and Cragg devices (rotating brushes).These devices use a rapidly spinning basket or brush to fragment the thrombus into small particles. The remaining particulate thrombus may be aspirated through a vascular sheath or embolized to the central venous circulation. Disadvantages of these devices include endothelial damage caused by wall contact and possible distal embolization of large particulate thrombi prior to adequate maceration with the device. In addition, these devices may suffer reduction in rotational speed when used across sharp corners, such as in loop grafts.

Hydrodynamic devices include the Possis, Oasis and Thrombex PMT devices. These devices create a hydrodynamic vortex using powerful saline jets or a rotating high-speed micropropeller. Because the pressure is lower in a moving fluid than in a stationary fluid, flowing objects (i.e., thrombi) will be sucked into the vortex. The vortex converts the thrombus into a thick slurry that is then aspirated through the catheter. The advantage of these devices is that the thrombus is aspirated and not embolized to lungs. A disadvantage of these devices is that if partial flow is restored to the graft, further thrombectomy will be suboptimal, as blood as opposed to thrombus will be drawn into the vortex.

The most commonly used devices in United States are the Arrow-Trerotola device and the Possis device. The Arrow device is disposable and comes with its own handheld motor apparatus. The Possis device requires an expensive stationary pump unit with a disposable catheter.

Fresh thrombus is easily treated with all available devices. Thrombus within pseudoaneurysms tends to be chronic in nature and resistant to fragmentation with hydrodynamic devices. The Arrow device is useful in this setting particularly when the pseudoaneurysm is compressed while the device is activated [38]. This maneuver allows contact of the basket wires with the entire extent of the thrombus. Residual particulate matter should be aspirated through the introducer sheath.

Both devices may be deployed over guidewires that are especially helpful in grafts with multiple pseudoaneurysms or tortuous segments. The over-the-wire Arrow device requires introduction through a 7-french sheath (6 french for the standard device) while the Possis Xpedior catheter may be placed through a 6-french sheath. The thrombectomy device is advanced to the venous end of the graft, activated and slowly withdrawn. The sheath may be aspirated following each pass of the catheter. Multiple passes may be performed until the limb is clear of thrombus. A sheath may then be placed aiming towards the arterial graft limb, allowing clearance of thrombus from this limb using the thrombectomy device. Alternatively, if only a small amount of thrombus is identified within this limb, residual clot may be macerated with an angioplasty or Fogarty balloon. Native venous thrombus, whether present initially or following manipulation, is best treated with the Possis device.

Aspiration Thrombectomy

Aspiration thrombectomy is the preferred method of thrombus removal in our practice. A 6-french MPA guiding catheter (Cordis, Miami, Fla., USA) is advanced through the sheath to the venous anastomosis. Continuous aspiration is performed using a 60-ml syringe. The catheter is then removed and cleared of the thrombus, which is flushed onto sterile gauze and examined. Alternatively, rapid, intermittent aspiration may be performed allowing the clot to be 'milked' out of the graft. Two or three catheter passes are usually required to clear the graft of thrombus. If residual thrombus is noted within the arterial graft limb, a crossing 6-french sheath may be introduced and thrombus aspirated from this graft limb. Alternatively, a smaller sheath may be placed, and the thrombus displaced or macerated with the arterial plug.

Angioplasty of Venous Lesion

Treatment of the venous outflow lesion should proceed following thrombus removal. In 85% of cases, a single lesion at or just beyond the venous anastomosis is identified. Multiple angiographic views may be required to delineate the site of stenosis if several overlapping vessels are present. The lesion is then dilated with the angioplasty balloon. Resilient lesions require dilatation with a high-pressure balloon (we routinely use high-pressure balloons for all venous outflow lesions in our practice). A postangioplasty fistulagram performed in the angioplasty site is reevaluated. If greater than 30% residual stenosis is noted, or if the graft is still pulsatile (poor/no thrill palpated) the lesion may be redilated with a larger balloon (1 mm larger). Lesions which are resistant to high-pressure balloon inflation may be treated with 'buddy' wire technique or with a cutting balloon as described in the previous section.

Dislodgement and/or Maceration of the Arterial Plug

Dislodgement and maceration of the arterial plug represent the final step of graft recanalization. A rubbery, lysis-resistant, tubular plug of densely packed red blood cells and fibrin is invariably present at the arterial anastomosis. The volume of the plug is typically less than 0.5 ml representing minimal risk if embolized to the lungs. The plug is dislodged using a 3- to 5-french Fogarty embolectomy catheter (Baxter, Irvine, Calif., USA) that is advanced beyond the AV anastomosis into the native artery, gently inflated with dilute contrast and slowly withdrawn into the graft. Compliant balloons are less traumatic to the artery and allow variable expansion that permits a better 'pull' on the plug. Noncompliant (angioplasty) balloons are preferred by some interventionalists but should be used carefully as excessive shear stress at the AV anastomosis may predispose to vascular injury. If kinking, tortuosity or pseudoaneurysm is present adjacent to the AV anastomosis, it may be difficult to cross with the Fogarty balloon. The anastomosis should then be crossed with a hydrophilic guidewire and angled catheter. The catheter may be exchanged for an over-the-wire Fogarty balloon catheter, which will allow maintenance of guidewire position during balloon passes.

If graft inflow is poor following several passes with the balloon, residual adherent thrombus at the AV anastomosis should be suspected. Although it has been estimated that approximately 5% of thrombosed grafts will have an underlying arterial anastomotic lesion, several authors suspect that these 'stenoses' may represent adherent clot. We routinely use the Fogarty 'adherent-clot' catheter (Baxter, Irvine, Calif., USA) in these situations. This catheter has a wire coated with latex at its tip which forms a stiff coil when deployed. The catheter must be deployed through a 6- to 7-french sheath. Care should be taken when using this device as vigorous manipulation with it may predispose to vascular injury. A 5- or 6-mm angioplasty balloon may also be used for treatment of these lesions.

After this step is completed, angiographic evaluation of the arterial inflow through the central venous outflow is performed. All significant lesions should be treated prior to termination of the procedure to prevent early graft rethrombosis. Khan and Vesely [39] have shown that up to 20% of patients with repeated graft thrombosis may have underlying proximal arterial inflow lesions. A palpable thrill should be present within the graft without significant pulsatility. When the venous anastomosis is compressed, the intensity of the pulse palpated within the graft should increase. If it does not, a persistent venous anastomotic stenosis should be suspected. Pressure measurements may be performed to confirm adequate correction of flow-limiting lesions. The ratio of upper extremity systolic cuff pressure to systolic pressure within the venous graft limb should be no greater than 33% while the ratio to arterial limb pressure should be no greater than 50% [40]. Intraprocedural blood flow measurement has been reported but the apparatus is not yet commercially available.

Once the final fistulagram is performed, the sheath is removed. Hemostasis is achieved using manual compression at the site for approximately 15 min. A purse string monofilament suture may also be used and compression applied for 1–2 min following suture placement. Sutures should be removed within 72 h following placement. Manual compression may also be aided by gelfoam or thrombotic patches (Syvec patch) applied to the puncture site.

Complications

Arterial embolism is the most serious complication of graft recanalization and occurs in 1/50–100 cases. The patient may be asymptomatic, may experience mild discomfort or numbness within the hand, or may experience severe, unrelenting forearm and hand pain associated with acute motor or sensory loss within the distal extremity. Physical examination demonstrates a cool or cold hand with loss of distal radial and/or ulnar pulses. Treatment includes adequate heparinization to prevent thrombosis of the distal vascular bed. If the graft is patent, the 'backbleeding' technique may be performed to dislodge the thrombus [41]. This technique relies on the principle of backbleeding via collateral vessels to 'reflux' the embolus back into the graft. A compliant balloon is advanced into the inflow artery proximal to the anastomosis and inflated. The patient exercises his hand for approximately 1 min, the balloon is then deflated and repeat angiography is performed. Our preference is to treat emboli by pulling the clot into the graft using an over-the-wire Fogarty balloon or via thromboaspiration with a 5-french open-ended guiding catheter. Care should be taken during advancement of the balloon to avoid further fragmentation and more distal displacement of the embolus. If the clot-containing vessel cannot be accessed from the graft, antegrade brachial artery puncture may be performed and the clot withdrawn to a more proximal location with a Fogarty balloon. (fig. 6) The thrombus can then be withdrawn into the graft using standard techniques. If the embolus cannot be withdrawn with these maneuvers, patient

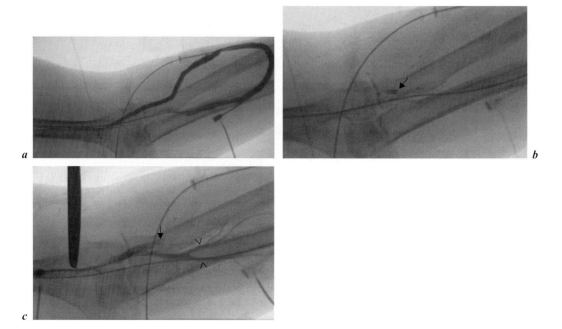

Fig. 6. Angiographic images following recanalization of left forearm loop graft in patient with known radial artery occlusion. Patient complained of pain and numbness in her hand following graft declotting. *a* Fistulagram demonstrates wide patency of graft and venous outflow. *b* Delayed image demonstrates stagnant contrast outlining a meniscoid filling defect within the brachial artery consistent with an embolus (arrow). Attempts to cannulate the brachial artery distal to the graft were unsuccessful, secondary to sharp angulation at the anastomotic site. *c* Antegrade brachial artery puncture was performed and a sheath placed. The embolus was withdrawn into the graft using a 4-french over-the-wire Fogarty balloon. Note occlusion of graft by the embolus (arrow). (This was macerated with an angioplasty balloon.) Ulnar and interosseous arteries are widely patent (arrowheads). Patient's symptoms resolved.

symptomatology should determine further treatment. If the patient is asymptomatic, anticoagulation therapy may be adequate. If the patient is moderately symptomatic thrombolytic therapy should be considered. If the patient is severely ischemic, she should be referred for emergent surgical embolectomy.

Venous rupture or perforation following balloon angioplasty is of little immediate consequence if antegrade blood flow has not been restored within the graft. If blood flow has been restored, and no alternative venous outlet is present, the site of perforation may represent the only available outlet to blood flow and an expanding hematoma may develop rapidly. Careful attention should

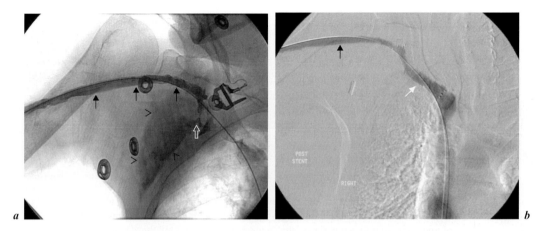

Fig. 7. 65-year-old female presents with a thrombosed right upper arm brachiocephalic fistula. Following aspiration thrombectomy with a 6-french open-ended catheter, contrast fistulagram (not shown) uncovered long segment narrowing of cephalic vein within the upper arm. Percutaneous angioplasty of the cephalic vein was performed with a 7 mm × 10 cm balloon. *a* Following balloon deflation, the patient complained of right shoulder pain. Repeat fistulagram demonstrates patency of cephalic vein (arrows) with extravasation of contrast into the soft tissues of the axilla (arrowheads). Open arrow denotes site of venous rupture. The site was redilated submaximally with a 5-mm balloon with resolution of extravasation, but with persistent obstruction to antegrade blood flow. *b* Final angiogram following deployment of 12 × 60 mm Luminex Nitinol Stent (Bard) across the cephalic arch extending into the subclavian vein (white arrow) demonstrates wide patency of the fistula (arrows) with no further contrast extravasation.

be made to maintain guidewire position across the lesion as it will be difficult to recross the lesion following perforation. Initial treatment should include prolonged, submaximal balloon inflation (inflate for 5- to 10-min intervals with periodic deflation to avoid graft rethrombosis). Uncovered metallic stents have been used to successfully treat these lesions by directed blood flow through the low-resistance stent lumen and allowing the perforation site to heal (fig. 7). We have also used PTFE-coated VIABAHN (W.L. Gore and Associates, Newark, Del., USA) stents to treat these lesions, although no large studies have documented prolonged venous patency associated with this device.

Although studies have shown that the incidence of asymptomatic pulmonary embolism following percutaneous recanalization of dialysis grafts may be as high as 50%, symptomatic pulmonary embolism remains the most feared complication of this procedure. Symptoms range from mild dyspnea to frank unresponsiveness with cardiovascular collapse. Oxygen should be administered via a 100% nonrebreathing mask and intravenous fluid administered. Additional

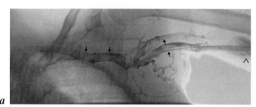 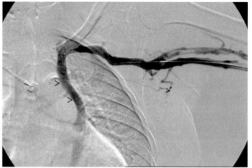

Fig. 8. Angiographic images from the study of a patient who presented with thrombosis of her left forearm loop dialysis graft. Following manipulation to control a minor venous rupture at a venous angioplasty site extensive thrombosis of the venous outflow ensued. *a* Note multiple filling defects (arrows) throughout the brachial and axillary veins consistent with thrombi. Also note contrast extravasation (arrowhead) at venous rupture site. Several passes with Xpedior (AngioJet) Thrombectomy device (not shown) were performed. *b* Postthrombectomy images demonstrate complete resolution of thrombus. Incidentally noted is a left-sided superior vena cava (arrowhead).

intravenous heparin should be administered. An emergency resuscitative team should be called immediately if the patient becomes hemodynamically compromised. The best way to avoid this complication is to refer patients with compromised cardiorespiratory function for surgical thrombectomy.

Acute respiratory insufficiency may also occur in a dialysis patient who is fluid overloaded and is placed in the supine position for several minutes. Fluid redistribution within the lungs may result in frank pulmonary edema. The patient will complain of dyspnea and will demand to sit up. The patient should be immediately placed into the sitting position and 100% oxygen should be administered via a nonrebreathing mask. Anesthesiology support should be obtained if the patient requires intubation with mechanical ventilation. Emergent or semiemergent hemodialysis will generally be required.

Thrombosis of the venous outflow may be the result of inadequate heparinization or embolization during the procedure. It should be treated with standard percutaneous thrombectomy and thrombolytic techniques. We have had excellent success with the use of the Possis thrombectomy device in these situations (fig. 8). If significant thrombus is lodged by a central venous stenosis, the stenosis should not be dilated until the thrombus is removed to prevent embolization to the lungs following dilatation.

A pseudoaneurysm may develop within a native artery secondary to overinflation or manipulation with a Fogarty balloon (fig. 9). This lesion may

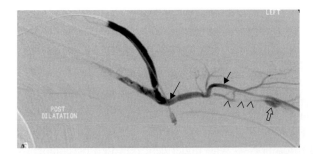

Fig. 9. 'Reflux' angiogram following recanalization of thrombosed left upper arm loop dialysis graft demonstrates patent brachial (large arrow) and radial (small arrow) arteries. A rounded collection of contrast (open arrow) that persists on delayed images is identified overlying the interosseous artery. This is consistent with a pseudoaneurysm secondary to overinflation of the Fogarty balloon within the artery. Note spasm versus dissection within the interosseous artery proximal to the pseudoaneurysm (arrowheads).

thrombose spontaneously, may be treated with via deployment of a covered stent across it or may require surgical repair. Treatment should be determined by the size of the lesion and patient symptomatology.

Other complications include reactions to iodinated contrast media, arterial dissection, perforation or occlusion, angioplasty balloon rupture and inability to deflate the balloon following dilatation.

Results

Most series report primary patency in the range of 70% at 1 month, 40% at 3 months, and 25% at 6 months. Secondary patencies are reported in the range of 63–95% at 1 year. Beathard et al. [42] reported a large series of 1,176 percutaneous mechanical thrombolysis procedures with a high technical success of 95% and a low minor complication rate of 3%. Primary patency rates at 30, 90 and 380 days were 74, 52 and 17%, respectively. Although these long-term results initially appear poor, comparison with surgical thrombectomy reveals a 1-year primary patency of 36% [43]. The average primary patency of any graft prior to its first episode of thrombosis is less than 1 year and the average life span of a graft is less than 3–4 years. In view of these facts and the relative paucity of available access sites for each patient, prolongation of access life via percutaneous methods is justified. Surgeons have advocated surgical revision following the second episode of graft thrombosis. As opposed to surgical procedures (surgical revision, jump graft or new graft placement) which compromise remaining, available veins for access with each procedure, percutaneous methods do not. Beathard [44], in a study of 466 patients with dialysis graft thrombosis, randomized patients to surgical versus radiological treatment in a 12-month period. Thrombolysis reduced the need for graft revision by two thirds and did not increase the episodes of graft thrombosis. DOQI guidelines recommend a higher standard (50% 6-month and 40% 1-year unassisted patency rate) following surgical revision as opposed to radiological intervention (40% 3-month unassisted patency) [5, guideline 21 E].

Some interventionalists recommend surgical revision if a graft rethromboses rapidly following percutaneous recanalization. Murray et al. [45] studied 39 patients with early (<1 month) rethrombosis of their dialysis graft following pharmacomechanical thrombolysis who underwent repeated percutaneous recanalization. They uncovered unsuspected lesions in 18%, used a larger balloon in 41% and deployed stents in 18% of cases. They reported a 35% primary patency at 3 months, which is comparable to grafts without early failure. In our practice, we recommend surgical revision for patients who have undergone three percutaneous thrombectomy procedures in 3 months, patients who have long segment venous stenoses which are not amenable to angioplasty or stenting or recoiling stenoses which are easily amenable to surgical revision.

The method of clot removal has not been shown to correlate to long-term graft patency. Smits et al. [46] compared thrombectomy with the Cragg brush, the Hydrolyser and the Arrow-Trerotola device. Technical success (85–95%), 30-day (55–73%), 60-day (49–61%) and 90-day (40–49%) patencies were not significantly different with each device. Vogel et al. [47] compared percutaneous treatment of thrombosed dialysis grafts with 'lyse and wait' thrombolysis with urokinase and 'lyse and wait' technique versus mechanical thrombectomy. Although the mean procedure time was shorter with lyse and wait urokinase versus mechanical thrombectomy (34 vs. 45 min) and there was a slightly increased bleeding complication rate with the 4-mg TPA dose, patency rates were similar in each group. The only variable which was of predictive value in determining graft patency was the result of percutaneous angioplasty. It is clear that a high caliber screening program before and after percutaneous interventions is essential to prolong access life.

Percutaneous Angioplasty of Failing Native Dialysis Fistulae

Physical Examination

Physical examination of a native fistula may require some experience. True aneurysms may be identified along the course of the outflow vein particularly at sites of repeated dialysis puncture. In a normally functioning fistula, a prominent thrill is palpated at the AV anastomosis which becomes less prominent quite rapidly along the course of the outflow vein. The thrill will be prominent within venous aneurysms and at sites of stenoses.

Manual palpation of the outflow vein may uncover stenotic segments. Normal venous segments are soft and pliable while stenotic segments are palpated as tough cords. If a tourniquet is applied upstream to the stenosis, the normal venous segment will distend while the stenotic segment will not.

Venous outflow stenoses result in a distended outflow vein proximal to the stenosis. Although this venous segment may be easy to puncture for the hemodialysis staff, it will predispose to the formation of venous aneurysms and to increased compression times following hemodialysis. Dilated collateral channels branching from or coursing adjacent to the main outflow vein should be noted as they are indicative of a downstream stenosis. Prominent collaterals may predispose to distal extremity edema if they are insufficiently developed to compensate for the upstream stenosis or if flow is retrograde down them into the hand.

The presence of aneurysms within the main outflow vein is also indicative of an underlying pathology. A distended aneurysm indicates an outflow lesion whereas a collapsed aneurysm is indicative of an inflow lesion. If a stenosis develops between dialysis puncture sites, the upstream aneurysm will be distended while the downstream aneurysm will collapse.

If the limb is placed into the upright position, and the outflow vein collapses, an arterial inflow lesion should be suspected. If the outflow vein remains distended, a venous outflow stenosis should be suspected. If a tourniquet is placed at the elbow, distention of the outflow vein is suggestive of an inflow lesion while if there is no change, an outflow lesion may be suspected.

Doppler ultrasound examination is an excellent supplement to physical examination and is routinely used in our practice. Ultrasound can also play a role in the triage of patients for surgery or for percutaneous recanalization techniques.

Contraindications

Contraindications to percutaneous treatment of native AV fistulae stenoses are similar to those of dialysis bypass graft stenoses and include suspected infection of the fistula or adjacent soft tissues, vascular steal syndrome, and an anastomotic lesion within a fistula which is less than 6 weeks old.

Technique

As opposed to grafts, 50% of forearm fistulae develop stenoses at or just beyond the AV anastomosis (fig. 10). The juxta-anastomotic region represents the surgical mobilization or 'swing' point which may explain the propensity to develop stenoses in this segment [48]. Stenoses also occur within the outflow cephalic vein between dialysis puncture sites. Upper arm fistulae develop stenoses along the course of the outflow cephalic vein, particularly its most

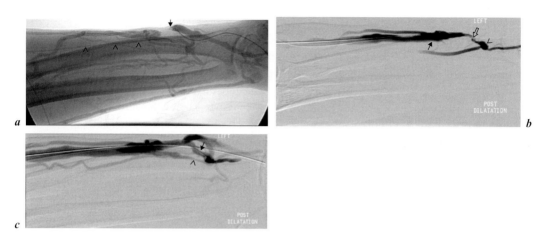

Fig. 10. Angiographic images from study of a patient referred for evaluation of a failing left forearm radiocephalic native fistula. Physical examination demonstrated a collapsed outflow vein with no pulse palpable within it. *a* Small catheter placed into cephalic outflow vein which occludes approximately 4 cm beyond AV anastomosis (arrow). Occlusion could not be crossed in antegrade fashion; retrograde puncture of the collapsed outflow vein was performed under ultrasound guidance (not shown) and a catheter placed (arrowhead). Note catheter tip in collateral channel. *b* The occlusion was crossed and dilated with an 8-mm angioplasty balloon. Postangioplasty angiogram demonstrates wide patency of the outflow vein (arrow). A juxta-anastomotic stenosis is uncovered (open arrow). Note small aneurysm at AV anastomosis (arrowhead). *c* Result following angioplasty with a 6-mm balloon (arrow). Note minimal spasm within the radial artery. Good thrill palpated throughout the fistula.

central portion at its junction with the axillary vein, as well as at or just beyond the AV anastomosis (fig. 11). Transposed brachiobasilic fistulae develop stenoses within the proximal and distal segments of the transposed basilica vein (fig. 12).

Some interventionalists recommend tailoring the access site for the outflow vein to the patient's suspected lesion. If an AV anastomotic lesion is suspected, retrograde puncture of the outflow vessel should be performed at least 3 cm beyond the anastomosis while antegrade puncture of the outflow vein beyond the AV anastomosis is performed for venous outflow lesions. In our practice, we routinely access the cephalic vein at the elbow to allow treatment of AV anastomotic and cephalic outflow lesions within the forearm through one puncture site. For upper arm fistulae, we generally perform antegrade puncture of the cephalic vein several centimeters beyond the AV anastomosis for treatment of outflow venous lesions. A second, retrograde puncture is performed if an AV anastomotic lesion is identified and requires treatment.

Outflow veins which are immature or poorly distended may be difficult to access initially. A tourniquet may be tightened across the arm to promote venous

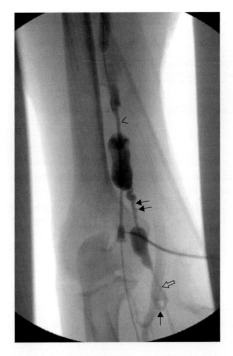

Fig. 11. Digital image from fistula-gram of a patient who presents with increasing recirculation in his right upper arm brachiocephalic fistula. Note stenoses at the AV anastomosis (single arrow), in the juxta-anastomosis region (open arrow), between dialysis puncture sites (double arrow) and within the outflow cephalic vein. These lesions were successfully treated with balloon angioplasty with good results.

distention. The vein may also be easily accessed under real-time ultrasound guidance using a 7- to 10-MHz linear transducer. The vein should be accessed with a 21-gauge micropuncture (Cook) or similar access needle. After placing a 6-french vascular sheath into the vessel, 3,000 to 5,000 units of intravenous heparin are administered. A 4-french Berenstein glide catheter (Boston Scientific, Natick, Mass., USA) is advanced through the sheath, guided beyond the AV anastomosis, and positioned within the distal radial artery. Angiography is performed with visualization of the arterial inflow through the entire venous outflow including the central veins. If prominent collateral channels are present adjacent to the AV anastomosis, it may be difficult to identify the actual anastomotic vein. If the catheter can be advanced upstream to the collaterals, compression of the outflow vein during contrast injection may opacify the anastomotic vein via retrograde contrast flow. Examination of the fistula with placement of radiopaque marker over the external course of the vein may also be helpful. If these maneuvers are unsuccessful or if one encounters an AV anastomotic or native arterial lesion that cannot be crossed, antegrade brachial artery puncture may be performed (fig. 13).

In patients with mature fistulae, the brachial and radial arteries are dilated and easy to access. If no intervention via the arterial approach is planned, a small

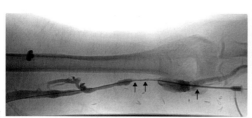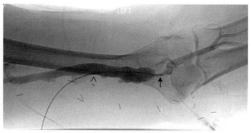

a   *b*

Fig. 12. 60-year-old hemodialysis patient presents with increased recirculation in her left upper arm transposed brachiobasilic fistula. *a* Fistulagram demonstrates high-grade stenosis within the distal segment of the transposed vein (arrows). Note overlapping of aneurysm and proximal venous segment on this image (arrowhead). *b* Following angioplasty of distal venous segment with a 9 mm × 4 cm balloon, wide patency of this segment is noted (arrowhead). However, a tight juxta-anastomosic stenosis is uncovered on this oblique view. Multiple views may be required to evaluate overlapping segments.

access catheter should be used to minimize puncture site size. The vessel may be accessed with a 20-gauge Angiocath or with a 21-gauge micropuncture needle which may be exchanged for the 2.5-french inner cannula of the tapered dilator which accompanies this system. The AV anastomosis may be visualized via angiography performed through these catheters. If intervention via this route is planned, a 4-french vascular sheath is placed. A 4-french Berenstein catheter is advanced through the sheath, the radial artery is selected, and the catheter advanced beyond the AV anastomosis into the outflow vein. Whether from ante-grade arterial or retrograde venous approaches, we prefer 0.018-inch gold-tipped glide wires (Boston Scientific, Natick, Mass., USA) for atraumatic passage through AV anastomotic stenoses. Once the guidewire has been advanced into the vein, 'through and through' access (both ends of the guidewire exit the skin) may be obtained by snaring the tip of the wire with a 10- to 15-mm loop snare (Microvena, White Bear Lake, Minn., USA) or by advancing the wire tip into the venous sheath, removing the sheath and grabbing the wire. This will allow balloon dilatation to be performed via the venous sheath without requiring upsizing of the arterial sheath. Alternatively dilatation may be performed through the 4-french arterial sheath using small vessel balloons.

Once an AV or juxta-anastomotic stenosis is crossed via the standard venous route all attempts should be made to advance the wire into the inflow artery proximal to the AV anastomosis. This is important as balloon dilatation adjacent to the anastomosis may lift a dissection flap which partially occludes the anastomosis. With the wire across the anastomosis, dissection will preferen-tially occur within the distal radial artery which usually is of little consequence.

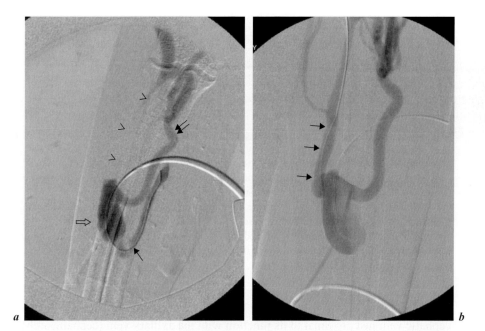

Fig. 13. Patient with failing right forearm radiocephalic fistula. Dialysis nurse could not access the outflow cephalic vein. Cephalic vein is collapsed beyond an aneurysm located just beyond the AV anastomosis. *a* Angiogram performed with catheter tip in the radial artery demonstrates wide patency of the AV anastomosis (single arrow). The cephalic vein occludes beyond the aneurysm (arrowheads denote course of vein). Fistula outflow is via a deep, non-palpable collateral (double arrows) which drains into the antecubital vein. Attempt to cross the occlusion in antegrade fashion was unsuccessful. Venogram (not shown) performed via retrograde puncture of the cephalic vein at the elbow demonstrates focal occlusion of the vein adjacent to the aneurysm. Occlusion was crossed with a hydrophilic guidewire and was dilated with an 8-mm angioplasty balloon. *b* Final angiogram demonstrates wide patency of the outflow vein (arrows).

Additionally, if the fistula thromboses during manipulation, it will facilitate rapid recanalization maneuvers.

We routinely dilate juxta-anastomotic stenoses with standard 7- to 8-mm balloons. If the lesion involves or extends to within 2 cm of the AV anastomosis, we will use 5–7 mm × 4 cm low-profile Symmetry balloons over a 0.018-inch guidewire. The balloon is positioned overlapping the distal radial artery and the outflow vein. Although slightly more expensive than standard balloons, they track easily across acutely angled anastomoses and do not 'buckle' as most standard balloons. Dilatation of these lesions may be quite painful and adequate sedative medication should be administered.

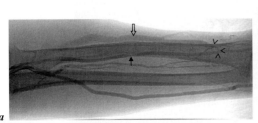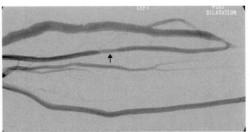

a   *b*

Fig. 14. 54-year-old male presents with poor arterial inflow into his left radiocephalic fistula. Ultrasound examination demonstrated a radial artery stenosis in the forearm. *a* Brachial artery angiogram demonstrates focal stenosis of radial artery in the mid portion of the forearm. Note mild narrowing at the AV anastomosis of the fistula (arrowheads). Cephalic outflow vein (open arrow) is widely patent. *b* Following angioplasty with 3- and 4-mm angioplasty balloons, much improved flow is seen through the vessel (arrow). 1-year follow-up study (not shown) demonstrated no change in the appearance of the vessel.

Venous outflow lesions should be treated with high-pressure balloons. Care should be taken when dilating lesions within the distal segment of the cephalic vein just proximal to its junction with the axillary vein (cephalic arch) as this segment is prone to dissection and perforation. If a venous occlusion cannot be crossed in an antegrade fashion, vessel recanalization via the retrograde route may be attempted (fig. 10, 14).

Following angioplasty, repeat angiography is performed. Radiographic and clinical endpoints include rapid flow through the fistula with no evidence of contrast hold-up, <30% residual stenosis at angioplasty sites, and palpation of a continuous thrill within the outflow vein. If angiography demonstrates a raised dissection flap at the angioplasty site which is flow limiting, submaximal prolonged inflation with the same or smaller angioplasty balloon should be performed. If >30% residual stenosis is present, the stenosis may be redilated with a larger balloon (1 mm greater in diameter) assuming no perforation is present. Recoiling stenoses should initially be treated with redilatation and if not responsive, stent placement or surgical revision should be considered. We avoid stent placement across the AV anastomosis of forearm and brachiocephalic fistulae at dialysis puncture sites or at the elbow. Some authors have advocated the use of 'wide-mesh' stents (Symphony, Meditech or ZA, Cook) if deployment across a cannulation site is required [49].

Complications

Complications are similar to those encountered with percutaneous angioplasty of dialysis grafts. Venous rupture is suspected if the patient complains of persistent pain following deflation of the angioplasty balloon or if an expanding hematoma develops at the angioplasty site. Rupture should be treated with intermittent, prolonged (5- to 10-min) submaximal balloon inflation at the rupture site. If unsuccessful, covered or uncovered stents may be used to treat this lesion.

Severe venospasm may occur during manipulation within the native vein which may predispose to acute vessel thrombosis. Adequate heparinization should be confirmed by activated clotting time measurement and additional heparin administered if needed. Spasm may be treated with administration of 200 µg of nitroglycerin administered directly into the vein. Repeated doses may be administered assuming the patient's blood pressure is stable. Waiting about 10–15 min may result in spontaneous resolution of the spasm. If the spasm persists, submaximal dilatation with a small (4- to 5-mm) angioplasty balloon may 'break' it.

Thrombosis of the fistula may occur during intravascular manipulation, particularly when inadequate heparin is administered. Maintenance of guidewire access across the AV anastomosis will facilitate rapid recanalization of the fistula using standard percutaneous techniques.

Infection is much less common in fistulae than in grafts. Perivascular cellulitis is the most common infection and is characterized by localized erythema, swelling and tenderness to palpation. Cellulitis is generally easily treated with antibiotics. Septic phlebitis, abscess formation within a thrombosed aneurysm and superinfection of a perivenous hematoma are rare but serious complications. If suspected, the patient should be referred to a vascular surgeon for drainage with possible venous excision.

Results

Few large series have been published with results of percutaneous angioplasty of native dialysis fistulae. In addition, many series combine thrombosed with patent fistulae, and do not separate forearm and upper arm fistulae in their evaluation. Turmel-Rodrigues et al. [49] evaluated percutaneous procedures in 209 patients with forearm AV fistulae, 74 upper arm AV fistulae and 156 synthetic grafts. 726 angioplasties, 135 stents, and 257 declotting procedures were performed in these patients. Technical success was 78–98% and the complication rate was 2%. 1-year primary patency rates for the failing forearm fistula was 50%, upper arm fistula 34% and synthetic graft was 25%. 1-year secondary patency rates were similar for the failing versus thrombosed forearm fistula (85 vs. 80%), 82 versus 65% for the failing versus thrombosed upper arm fistula, and 92 versus 75% for the failing versus thrombosed graft. 4-year secondary patency rates of 51–77% were obtained for all the native fistulae compared to 24% for the initially thrombosed graft. They noted that 1.9 interventions were required to attain a 79% 3-year patency with fistulae while 4.5 interventions were required to attain a 73% secondary patency in grafts.

Manninen et al. [50] reported on 103 interventions in 53 fistulae. Technical and clinical success was obtained in 95 and 92% although anatomic success (<30% residual stenosis) was only achieved in 76%. Primary patency at 6,12, 24 and 36 months was 58, 44, 40 and 32%, respectively, while secondary patency was 90, 85, 79 and 79%, respectively. Clark et al. [51], in analyzing prognostic factors affecting long-term patency, noted that lesion length >2 cm was highly correlated with necessity of repeated interventions and decreased patency. Rajan et al. [52] identified cephalic arch stenosis as a frequent cause of fistula dysfunction in upper arm fistula (39 vs. 2% of forearm fistulae in their series). The cephalic arch is the perpendicular portion of the cephalic vein in the region of the deltopectoral groove proximal to its junction with the axillary vein. They noted a requirement of high-pressure balloons to treat these resistant lesions and a high venous rupture rate of 6% (1.7–2.8% normally). 6-month patency was poor at 42%.

Stents were used in 5–20% of interventions in these series. As it is more difficult to repair outflow venous stenoses of native fistulae surgically, it is expected that stent placement will become more common with increasing predominance of native fistulae.

Percutaneous Treatment of the Thrombosed Native AV Fistula

There are several major differences between the thrombosed dialysis bypass graft and the native AV fistula which make percutaneous treatment of native fistulae more challenging. First, a thrombosed mature fistula, particularly one with multiple aneurysms, contains a large amount of thrombus within it. Second, aneurysms may contain layered, mature thrombus along its walls which is resistant to thrombolysis. Third, as opposed to grafts, thrombus may become rapidly adherent to the vessel wall making early treatment (preferably <1–2 days and generally <3 weeks) essential. Fourth, aneurysms and tortuous venous segments may make guidewire traversal through the outflow vein more difficult.

Physical examination and contraindications have already been discussed in previous sections (please refer to Physical Examination section of Percutaneous Angioplasty of Failing Native Dialysis Fistulae). Of note, thrombosis of a native vein may induce a reactive phlebitis which should not be mistaken for an infection. The skin over the vein may be minimally erythematous and warm to touch. The site may be tender to palpation and a cord may be palpated. No fluctuance or edema should be noted and the patient should be afebrile. These patients may be exquisitely sensitive to endovascular manipulation within this vein and should be given appropriate medication for pain control.

Technique

As the outflow vein of the fistulae is rarely completely thrombosed, applying a tourniquet to the arm will promote distention of the outflow vein. The outflow vein is punctured at its most distal, palpable site (near the elbow for forearm fistulae) aiming towards the AV anastomosis using a 21-gauge micropuncture needle. Ultrasound guidance may be of assistance in accessing small, poorly palpable veins. A 6-french vascular sheath is placed. 3–5,000 units of intravenous heparin are administered. A formal venogram is performed to evaluate the extent of the thrombus and the venous outflow. Contrast should be injected gently to avoid reflux of clot into the native artery. In up to 50% of cases, no or minimal thrombus is seen within the outflow vein with only a tight stenosis present. Treatment of this lesion should then proceed as with any open shunt. If thrombus is present, thrombus removal should proceed using the operators preferred method. If the outflow vein cannot be crossed or if thrombus cannot be adequately removed from the fistula from the single puncture site, the vein should be punctured approximately 2–3 cm beyond the AV anastomosis aiming cephalad. After sheath placement, a catheter is advanced through the outflow vein which may then be dilated with an angioplasty balloon. If the venous outflow is severely and diffusely diseased with no other outflow channel present and cannot be crossed with a guidewire, consideration should be made to abandoning the access.

Thrombus removal may be accomplished via injection of a thrombolytic agent, mechanical thrombectomy, thrombectomy using a rotating pigtail catheter or aspiration thrombectomy [53]. We prefer using aspiration thrombectomy supplemented with mechanical thrombectomy for problem cases. A 6- to 8-french MPA guiding catheter (Cordis, Miami, Fla., USA) is advanced through an appropriately sized sheath and embedded into the thrombus. We generally use the 6-french catheters for normal sized veins and the larger catheters for large veins with aneurysms. Aspiration is performed via continuous suction applied to the catheter using a 60-ml syringe. The catheter is removed, cleared of thrombus and the sequence repeated until all thrombus is removed. Aneurysms should be manually compressed during aspiration to facilitate thrombus removal. If flow is restored into the fistula, large amounts of blood will be aspirated through the catheter with minimal thrombus. To minimize blood loss, antegrade blood flow should not be restored until thrombus is cleared, if possible. If adherent thrombus, common within aneurysms, cannot be aspirated or dislodged, maceration with a mechanical thrombectomy may be helpful. The over-the-wire, 7-french Arrow-Trerotola or the 6-french Xpedior device may be used to macerate this thrombus while the aneurysm is manually compressed. If the Arrow-Trerotola device is used, thrombus fragments should be aspirated through the introducer sheath.

It is essential to maintain guidewire access across the artery and vein during these manipulations as recrossing tortuous, aneurysmal venous segments may be challenging. A 'safety' wire may be useful in this situation [53]. After placing a long sheath through the vessel, a second guidewire is advanced through the sheath. The sheath is then removed and readvanced over a single wire, leaving the second wire exiting the skin outside the sheath. If the wire access is lost during thromboaspiration or another manipulation, the sheath can be rapidly advanced over the second wire.

If the AV anastomosis cannot be crossed from a retrograde approach, brachial artery puncture may be performed and the lesion crossed from the arterial approach. Some authors advocate brachial artery access as the primary access site for native fistula angioplasty and recanalization [50]. However, when using 5- and 6-french sheaths, they reported an 8% major complication rate with 4 patients requiring emergent surgery for brachial artery pseudoaneurysms and uncontrollable bleeding. Most manipulations, including balloon dilatation and advancement of a 4-french Fogarty balloon across the AV anastomosis, may be performed through a 4-french arterial sheath which will minimize the risk of complication.

Once thrombus is removed, directed contrast venography should further delineate any underlying stenoses. Stenoses should be treated with balloon dilatation as described in the preceding section.

After treatment of stenotic lesions, the arterial plug, if present, is dislodged with a 4- or 5.5-french over-the-wire Fogarty balloon. Once dislodged, it may be macerated with an angioplasty balloon or pushed centrally using the Fogarty balloon. Angiographic evaluation should then be performed encompassing examination of the arterial inflow through and including the central venous outflow. If rapid flow is not identified within the fistula, remaining stenoses or thrombi must be identified and treated. Minimal vessel irregularity or small thrombi are acceptable if brisk flow is identified throughout the fistula.

Stents may be required for treatment of lesions that are poorly responsive to angioplasty, chronically recurring or recoiling lesions and for treatment of balloon-induced vessel ruptures. They may be of particular use for the treatment of adherent thrombus within an aneurysm of the outflow vein which cannot be aspirated or macerated mechanically. A stent may be deployed across the aneurysm, trapping the thrombus (for a discussion of stent use, please refer to the preceding section). We have not had significant experience with this technique.

Complications
Complications include venous rupture, venous outflow thrombosis, arterial embolism, infection and pulmonary embolism (please refer to the Complications section of Treatment of the Thrombosed Dialysis Bypass Graft for a discussion on the management of these complications).

Results

As noted regarding angioplasty of native fistulae, there is a paucity of literature regarding recanalization of occluded native hemodialysis fistulae. Haage et al. [54] reported an 89% technical success rate in a series of 81 procedures in 54 patients with primarily forearm fistulae, three quarters of whom had long segment thrombus, using primarily mechanical declotting methods. 11% rethrombosed within 2 weeks and required a repeat procedure. Primary patency at 1, 3, 6 and 12 months was reported as 74, 63, 52 and 27%, respectively, while secondary patency at 3, 6,12 and 24 months was reported as 75, 65, 51 and 22%, respectively. Turmel-Rodrigues et al. [55] subdivided forearm and upper arm fistulae and reported a significant difference in technical success (93 vs. 79%) and 1-year primary patency (49 vs. 9%) between fistulae at both sites. They attribute the poorer outcome with upper arm fistulae to problems with the treatment of cephalic arch stenoses. Other authors have not noted these differences but the studies are smaller [56]. Clearly, studies with larger numbers of patients with upper arm fistulae are required to clarify this issue.

Technical success is slightly decreased in fistulae as compared to grafts (79–93 vs. 94–100%) and procedure times are generally double that of graft declotting (36–68 vs. 120 min). However, though it is more challenging to recanalize an occluded fistulae, the operator is rewarded for his effort with a significant increase in the primary patency of the treated fistula in comparison to grafts, as well as a greater maintenance-free interval before reintervention (19.6 months for forearm fistulae vs. 6.4 months for grafts).

A nonmaturing fistulae is another potential area for interventional therapy. Beathard et al. [57] reported an 82.5% salvage rate for nonmaturing fistulae using angioplasty of venous stenoses in combination with surgical ligation of accessory veins. Turmel-Rodrigues et al. [58] reported a 97% technical success rate with angioplasty or stenting of underlying stenoses without ligation of collateral veins. In a series of 69 cases including 17 occluded fistulae, they reported primary and secondary 1-year patency rates of 39 and 79%, respectively.

Conclusion

Endovascular interventions have revolutionized the treatment of dialysis access failure. These percutaneous therapies allow rapid, outpatient treatment of the most frequent complications associated with dialysis access. Screening programs are essential to detect the failing access prior to thrombosis and to confirm adequate interventional treatment. As more native fistulae are constructed in response to DOQI recommendations, further experience and innovation will be developed for the treatment of failing, failed and immature native fistulae.

Acknowledgment

The author thanks Dr. James Silberzweig for his assistance in editing this manuscript.

References

1   Mayers JD, Markell MS, Cohen LS, Hong J, Lundin P, Friedman EA: Vascular access surgery for maintenance hemodialysis. Variables in hospital stay. ASAIO J 1992;38/2:113–115.
2   Feldman HI, Held PJ, Hutchinson JT, Stoiber E, Hartigan MF, Berlin JA: Hemodialysis vascular access morbidity in the United States. Kidney Int 1993;43:1091–1096.
3   Roberts AB, Sullivan KL, Ross RP, et al: Graft surveillance and angioplasty prolongs dialysis graft patency. J Am Coll Surg 1996;183:486–492.
4   Safa AA, Valji K, Roberts AC, Ziegler TW, Hye RJ, Oglevie SB: Detection and treatment of dysfunctional hemodialysis access grafts: Effect of a surveillance program on graft patency and the incidence of thrombosis. Radiology 1996;199:653–657.
5   III. NKF-K/DOQI: Clinical Practice Guidelines for Vascular Access: Update 2000. Am J Kidney Dis 2001;37(suppl 1):S137–S181.
6   Schwab SJ, Raymond JR, Saeed M, Newman GE, Dennis PA, Bollinger RR: Prevention of hemodialysis fistula thrombosis. Early detection of venous stenoses. Kidney Int 1989;36:707–711.
7   Sands JJ, Jabyac PA, Miranda CL, Kapsick BJ: Intervention based on monthly monitoring decreases hemodialysis access thrombosis. ASAIO J 1999;45/3:147–150.
8   Schackelton CR, Taylor DC, Buckley AR, Rowley VA, Cooperberg PL, Fry PD: Predicting failure in polytetrafluoroethylene vascular access grafts for hemodialysis: A pilot study. Can J Surg 1987; 30:442–444.
9   Strauch BS, O'Connell RS, Geoly KL, Grundlehner M, Yakub YN, Tietjen DP: Forecasting thrombosis of vascular access with Doppler color flow imaging. Am J Kidney Dis 1992;19: 554–557.
10 Smits JH, van der Linden J, Hagen EC, Modderkolk-Cammeraat EC, Feith GW, Koomans HA, van den Dorpel MA, Blankestijn PJ: Graft surveillance: Venous pressure, access flow, or the combination? Kidney Int 2001;59:1551–1558.
11 Smits JH, Blankestijn PJ: Haemodialysis access: The case for prospective monitoring. Curr Opin Nephrol Hypertens 1999;8:685–690.
12 Hathaway PB, Vesely TM: The apex-puncture technique for mechanical thrombolysis of loop hemodialysis grafts. J Vasc Interv Radiol 1999;10:775–779.
13 Gray RJ: Percutaneous intervention for permanent hemodialysis access: A review. J Vasc Interv Radiol 1997;8:313–327.
14 Bittl JA, Feldman RL: Cutting balloon angioplasty for undilatable venous stenoses causing graft failure. Catheter Cardiovasc Interv 2003;58:524–526.
15 Ryan JM, Dumbleton SA, Smith TP: Technical innovation. Using a cutting balloon to treat resistant high grade dialysis graft stenosis. AJR Am J Roentgenol 2003;180:1072–1074.
16 Gray RJ, Dolmatch BL, Buick MK: Directional atherectomy treatment for hemodialysis access: Early results. J Vasc Interv Radiol 1992;3:497–503.
17 Haage P, Vorwerk D, Piroth W, et al: Treatment of hemodialysis-related central venous occlusion: Results of primary Wallstent placement and follow-up in 50 patients. Radiology 1999;212:175–180.
18 Glanz S, Gordon D, Butt KM, et al: Dialysis access fistulas: Treatment by transluminal angioplasty. Radiology 1984;152:637–642.

19 Beathard GA: Percutaneous transvenous angioplasty in the treatment of vascular access stenosis. Kidney Int 1992;42:1390–1397.

20 Aruny JE, Lewis CA, Cardella JF, et al: Quality improvement guidelines for percutaneous management of thrombosed or dysfunctional dialysis access. Standards of Practice Committee for the SCVIR. J Vasc Interv Radiol 1999;10:491–498.

21 Schwab SJ, Oliver MJ, Suhocki P, McCann R: Hemodialysis arteriovenous access: Detection of stenosis and response to treatment by vascular access blood flow. Kidney Int 2001;59:358–362.

22 van der Linden J, Smits JHM, Assink JH, et al: Short and long term effects of percutaneous transluminal angioplasty in hemodialysis vascular access. J Am Soc Nephrol 2002;13:715–720.

23 Funaki B, Kim R, Lorenz J, et al: Using pullback pressure measurements to identify venous stenoses persisting after successful angioplasty in failing hemodialysis access grafts. AJR Am J Roentgenol 2002;178:1161–1165.

24 Beathard GA: Thrombolysis versus surgery for the treatment of thrombosed dialysis access grafts. J Am Soc Nephrol 1995;6:1619–1624.

25 Schuman E, Quinn S, Standage B, Gross G: Thrombolysis versus thrombectomy for occluded hemodialysis grafts. Am J Surg 1994;167:473–476.

26 Cynamon J, Pierpont CE: Thrombolysis for the treatment of thrombosed hemodialysis access grafts. Rev Cardiovasc Med 2002;3(suppl 2):S84–S91.

27 Goldberg JP, Contiguglia SR, Mishell JL, Klein MH: Intravenous streptokinase for thrombolysis of occluded arteriovenous access. Its use in patients undergoing hemodialysis. Arch Intern Med 1985;145:1405–1408.

28 Davis GB, Dowd CF, Bookstein JJ, Maroney TP, Lang EV, Halasz N: Thrombosed dialysis grafts: Efficacy of intrathrombic deposition of concentrated urokinase, clot maceration, and angioplasty. AJR Am J Roentgenol 1987;149/1:177–181.

29 Valji K, Bookstein JJ, Roberts AC, Davis GB: Pharmacomechanical thrombolysis and angioplasty in the management of clotted hemodialysis grafts: Early and late clinical results. Radiology 1991; 178/1:243–247.

30 Valji K, Bookstein JJ, Roberts AC, Oglevie SB, Pittman C, O'Neill MP: Pulse-spray pharmaco-mechanical thrombolysis of thrombosed hemodialysis access grafts: Long-term experience and comparison of original and current techniques. AJR Am J Roentgenol 1995;164:1495–1503.

31 Beathard GA: Mechanical versus pharmacomechanical thrombolysis for the treatment of thrombosed dialysis access grafts. Kidney Int 1994;45:1401–1406.

32 Cynamon J, Lakritz PS, Wahl SI, Bakal CW, Sprayregen S: Hemodialysis graft declotting: Description of the 'lyse and wait' technique. J Vasc Interv Radiol 1997;8:825–829.

33 Falk A, Mitty H, Guller J, Teodorescu V, Uribarri J, Vassalotti J: Thrombolysis of clotted hemodialysis grafts with tissue-type plasminogen activator. J Vasc Interv Radiol 2001;12:305–311.

34 Falk A, Guller J, Nowakowski FS, Mitty H, Teodorescu V, Uribarri J, Vassalotti J: Reteplase in the treatment of thrombosed hemodialysis grafts. J Vasc Interv Radiol 2001;12:1257–1262.

35 Duszak R Jr, Sacks D: Dialysis graft declotting with very low dose urokinase: Is it feasible to use 'less and wait'? J Vasc Interv Radiol 1999;10/2:123–128.

36 Trerotola SO, Vesely TM, Lund GB, Soulen MC, Ehrman KO, Cardella JF: Treatment of thrombosed hemodialysis access grafts: Arrow-Trerotola percutaneous thrombolytic device versus pulse-spray thrombolysis. Arrow-Trerotola Percutaneous Thrombolytic Device Clinical Trial. Radiology 1998;206:403–414.

37 Sharafuddin MJ, Hicks ME: Current status of percutaneous mechanical thrombectomy. II. Devices and mechanisms of action. J Vasc Interv Radiol 1998;9/1:15–31.

38 Hein AN, Vesely TM: Use of the percutaneous thrombolytic device for the treatment of thrombosed pseudoaneurysms during mechanical thrombectomy of hemodialysis grafts. J Vasc Interv Radiol 2002;13/2:201–204.

39 Khan FA, Vesely TM: Arterial problems associated with dysfunctional hemodialysis grafts: Evaluation of patients at high risk for arterial disease. J Vasc Interv Radiol 2002;13:1109–1114.

40 Sullivan KL, Besarab A, Bonn J, Shapiro MJ, Gardiner GA Jr, Moritz MJ: Hemodynamics of failing dialysis grafts. Radiology 1993;186:867–872.

41 Trerotola SO, Johnson MS, Shah H, Namyslowski J: Backbleeding technique for treatment of arterial emboli resulting from dialysis graft thrombolysis. J Vasc Interv Radiol 1998;9/1:141–143.

42   Beathard GA, Welch BR, Maidment HJ: Mechanical thrombolysis for the treatment of thrombosed hemodialysis access grafts. Radiology 1996;200:711–716.

43   Hodges TC, Fillinger MF, Zwolak RM, Walsh DB, Bech F, Cronenwett JL: Longitudinal comparison of dialysis access methods: Risk factors for failure. J Vasc Surg 1997;26:1009–1019.

44   Beathard GA: Angioplasty for arteriovenous grafts and fistulae. Semin Nephrol 2002;22/3:202–210.

45   Murray SP, Kinney TB, Valji K, Roberts AC, Rose SC, Oglevie SB: Early rethrombosis of clotted hemodialysis grafts: Graft salvage achieved with an aggressive approach. AJR Am J Roentgenol 2000;175:529–532.

46   Smits HF, Smits JH, Wust AF, Buskens E, Blankestijn PJ: Percutaneous thrombolysis of thrombosed haemodialysis access grafts: Comparison of three mechanical devices. Nephrol Dial Transplant 2002;17:467–473.

47   Vogel PM, Bansal V, Marshall MW: Thrombosed hemodialysis grafts: Lyse and wait with tissue plasminogen activator or urokinase compared to mechanical thrombolysis with the Arrow-Trerotola Percutaneous Thrombolytic Device. J Vasc Interv Radiol 2001;12:1157–1165.

48   Falk A, Teodorescu V, Lou WY, Uribarri J, Vassalotti JA: Treatment of 'swing point stenoses' in hemodialysis arteriovenous fistulae. Clin Nephrol 2003;60:35–41.

49   Turmel-Rodrigues L, Pengloan J, Baudin S, Testou D, Abaza M, Dahdah G, Mouton A, Blanchard D: Treatment of stenosis and thrombosis in haemodialysis fistulas and grafts by interventional radiology. Nephrol Dial Transplant 2000;15:2029–2036.

50   Manninen HI, Kaukanen ET, Ikaheimo R, Karhapaa P, Lahtinen T, Matsi P, Lampainen E: Brachial arterial access: Endovascular treatment of failing Brescia-Cimino hemodialysis fistulas – Initial success and long-term results. Radiology 2001;218:711–718.

51   Clark TW, Hirsch DA, Jindal KJ, Veugelers PJ, LeBlanc J, Clark TW, Hirsch DA, Jindal KJ, Veugelers PJ, LeBlanc J: Outcome and prognostic factors of restenosis after percutaneous treatment of native hemodialysis fistulas. J Vasc Interv Radiol 2002;13/1:51–59.

52   Rajan DK, Clark TW, Patel NK, Stavropoulos SW, Simons ME: Prevalence and treatment of cephalic arch stenosis in dysfunctional autogenous hemodialysis fistulas. J Vasc Interv Radiol 2003;14:567–573.

53   Turmel-Rodrigues L, Raynaud A, Louail B, Beyssen B, Sapoval M: Manual catheter-directed aspiration and other thrombectomy techniques for declotting native fistulas for hemodialysis. J Vasc Interv Radiol 2001;12:1365–1371.

54   Haage P, Vorwerk D, Wildberger JE, Piroth W, Schurmann K, Gunther RW: Percutaneous treatment of thrombosed primary arteriovenous hemodialysis access fistulae. Kidney Int 2000;57:1169–1175.

55   Turmel-Rodrigues L, Pengloan J, Rodrigue H, Brillet G, Lataste A, Pierre D, Jourdan JL, Blanchard D: Treatment of failed native arteriovenous fistulae for hemodialysis by interventional radiology. Kidney Int 2000;57:1124–1140.

56   Rajan DK, Clark TW, Simons ME, Kachura JR, Sniderman K: Procedural success and patency after percutaneous treatment of thrombosed autogenous arteriovenous dialysis fistulas. J Vasc Interv Radiol 2002;13:1211–1218.

57   Beathard GA, Settle SM, Shields MW: Salvage of the nonfunctioning arteriovenous fistula. Am J Kidney Dis 1999;33:910–916.

58   Turmel-Rodrigues L, Mouton A, Birmele B, Billaux L, Ammar N, Grezard O, Hauss S, Pengloan J: Salvage of immature forearm fistulas for haemodialysis by interventional radiology. Nephrol Dial Transplant 2001;16:2365–2371.

Joseph Shams
Assistant Professor of Radiology,
Albert Einstein College of Medicine,
Division of Vascular and Interventional Radiology
Beth Israel Medical Center, New York, N.Y.
Tel. +1 212 870 9132, E-Mail jshams@bethisraelny.org

Ronco C, Levin NW (eds): Hemodialysis Vascular Access and Peritoneal Dialysis Access.
Contrib Nephrol. Basel, Karger, 2004, vol 142, pp 323–349

....

Quality Assurance and Continuous Quality Improvement Programs for Vascular Access Care

Brian A.J. Walters[a,b], *Phillip Pennell*[b], *Juan P. Bosch*[a]

[a]Gambro Healthcare, Scientific Affairs and Clinical Research, Ft. Lauderdale,
Fla., and [b]Division of Nephrology and Hypertension, University of Miami,
Miami, Fla., USA

Introduction

In the United States, the National Kidney Foundation (NKF) published clinical practice guidelines for vascular access in 1997 and updated them in 2001 [1, 2]. The Kidney Disease Outcomes Quality Initiative (K/DOQI) introduced 38 clinical practice guidelines based on evidence or expert opinion to improve outcomes associated with vascular access [1, 2]. Similar clinical practice guidelines were introduced in Canada, and guidelines for Europe are expected in the next year [3, 4]. These guidelines recognized that the effective establishment of a quality program aimed at maintaining the patency and life of an adequately functioning vascular access was critical to the survival and quality of life for hemodialysis patients [5, 6]. The critically important issues cited by these vascular access clinical practice guidelines include early identification of patients with chronic kidney disease (CKD), early referral to a nephrologist, early identification and protection of vessels suitable for creation of a native fistula, patient education, timely placement of an appropriate permanent access, maximizing use of native arteriovenous fistulas (AVFs) and minimizing use of grafts and vascular catheters, minimizing complications (infections, stenosis, thrombosis, aneurysms, and ischemia of limbs), and optimizing the functional life of the access [1, 2].

While programs aimed at improving vascular access management in prevalent hemodialysis patients are important, it is becoming clear that the success of any vascular access quality program requires an impact on the predialysis medical community to reduce the number of patients beginning dialysis with a

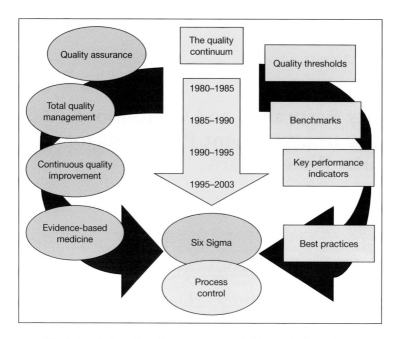

Fig. 1. Evolution of quality management [with permission, 13].

catheter owing to late referral to nephrology and delay of vascular access planning. The recent publication of clinical practice guidelines for the care of CKD patients prior to dialysis initiation will help to bring vascular access planning issues to the attention of physicians not routinely involved in dialysis care [7]. However, it is essential that renal physicians actively expand their spheres of influence within the larger medical community and proactively advocate access planning during CKD stage 4, as proposed by peer review organizations [5, 7]. Once the access is created, the quality program should ensure that each patient has an individualized proactive vascular access plan, a surveillance program to detect access dysfunction, and interventions to maintain access patency.

Our purpose is to describe the essential elements of structured quality assurance (QA) and continuous quality improvement (CQI) programs for vascular access that will lead to optimizing clinical outcomes and quality of life for hemodialysis patients. We believe that this is possible by integration of the theories of total quality management (TQM) with evidence-based medicine (EBM) through the process of CQI refined by the application of Six Sigma theory. The evolution of these theories in quality management is outlined in figure 1. To have an impact, the program must involve the surgical team during the predialysis period and promote the use of AVFs [8]. The program also needs

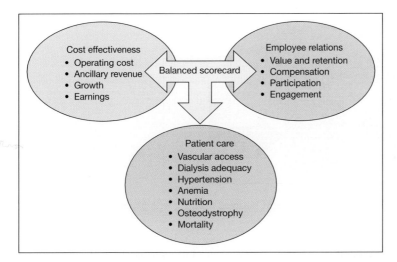

Fig. 2. Three components of quality that must function in harmony for ESRD quality objectives to succeed [with permission, 13].

to be tailored for each individual patient and to involve the patient in decisions that obviously will have a profound impact on self-perception, mental health, quality of life as well as mortality.

Quality Management Theory

As the hemodialysis population continues to increase at a rate of 5–10% each year around the world, there needs to be a structured process of monitoring quality that is combined with a disciplined approach to solving clinical problems and improving outcomes for patients. A process is required that focuses on the welfare of the patient and draws upon the leadership of the physician while empowering all healthcare personnel within the dialysis facility to participate and contribute to improving care. The process that we propose recognizes that medical quality is defined as the adherence to recognized appropriate medical standards of peer-reviewed practices that consistently have been associated with the best patient outcomes. Medical standards of care address the extent to which a particular procedure, treatment, test or service is efficacious, is clearly indicated for the patient, and is neither deficient nor excessive in meeting the patients' needs. In order to achieve CQI, three important areas of quality must operate in harmony, patient care, employee relations, and cost effectiveness (fig. 2). These three areas of quality may be condensed into a balanced scorecard, based upon

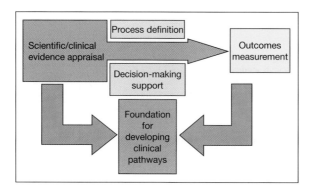

Fig. 3. Four components of EBM [adapted from 10; with permission, 13].

instantaneous data, that engages management, physicians and healthcare employees in a long-term binding strategy to create innovation, sustain quality and retain customer (patient) satisfaction [9].

Both quality process and quality outcomes are best defined on the basis of EBM and expert opinion. Such a process has been utilized by the NKF to develop the K/DOQI guidelines for vascular access (as well as guidelines for adequacy of hemodialysis and peritoneal dialysis, anemia, nutrition, dyslipidemia, osteodystrophy, and the care of CKD patients). In practice, such a process involves forming a healthcare team to convert problems into answerable questions and to search the medical literature for the best evidence upon which to answer the questions. After reviewing the evidence for accuracy, validity and integrity, the results of the EBM process are applied to modify routine clinical practice so that subsequent outcomes can be evaluated in order to confirm the value of the modifications before communicating back to the team and colleagues (fig. 3) [10]. Unfortunately, EBM does not take into consideration factors outside of medical control that also impact on successful outcomes. These factors include a variety of dialysis facility issues that can only be addressed locally by a team of committed individuals through the processes of QA and CQI. Both of these processes also are data driven and involve problem-solving techniques that draw upon leadership, planning, teamwork, process control and improvement.

Application of Quality Management Theory to CQI

Total Quality Management
When the concepts and principles of quality management are integrated into the internal structure of an entire organization or institution, the resultant

---

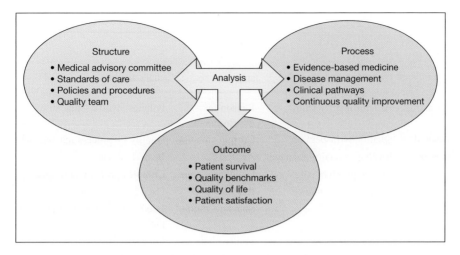

Fig. 4. Three components of TQM [with permission, 13].

culture that evolves is referred to as TQM. The concept of TQM, borrowed from business management theory, emphasizes the commitment to the customer (patient) by continually striving for improvement through data-driven, problem-solving solutions to issues that originate from and are implemented by empowered employees. To be successful, TQM requires an internal quality infrastructure consisting of defined standards of care, CQI programs, a team committed to process improvements, and flexibility within the institution to change and adjust to reengineering if necessary. The quality foundation is built from the analysis of data derived from delivery processes linked to outcomes (fig. 4). The application of TQM is a dynamic process that involves management and labor working harmoniously together in a positive interactive relationship to create a quality product at a reasonable cost (human and economic) that meets the customer's (patient's) needs and desires.

Quality Assurance

QA refers to the process of determining the extent to which a specific patient care outcome, or benchmark of quality outcome, is achieved in a specific clinical setting. The outcome benchmark ideally would be established by a consortium of multidisciplinary experts through the process of EBM, modified and extended by their expert opinion. Desired thresholds of compliance to the established benchmarks would be determined. Regardless of the specific clinical context (national, regional, or clinical facility), every quality program begins with and utilizes a QA surveillance process to identify areas of concern

Table 1. Differences between QA and CQI [with permission, 13]

QA		CQI	
steps	characteristics	steps	characteristics
Select a quality marker	Policies involve rules	Reason for improvement	Policies involve leadership
Determine threshold	Quality by inspection	Current situation	Quality by process management
Set survey frequency	Involves a quality manager	Analysis	Involves a team
Corrective actions	Simple problem solutions	Countermeasures	Complex problem solutions
Confirm effectiveness	Used for surveillance	Results	Used for improvement
		Standardization	Used as the basis for clinical pathways
		Future plan	Proactive

that consistently do not meet an achievable benchmark to prompt intervention through the CQI team. Outcomes below the established threshold would generate simple corrective actions, and results would be assessed after implementation by the healthcare team. The QA process tends to be a top-down process. Are benchmark goals being achieved? If not, will some corrective action achieve better outcomes?

Continuous Quality Improvement

The process of CQI is more complex in that it requires involvement of the entire multidisciplinary team in the process of analyzing the reasons for failing to meet the benchmark and designing countermeasures for improvement. The component steps of QA and CQI are listed in table 1 together with the essential differences between the two quality programs. CQI involves review of all pertinent processes operative in the local environment, including staffing issues and patient-specific factors such as acuity of illness, comorbidities, compliance issues, social support systems, as well as access issues such as insurance, medications, and transportation. In order for the CQI process within a dialysis facility to be successful, there must be support from the leadership, commitment to the CQI philosophy and process, and empowered health care personnel on the CQI team. The team is responsible for setting its own priorities regarding specific outcome benchmarks to investigate, identifying factors contributing to the problem under scrutiny, collecting and analyzing data, developing and implementing a correction plan, monitoring outcome performance, and reporting results to the entire healthcare team.

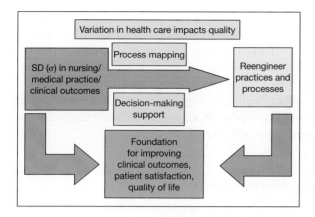

Fig. 5. Components of Six Sigma theory [with permission, 13].

Six Sigma

Once a high level of quality performance has been achieved through the QA/CQI process described above, further refinement in quality outcomes can be achieved by application of Six Sigma theory, also borrowed from business management [11]. The Six Sigma philosophy institutes a method of improving quality by reducing outcome variability, as reflected in the standard deviation (SD, sigma, σ) of the quality outcome mean, among a group of patients or between two groups of patients attending different facilities or the same facility [11]. The 'Six' refers to the goal of operating within a level of excellence where six SD from the mean to the nearest specification limit are achieved. This will result in 99.9997% of the population (patients/facilities) meeting the quality benchmark or only 3.4 patients/facilities in one million measurement opportunities not meeting the benchmark.

The Six Sigma quality concept first identifies an outcome specification such as the percent of patients beginning dialysis with an AVF or the access flow predictive of stenosis, sets a target specification/standard, and then monitors the frequency of not meeting the specification (fig. 5). The program identifies and corrects those process factors that exert pressure on the variability of the outcome specification, as indicated by large SD in the mean outcome benchmark. The notion is, for example, that referral for angioplasty for access flows below the target level is poor clinical practice and that referral for angioplasty for access flows above target is inefficient, or wasteful of clinical resources, and that low variability of the variance around the mean value represents maximum productivity with the least expenditure of resources. Interpatient variation (σ) expresses the ability of the healthcare team to deliver consistently high quality care to all patients within the facility, and intrapatient variation (σ) tests the ability of the healthcare team to reproduce this quality of care consistently in the same patient over time. Because Six Sigma is process oriented and driven, management must empower staff members to design and monitor the processes of both clinical performance and quality outcomes. Studies within our own Gambro Healthcare facilities suggest that variability in outcome performance, as determined by Six Sigma, is an important predictor of both medical outcomes and cost effectiveness.

The Quality Cost Continuum

Medical quality, as it is defined here, will always be directly linked to improving cost effectiveness, and vascular access quality programs are no exception [12, 13]. While different models of health care exist around the world, whether not for profit or for profit, there must be accountability and balance between spending and improved outcomes in order for quality to have meaning. There are fundamental choices available for appropriate vascular access care that impact on outcomes and cost. It is not surprising that choices in providing vascular access have an impact on the cost of providing care to dialysis patients. Hospitalization accounts for approximately 36% of the approximately USD 70,000 annual cost of taking care of a dialysis patient in the United States and the use of a catheter as the primary method of vascular access is the strongest predictor of hospitalization [14].

A native AVF using the patient's own endogenous vasculature is the preferred vascular access for hemodialysis owing to longevity of patency and low rate of complications, but success depends upon the physical attributes of the artery and vein selected as well as sufficient lead-in time for the fistula to mature. Arteriovenous grafts are the secondary preferred vascular access option, and grafts composed of polytetrafluoroethylene (PTFE) material are recommended over other synthetic material, or bovine grafts, because of their longer survival and surgical ease of construction and repair. The least desirable method of vascular access is a tunneled cuffed venous catheter, which is associated with high morbidity due to thrombosis and infection [1, 2, 15]. Infections, particularly linked to cuffed venous catheters, are second only to cardiovascular disease as a major cause of death and amplify the cost of managing patients with end-stage renal disease (ESRD) [16]. The results of the United States Renal Data System (USRDS) Morbidity and Mortality Study Wave 1 have clearly shown that adjusted relative risk for mortality is much higher in both diabetic and non-diabetic patients with a vascular catheter than in patients with an AVF, and grafts were associated with a higher mortality than AVFs in diabetic patients [17].

Catheters induce inflammatory responses from the immune system and contribute to the proinflammatory state, a characteristic of patients on dialysis that may have many adverse clinical effects, not the least of which is a decrease in the dose response to erythropoietin that escalates the cost of treating anemia [18–20]. Patients with catheters have more intradialytic complications, lower blood flows and significantly lower dialysis dose delivered than patients dialyzed through an AVF or graft [21]. Data from the United States Medicare dialysis program also indicate that the overall cost of care for dialysis patients with catheters or grafts is approximately 28 and 11% higher, respectively, than dialysis patients with an AVF [16].

In the United States, expenditures on vascular access have reached over 1 billion dollars per year and have prompted investment in interventional nephrology programs to improve care while at the same time reducing the cost of hospitalization owing to vascular access problems. There has been a movement towards developing dedicated access centers staffed by interventional nephrologists and such centers have been demonstrated to optimize the healthcare of hemodialysis patients and to have a positive impact on quality and cost [22].

Provision of renal replacement therapy for citizens with ESRD, regardless of the country of origin, is expensive and beyond affordable cost for almost any individual irrespective of the preferred healthcare system, be it for profit or not for profit, in the country of origin. The burden for supporting this therapy rests on tax-paying citizens. With the emerging global epidemic of diabetes, opportunities to be more cost effective cannot be ignored. The cost savings realized from a successful vascular access quality program may be invested in dialysis programs offering more frequent dialysis treatments, such as daily dialysis, or extending dialysis treatment times, both of which may provide added benefit to patients.

Vascular Access: The Current Situation

Any quality program must begin with the end in mind and with an appraisal of the benchmarks of vascular access quality, as they exist currently [23]. Across the world, there are differences in the use of AVFs, grafts and catheters among both incident patients and prevalent patients despite global acceptance by physicians of the value of reducing the use of catheters and increasing the use of AVFs [24].

As dialysis healthcare chains such as Gambro Healthcare and Fresenius Medical Care expand into the global marketplace, comparisons in vascular access outcomes between countries become possible. These data can be added to international outcome studies such as the Dialysis Outcomes and Practices

Patterns Study (DOPPS) that have pioneered global quality benchmarking in ESRD [24]. Surveillance data from Gambro Healthcare confirm that, among prevalent patients in the United States, the use of AVFs was 29% (DOPPS 24%) and catheters 20% (DOPPS 17%), while, in Europe, the use of AVFs was 81% (DOPPS 80%) and catheters 9% (DOPPS 8%) [24, 25].

There are also differences in vascular access rates among incident patients in the United States and Europe. Among 10,573 patients beginning dialysis within Gambro Healthcare facilities from 1998 through 2000, 58% initiated replacement therapy through a catheter and only 19.7% had a functioning AVF [25]. Surprisingly, there were no differences in the rates between patients who had private versus government-funded healthcare insurance, suggesting that the root causes of the problem were complex and deeply ingrained into the medical system. In Europe, the DOPPS found that 31% of incident patients began dialysis with a catheter although there was a broad spectrum among countries with Germany (15%) having the lowest incidence and United Kingdom (50%) the highest [24]. A similar broad spectrum of vascular access outcomes was found among the 18 regional networks in the United States in 2000, despite the introduction of clinical performance measures that require AVFs in 50% of incident patients and 40% of prevalent patients and a reduction in the use of catheters to 10% [26]. Vascular access data outlined above help to identify the extent of the problem and the extent to which the current situation deviates from peer-reviewed benchmarks.

Selecting a Quality Program

The program begins with the formation of a network of dialysis facilities that jointly recognize the value of comparative outcome data and are willing to share their data. In the United States this includes 18 regional networks but in other countries it may be facilities that jointly recognize the value of comparative outcome data. The facilities may be divided into geographic regions, as they are in the United States, but may also remain country specific such as in Europe and South America.

The next step is to form a peer review medical council, which should include physicians who consistently have achieved optimal outcomes in patient care, such as the least number of patients with catheters, the lowest vascular access complications and low vascular access-related hospitalization rates.

The QA process involves selecting a set of vascular access quality markers, setting a threshold of performance, monitoring compliance by setting a frequency of data collection, introducing corrective actions and confirming their effectiveness by follow-up surveillance. Point prevalent data, such as the percentage of patients in each facility dialyzed through a catheter or graft or AVF, are circulated throughout the network. The value of this initial approach is that it reveals the variations in practice patterns that exist among dialysis facilities in geographically similar regions [27]. Comparative data are compelling when organized in a hierarchical order from the facility with the highest percentage of catheters to that with the least [28]. Physicians are exposed to performance criteria from their peers and are provided with opportunities to examine reasons for the differences through their own internal QA programs.

This improvement by decree and inspection is the first step in providing visibility to vascular access standards of care and focuses attention on the issue. Unfortunately, this approach provides only one dimension to the quality continuum. Quality improvement is a multidimensional commitment by any healthcare program whether the program originates within a dialysis facility, group of facilities, corporation or country.

A multidisciplinary approach has been advocated in order to integrate and improve access care [29–31]. The program has the responsibility of coordinating the contribution of nephrologists, surgeons and interventionalists (surgeons, radiologists and nephrologists) with the dialysis healthcare team to provide leadership, improvements through process management, solutions to complex issues and the development of clinical pathways associated with optimal outcomes.

In order to expand on these principles and implement the guidelines advocated by peer review authorities, a vascular access care program (VACP) was developed by Gambro Healthcare and field-tested within the northeastern and southeastern United States in 1998 through 1999. It subsequently has been integrated within the Gambro Healthcare facilities, and our experiences with this program will be used to provide guidance as we negotiate the clinical pathway to optimal access care (see below).

Predialysis Vascular Access Quality Program (CKD Stage 2–4)

To have a maximum impact on vascular access outcomes, the vascular access quality program must proactively address access planning in CKD patients long before the need for permanent renal replacement therapy. Numerous studies demonstrate the relationship between early referral to a nephrologist and a higher likelihood of beginning dialysis with an autologous AVF [32–34]. Other studies have indicated that early referral does not fully explain the large regional variations in the percentage of AVFs in prevalent patients nor the failure of policies to increase the percentage of AVFs after initiation of dialysis, and late referral is now perceived as only one component in a complex chain of events that culminate in suboptimal vascular access care [35–37].

In the United States, nephrologists depend upon primary care physicians to refer CKD patients in sufficient time before dialysis initiation to coordinate surgical placement of the access. The reality is that this does not occur, and therefore catastrophic initiation of dialysis with a catheter is common. In an attempt to reverse this practice, major dialysis providers have developed pre-dialysis disease management programs.

In 2000, Gambro Healthcare developed a proprietary Connections© Program designed as a multidimensional QA program that focuses on improving predialysis patient outcomes through motivational educational programs that connect the patient to resources available in the community. A key component pertains to vascular access planning, including vessel site identification and preservation as well as vessel development through exercise. There are modules designed to motivate patients to practice healthy living behaviors such as compliance with medications, nutrition, and exercise. Other modules prompt clinical encounters at defined stages of kidney failure when medical interventions are appropriate.

Experience with the Gambro Healthcare Connections Program suggests that in order for education on the importance of vascular access to effectively impact clinical outcomes, encounters with the patient by the dialysis education team need to occur at CKD stage 2 (GFR 60–89 ml/min). The intention of the program is to prepare the patient for the acceptance of vascular access surgery by CKD stage 4 (GFR 15–29 ml/min). The Connections QA Program views the patient as having a central role in access planning and access planning as a fundamentally important component of the continuum of care in the predialysis period.

It is not the purpose of this review to describe the appropriate surgical evaluation of patients presenting for hemodialysis access. The surgical team, however, must be represented on the multidisciplinary vascular access CQI team to ensure that an algorithm for native AVF placement is appropriate and that interventions do not compromise future access planning. Such an algorithm developed by Huber et al. [38] is shown in figure 6. Essential components of the surgical QA algorithm include the physical examination process, non-invasive and invasive preoperative imaging practices, criteria used to determine the suitability of arteries and veins for AVF, and postoperative follow-up [39]. Each decision pathway in the algorithm should be documented preferably electronically in a vascular access medical history file for future reference and transfer to the dialysis facility medical files. The percentage of patients initiating dialysis with an AVF, graft or catheter should be documented and used to evaluate the predialysis vascular access quality program. While the goal is to achieve an AVF in at least 50% of all new patients, the most recent data from

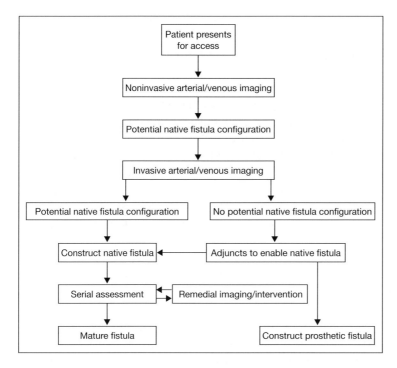

Fig. 6. Algorithm for the vascular access assessment and management of a patient prior to beginning hemodialysis [reproduced with permission, 38].

the United States regional networks indicate that only 27% of incident hemodialysis patients have an AVF [26].

Surveillance Data and Statistical Models

Surveillance data collection using electronic media have augmented and often replaced manual tools such as cause and effect diagrams, fishbone diagrams, cause and affect analysis, histograms, graphs, Pareto charts, scatter diagrams and use of a check sheet that lists all variables known to impact vascular access outcomes [40, 41]. The great value of constructing a vascular access database is that it facilitates the design of statistical models that enable hypotheses to be tested using univariate and multivariate regression analyses which identify the important variables contributing to suboptimal outcomes. The Cox proportional regression analysis is used to determine predictors of hazard such as mortality and vascular access failure [42–45]. These tools provide a level of insight into clinical pathways that was not possible in the preelectronic age. Statistical software packages for personal computers are available at low cost and allow predictive analyses to be performed by physicians and healthcare personnel with moderate expertise in statistical epidemiology. There are also sophisticated statistical software programs such as SAS version 6.12 (SAS Institute, Cary, N.C., USA) that incorporate program adjustments for facility level clustering and adjustments for random and nonrandom changes over time [45]. These tools, when added to the CQI matrix, enable resources to be quickly and efficiently directed to the root causes of suboptimal outcomes. Such a strategy can be used to identify the hierarchy of predictors of AVF, grafts or catheters in any patient cohorts.

Statistical models, for example, have shown that the predictors of having an AVF are similar between incident and prevalent hemodialysis patients. However, female patients are less likely to have an AVF despite recent evidence that anatomical differences are not a valid reason [24, 25, 28, 46, 47]. Obviously these data stress the need to correct the gender gap in appropriate vascular access care.

The Gambro Healthcare data, as well as those from the USA networks, suggest that the incidence of catheter use is increasing in both incident and prevalent patients, so the 'call to action' papers by opinion leaders in 1998 are equally applicable in 2003 and beyond [26, 48, 49]. Because the AVF may require several months to mature, access planning requires sufficient lead-in time to eliminate the need for temporary tunneled catheters. Indeed, according to the K/DOQI guidelines, patients should be referred to surgery for AVF placement within 1 year of anticipated initiation of dialysis therapy (or when creatinine clearance <25 ml/min or serum creatinine >4 mg/dl) [1, 2]. Data from the DOPPS study collected from approximately 5,000 HD patients in 145 US dialysis facilities and 101 dialysis facilities in Europe (France, Germany, Italy, Spain, and the United Kingdom) demonstrated that the strongest positive predictor for having an AVF, outside of geographical considerations, was being exposed to a predialysis care program [24].

These retrospective cross-sectional analyses are observational, not cause and effect, but they do provide a foundation upon which decisions regarding the appropriation of resources can be made. Prospective randomized controlled studies are used to show cause and effect. An advantage of observational studies is that the data are collected from a very large sample size and reflect the practices of physicians in the day-to-day care of patients. Controlled studies on the other hand are intended by their nature to reduce variations in clinical practice to the absolute minimum and may be very selective in their inclusion criteria. Therefore, the results of some controlled studies may not be directly applicable to clinical practice to the extent that some patients would not have been represented in the prospective controlled study owing to clinical parameters, such as comorbidity or compliance issues.

Vascular Access Care Program

The VACP is both the QA and CQI program for improving vascular access care and it should become an integral component of the dialysis facility's quality control team. The VACP is designed as a comprehensive proactive multidisciplinary team approach to survey and improve vascular access quality. An effective VACP requires a commitment to participatory leadership from the upper management of the facility, in particular the renal physician. The renal physician must participate as a team member and facilitate the multidisciplinary approach to solving problems.

The VACP team is educated in understanding the structure-process-outcome framework used in quality measurement (fig. 4). 'Structure' includes the table of organization within which the team functions and all of the policies and procedures developed within the organization to improve vascular access. It requires the team to understand the surgical and interventional programs that support the facility's VACP. Who are the surgeons responsible for access placement? Are they readily accessible for all patients? What services are offered? Are there data for surgeon-specific outcomes? What are the restraints under which the access placement program operates? Restraints might include factors ranging from access to operating room time to whether there is a regional predialysis CKD program, such as the Connections Program described earlier, that facilitates vascular access placement in a timely fashion prior to dialysis initiation. For example, studies within Gambro Healthcare suggest that the great variation in AVF placement in incident patients between facilities and within facilities is dependent on the nephrologist's involvement with surgical and medical colleagues in the medical community.

'Process' includes the execution of facility policies and procedures by the healthcare team to ensure success of the vascular access program. Process factors include flow charts and access surveillance protocols such as venous pressure monitoring and routine measurement of vascular access blood flow rate for the early detection of stenosis and risk for thrombosis. Also included are protocols to clear catheter blockage or to maintain optimal blood flow rates by using medications such as tissue plasminogen activator and urokinase [50, 51].

'Outcome' is measured at an optimal frequency and reported back to the quality control team to facilitate the early recognition of adverse trends and to document the value of interventions supported by the team. Quality has a time component that pertains to frequency of both monitoring and reporting as well as to documenting the achievement and maintenance of designated quality benchmarks. Once a quality benchmark has been reached, it should be maintained with as small a variation as possible, as measured by the SD of the mean. Applying the Six Sigma theory, facilities with lower SD in maintaining the specified benchmark are considered to have achieved a higher level of quality care than facilities maintaining the benchmark with higher SD.

At the level of a corporation or regional network management program, the VACP identifies facilities with suboptimal outcomes in vascular access and, through the application of CQI methodology, provides support to facility medical directors to improve outcomes. While appropriate benchmarks are determined by the corporate or network multidimensional team, at the facility level, realistic achievable improvements should be the primary focus of the CQI process rather than absolute target goals, or numbers, recommended by opinion leaders. To determine whether a facility is underperforming in relation to vascular access outcomes, the VACP team must compare vascular access point prevalence data with other facilities within the same geographic region. This requires sharing of data between independent facilities through a peer review body such as the Networks in the United States or the electronic communication of comparative data such as occurs within Gambro Healthcare. The facilities are arranged in descending order, for example, the facility having the lowest percentage of patients with a catheter as the only means of vascular access (no maturing AVF) at the top. Facilities in the lower quartile are then compared with facilities in the upper quartile regarding other quality markers for vascular access in an effort to determine the root cause of the problem. After analysis for confounding variables that may have impacted the results, facilities in the lower quartile are submitted to the VACP peer review committee for intervention. Confounders known to have an impact on quality differences among facilities include differences in illness acuity, abnormally high staff turnover, and a sudden influx of incident patients with catheters [52].

Such a process involves an open, honest dialogue with and within the facility identified. In some cases, this dialogue is between the peer review network physician or a regional quality council physician and the physician responsible for the facility. Experience has shown that, for the CQI process to be successful, there must be support from the medical leadership of the dialysis facility for the entire team that is responsible for instituting the VACP. Leadership includes commitment to the CQI philosophy by attending the vascular access team meetings, establishing a mission statement, and empowering the healthcare personnel on the CQI team. The team is responsible for identifying the patients affected, selecting the vascular access surveillance methodology, training the staff and instituting the correction plan through the application of countermeasures that correct the root causes of the suboptimal outcome. The team is also responsible for monitoring the outcome performance measures following institution of the correction plan and reporting results back to the entire facility healthcare team and the HD Network Committee. Following the success of the CQI program, the team is responsible for standardizing the corrective plan by incorporating it into the facility medical procedures and policies. Follow-up monitoring should be continued to ensure that the root causes for the suboptimal outcome do not reappear.

The QA/CQI process that we have described can be effective in addressing unexpected problems for which solutions might not be immediately apparent. Examples of such problems include the chronic occurrence of clotted AVFs or grafts despite an ongoing surveillance program, delivery of suboptimal dialysis dose resulting from undetected recirculation, and too few AVFs resulting from chronic issues within the predialysis program [53, 54]. To illustrate, in a vascular access program confronted with the problem of recurring access thrombosis, the first step taken was to evaluate the surveillance program that, in this case, involved clinical inspection and dynamic vascular pressure monitoring, referral for Doppler ultrasound and subsequent confirmation of the suspected stenosis by angiography, followed by percutaneous angioplasty or surgical revision. The program was not working because the surveillance process detected stenosis too late and there were delays in interventional and surgical procedures, and limited surgical repertoire augmented the incidence of access failure. Setting priorities as to which of the identified problems first ought to be addressed, the facility's VACP elected to invest in an alternative surveillance methodology that measured vascular access flow. As a result, access stenoses, particularly in grafts, were identified with sufficient lead-in time before occlusion so that angioplasty procedures effectively improved access survival for patients in the facility.

An effective strategy to improve vascular access outcomes within a corporation or regional network is to enlist the advice and counsel from physicians who have maintained a successful record of remaining in the upper quartile of vascular access outcome performance over an extended period of time. The Gambro Healthcare network has continued to identify facilities that maintain outcomes in the upper quartile for several years. It has been found, for example, that facilities with the highest percentages of AVFs inevitably are managed by renal physicians who participate early in the care of CKD patients. These nephrologists are involved in the community health programs that identify high-risk CKD patients, such as patients with diabetes and/or hypertension. They are actively engaged in strategies that delay kidney disease progression and have built strong collegial relationships among their peers in the community, always operating at the periphery of their own sphere of influence. Analysis of practice patterns and disease management strategies utilized by

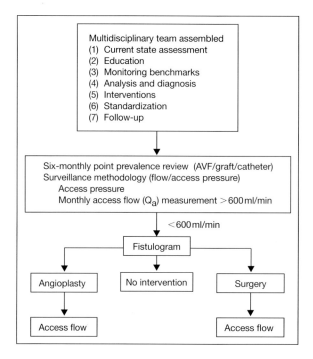

Multidisciplinary team assembled
(1) Current state assessment
(2) Education
(3) Monitoring benchmarks
(4) Analysis and diagnosis
(5) Interventions
(6) Standardization
(7) Follow-up

Six-monthly point prevalence review (AVF/graft/catheter)
Surveillance methodology (flow/access pressure)
  Access pressure
  Monthly access flow (Q_a) measurement > 600 ml/min

< 600 ml/min

Fistulogram

Angioplasty

No intervention

Surgery

Access flow

Access flow

Fig. 7. Components of the VACP.

physicians should become an important process used to foster improvement and excellence within the corporation or regional network VACP [55].

The following is a detailed example of an effective QA/CQI program in action that led to improvement of vascular access outcomes in 4 dialysis facilities in the northeastern United States and 6 facilities in the southeastern United States over a period of 3 years (1997 through 2000). Gambro Healthcare maintains a decentralized quality program that is supported by a central quality dataset known as the Nightingale Datamart® [11, 22]. Central surveillance data from the Nightingale Datamart indicated that the northeastern facilities had an incidence of catheter use significantly higher than other facilities in the same geographic region for four consecutive quarters. Trend analysis also indicated that catheter use was increasing over this time frame. In addition, vascular access hospitalization and noncompliance with the dialysis prescription frequency were significantly higher than in other facilities within that region, a characteristic of facilities with vascular access problems. The medical directors of the facilities assumed a leadership role in the ensuing months that the VACP was operating, a component essential to the success of the program. The 6 southeastern facilities were in the top quartile of vascular access outcomes and

Table 2. Quality metrics used to benchmark the success of the VACP

Quality marker	Target goal
Catheters[1]	10% reduction
AVF	10% increase
Graft	10% increase
Access-related hospitalization[2]	20% decrease
Access-related in-hospital days[3]	20% decrease
Access clotting[4]	20% decrease
Missed treatments for access-related problems[5]	20% decrease

[1]Catheters include patients using only catheter as primary means of vascular access.

[2]Access-related hospitalizations include total number of admissions to hospital for the cohort assessed.

[3]Access-related in-hospital days include total number of days spent in hospital by the cohort assessed resulting from access issues.

[4]Clotting events were confirmed by fistulogram and/or Doppler flow.

[5]Missed treatments include noncompliance caused by patients absenting themselves from the treatment because of access issues and do not include access-related hospitalization.

exceeded the benchmarks of the K/DOQI guidelines but, in this case, the medical director was not satisfied and believed that outcomes could be improved by implementing the same program.

The phases of implementation are shown in figure 7 and the details have been reported elsewhere [29, 30, 56, 57]. After monitoring the facilities for 6 months, the multidimensional team agreed upon a set of realistic achievable target goals for improving incidence of access thrombosis (table 2). Vascular access flow (Q_a) was assessed each month during dialysis using a Transonic HD01 hemodialysis monitor [30, 56]. This surveillance method had a sensitivity of 71% (true positive/true positive + false negatives × 100) and 100% specificity (true negatives/false positives + true negative × 100). Patients with measured access flow rates <600 ml/min were referred to radiology for confirmatory diagnosis by fistulogram. If a stenosis was detected, the patients were scheduled for angioplasty and/or surgery. Monitoring was continued on patients who were not confirmed to have a stenosis and patients who had access repair were followed to assess procedural effectiveness. Development of the program involved close collaboration between the radiology group and the surgical team. This multidisciplinary approach to improving vascular access outcomes has been reported by other workers [58].

Data collected over the first 6 months confirmed the value of using access flow rates to detect stenosis and to prevent clotting episodes (fig. 8). In the first

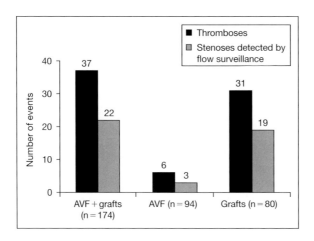

Fig. 8. Incidence of thromboses and stenosis detected by flow surveillance at Q_a <600 ml/min in a large inner city dialysis facility over 6 months after instituting a multidisciplinary VACP.

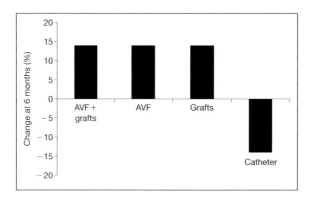

Fig. 9. Improvement in vascular access outcomes in a large inner city dialysis facility 6 months after instituting multidisciplinary VACP (n = 242).

6 months of instituting the program, there was a significant increase in both AVF and grafts as well as a reduction in the use of catheters (fig. 9). In the southeast, over the time frame that the program was being actively practiced, there was a 25% reduction in incident patients with catheters and an increase to 44% of incident patients with an AVF. This phenomenon of the mere presence of policies addressing vascular access resulting in more AVFs being placed has been reported in other studies [35, 56]. The shift in vascular access placement was accompanied by a decrease in the rates of radiological and surgical

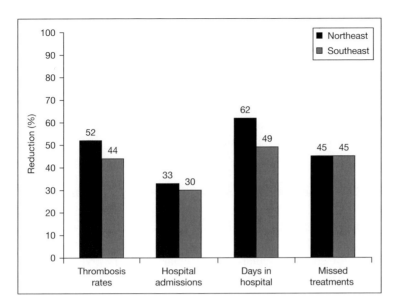

Fig. 10. Reduction in thrombosis rates (patient/month), hospital admissions for vascular access, number of days in hospital and missed treatments due to vascular access 2 years after instituting multidisciplinary VACP.

interventions performed: thrombectomies declined from 8.7 to 4.8% while fistulograms increased by 31% and angioplasties by 142%. As a consequence of implementing the QA/CQI process, the healthcare personnel in both regions of the country became highly skilled in recognizing vascular accesses that required intervention. Following the VACP being in place for 2 years, the success of the program was confirmed by reductions in thrombosis rate, vascular access hospitalizations, including length of stay, and missed treatments resulting from access problems (fig. 10).

The repetitive monitoring of selected vascular access quality benchmarks within any given year, such as biannually in the Core Indicators Project [26], has the important benefit of allowing conclusions to be reached by HD networks regarding the consistency of their access quality programs. Consistent quality over time and minimizing the variability in achieving quality benchmarks should become part of the HD network culture. As each facility in the lower quartile improves resulting from the CQI program, the benchmark means improve, the outcomes of facilities in the lower quartiles come closer to the outcomes of facilities in the highest quartile, and a culture of collaboration and mutual respect spreads within the network. Productivity improves and staff satisfaction with their responsibilities within the facility also improves.

When this level of quality performance is reached, one might consider shifting to the Six Sigma approach to monitoring SD in quality outcome means. Studies within Gambro Healthcare facilities suggest that variability in outcome performance is an important predictor of not only medical outcomes but also cost effectiveness. Facilities in the highest quartile of outcome performance that have the lowest SD in achieving specific outcome benchmarks usually have the lowest mortality and hospitalization rates and operate at lower cost than facilities with higher SD in outcome performance.

Infection Control and the Vascular Access Quality Program

An active infection control program within the dialysis facility augments the success of the vascular access quality program [59]. Infections are much more common with cuffed percutaneous vascular catheters and least often associated with AVFs. Variation in the type of vascular access being used among facilities influences the frequency of bloodstream infections encountered within the patient population and often the surveillance of bacteremias can be used as a tool to monitor the effectiveness of the vascular access quality program [60].

Primary bloodstream infections, where the pathogen was introduced directly into the patient's bloodstream from an external source, indicate either a break in infection control procedures or contamination of a medical device with direct access to the patient's bloodstream [61, 62]. The majority of secondary bloodstream infections occurring in hemodialysis patients originate from vascular percutaneous catheters [63].

The infection control program includes several components: active prospective surveillance of infections, staff and patient education about optimal antisepsis agents and techniques, prophylactic use of antimicrobial agents to eradicate nasal carriage of Staphylococcus, and policies that reduce the indiscriminate use of broad spectrum antibiotics [64–66]. Opportunities for the emergence of multiple resistant microbial pathogens are very high in long-term dialysis patients with underlying chronic disease, multiple episodes of infection and a history of antibiotic exposure [67].

Future Considerations

All vascular accesses have a limited life span. While it is not the purpose of this chapter to discuss future innovations in providing vascular access, it is worth mentioning that there have been significant advances in biocompatible flexible plastics coated with Teflon® polymers allowing endothelial cells rapidly to colonize the internal walls and mimic an autologous fistula [68]. Other new prosthetic devices discussed in another paper have reported encouraging results in clinical trials and these devices may have additional value where cannulation frequency is increased such as in daily short dialysis prescriptions [69].

The future success of vascular access quality programs may reside in the renal physicians gaining credentials as interventional nephrologists. The American Society for Diagnostic and Interventional Nephrology was founded in 2000 to promote training and certification for nephrologists in procedures related to hemodialysis catheters, peritoneal dialysis catheters, endoluminal procedures on hemodialysis accesses, and sonography of the kidneys and bladder [70]. Having an interventional nephrologist as an integral part of the healthcare team would be expected to have many benefits: improve the fragmented care of dialysis patients that results from delays in performing access interventions, lengthen survival time of accesses at risk, diminish hospitalizations for access procedures, enhance the development of a vascular access life plan for each patient by more frequent use of venous mapping, and support the development of an effective access care program [71–73]. Recent data from the USRDS suggests that the 25% reduction in vascular access-related hospitalizations between 1991 and 2000 among all age, gender, race, and primary diagnosis groups reflects the rising number of vascular access-related procedures performed in an outpatient setting [74]. It is expected that this new subspecialty of nephrology will expand into other areas of vascular access care traditionally reserved for vascular surgeons and radiologists, particularly the surgical placement of AVFs in a well-planned and timely manner. An essential component of this innovative approach will be having the QA/CQI program monitor patient outcomes as well as cost and patient satisfaction with the service. The development of interventional nephrology is an important approach to solving the predominant deficiencies in access care, particularly the timely recognition, diagnostic intervention and endoluminal correction of a failing access. The addition of this subspeciality to the already expanding knowledge and competency of renal physicians in managing vascular access planning and care will contribute to the ongoing success of renal replacement therapy.

References

1   NKF-DOQI clinical practice guidelines for vascular access. National Kidney Foundation-Dialysis Outcomes Quality Initiatives. Am J Kidney Dis 1997;30:S150–S190.
2   NKF-K/DOQI clinical practice guidelines for vascular access. National Kidney Foundation-Dialysis Outcomes Quality Initiatives. Am J Kidney Dis 2001;37(suppl 1):S137–S181.

3   Jindal KK, Ethier JH, Lindsay RM, Barre PE, Kappel JE, Carlisle EJF, Common A: Clinical Practice Guidelines for Vascular Access. Clinical Practice Guidelines of the Canadian Society of Nephrology for Treatment of Patients with Chronic Renal Failure. J Am Soc Nephrol 1999;10: S297–S305.

4   Di Giulio S, Meschini L, Triolo G: Dialysis outcome quality initiative (DOQI) guideline for hemodialysis adequacy. Int J Artif Organs 1998;21:757–761.

5   Schwab SJ, Beathard GA: The hemodialysis catheter conundrum: Hate living with them, but can't live without them. Kidney Int 1999;56:1–17.

6   Wu AW, Fink NE, Cagney KA, Bass EB, Rubin HR, Meyer KB, Sadler JH, Powe NR: Developing a health-related quality of life measure for end-stage renal disease: The CHOICE Health Experience Questionnaire. Am J Kidney Dis 2001;37:11–21.

7   NKF-K/DOQI clinical practice guidelines for chronic kidney disease: Evaluation, classification and stratification. Am J Kidney Dis 2002;37(suppl 1):S1–S266.

8   Sidawy AN, Gray R, Besarab A, Henry M, Ascher E, Silva M Jr, Miller A, Scher L, Trerotola S, Gregory RT, Rutherford RB, Kent KC: Recommended standards for reports dealing with arteriovenous hemodialysis accesses. J Vasc Surg 2002;35:603–610.

9   Kaplan RS, Norton DP: The Balanced Scorecard: Translating Strategy into Action. Boston, Harvard Business School Press, 1996.

10 Sackett DL: Evidence-Based Medicine: How to Practice and Teach EMB. New York, Churchill Livingstone, 1997.

11 Eckes G: The Six Sigma Revolution. New York, Wiley, 2001.

12 Eggers P, Milan R: Trends in vascular access procedures and expenditures in Medicare ESRD program; in Henry ML (ed): Vascular Access for Hemodialysis. Part VII. New York, Gore, 2001, pp 133–143.

13 Bosch JP, Walters BA: Continuous quality improvement for a hemodialysis network. Contrib Nephrol 2002;137:300–310.

14 Anel RL, Yevzlin AS, Ivanovich P: Vascular access and patient outcomes in hemodialysis: Questions answered in recent literature. Artif Organs 2003;27:237–241.

15 Pastan S, Soucie JM, McClellan W: Vascular access and increased risk of death among hemodialysis patients. Kidney Int 2002;62:620–626.

16 US Renal Data System: Excerpts from the USRDS 2001 Annual Data Report: Atlas of end stage renal disease in the United States. Am J Kidney Dis 2001;38(suppl 3):S1–S248.

17 Dhingra RK, Young EW, Hulbert-Shearon TE, Leavey SF, Port FK: Type of vascular access and mortality in US hemodialysis patients. Kidney Int 2001;60:1443–1451.

18 Ayus JC, Sheikh-Hamad D: Silent infection in clotted hemodialysis access grafts. J Am Soc Nephrol 1998;9:1314–1321.

19 Kaysen GA: Role of inflammation and its treatment in ESRD patients. Blood Purif 2002;20: 70–80.

20 Walters BAJ, Carter WB, Augustine BA, Bander SJ: Central venous catheters contribute to low blood hemoglobin in hemodialysis patients (abstract). J Am Soc Nephrol 2000;11:295A.

21 Ravani P, Marcelli D, Malberti F: Vascular access surgery managed by renal physicians: The choice of native arteriovenous fistulas for hemodialysis. Am J Kidney Dis 2002;40:1264–1276.

22 Arnold WP: Improvement in hemodialysis vascular access outcomes in a dedicated access center. Semin Dial 2000;13:359–363.

23 Bosch JP, Walters BAJ: Quality assurance and continuous quality improvement in the management of vascular access; in Ronco C, La Greca G (eds): Hemodialysis Technology. Contrib Nephrol. Basel, Karger, 2002, vol 137, pp 60–69.

24 Pisoni RL, Young EW, Dykstra DM, Greenwood RN, Hecking E, Gillespie B, Wolfe RA, Goodkin DA, Held PJ: Vascular access use in Europe and the United States: Results from the DOPPS. Kidney Int 2002;61:305–316.

25 Walters BAJ, Chan WW, Klasson PS, Ryu S, Bosch JP: Characteristics of patients beginning dialysis in the United States on government-funded vs. privately funded health insurance coverage. Dial Transplant 2002;31:735–750.

26 Center for Medicare and Medicaid Services: 2001 Annual Report: End Stage Renal Disease Clinical Performance Measures Project. Am J Kidney Dis 2002;39(suppl 2):S1–S98.

27 Allon M, Ornt BD, Schwab SJ, Rasmussen C, Delmez JA, Green T, Kusek JW, Martin AA, Minda S: Factors associated with the prevalence of arteriovenous fistulas in hemodialysis patients in the HEMO study. Kidney Int 2000;58:2178–2185.
28 Theelen B, Rorive G, Krzesinski JM, Collart F: Belgian peer review experience on the Achilles' heel in haemodialysis care: Vascular access. EDTNA ERCA J 2002;28:164–166.
29 Spergel LM: Improving outcomes in the face of managed care and capitation: One surgeon's perspective. Nephrol News Issues 1997;11/3:26–35.
30 Duda CR, Spergel LM, Holland J, Tucker T, Bander SJ, Bosch JP: How a multidisciplinary vascular access care program enables implementation of the DOQI guidelines. Nephrol News Issues 2000;14:13–17.
31 Burton B, Gross S, Vilchek DL: A CQI approach to improved vascular access outcomes. Nephrol News Issues 1995;9:33–36.
32 Arora P, Obrador GT, Ruthazer R, Kausz AT, Meyer KB, Jenuleson CS, Pereira BJ: Prevalence, predictors and consequences of late referral at a tertiary care center. J Am Soc Nephrol 1999;10: 1281–1286.
33 Goransson LG, Bergrem H: Consequences of late referral of patients with end-stage renal disease. J Intern Med 2001;250:154–159.
34 Avorn J, Winkelmayer WC, Bohn RL, Levin R, Glynn RJ, Levy E, Owen W Jr: Delayed nephrologist referral and inadequate vascular access in patients with advanced chronic kidney failure. J Clin Epidemiol 2002;55:711–716.
35 Besarab A: Preventing vascular access dysfunction: Which policy to follow. Blood Purif 2002;20: 26–35.
36 Allon M, Robbin ML: Increasing arteriovenous fistulas in hemodialysis patients: Problems and solutions. Kidney Int 2002;62:1109–1124.
37 Besarab A, Adams M, Amatucci S, Bowe D, Deane J, Ketchen K, Reynolds K, Tello A: Unravelling the realities of vascular access: The Network 11 experience. Adv Ren Replace Ther 2000; 4(suppl 1):S65–S70.
38 Huber TS, Ozaki CK, Flynn TC, Lee WA, Berceli SA, Hirneise CM, Carlton LM, Carter JW, Ross EA, Seeger JM: Prospective validation of an algorithm to maximize native arteriovenous fistulae for chronic hemodialysis access. J Vasc Surg 2002;36:452–459.
39 Huber TS, Seeger JM: Approach to patients with 'complex' hemodialysis access problems. Semin Dial 2003;16:22–29.
40 Allon M, Ornt BD, Schwab SJ, Rasmussen C, Delmez JA, Green T, Kusek JW, Martin AA, Minda S: Factors associated with the prevalence of arteriovenous fistulas in hemodialysis patients in the HEMO study. Kidney Int 2000;58:2178–2185.
41 Astor BC, Eustace MB, Powe NR, Klag MJ, Sadler JJH, Kink NE, Coresh J: Timing of nephrologist referral and arteriovenous use: The CHOICE study. Am J Kidney Dis 2001;38:494–501.
42 Le CT: Applied Categorical Analysis. New York, Wiley, 1998.
43 LE CT: Applied Survival Analysis. New York, Wiley, 1998.
44 Fisher LD, Van Belle V: Biostatistics: A Methodology for the Health Sciences. New York, Wiley, 1993.
45 Klein JP, Moeschberger ML: Survival Analysis Techniques for Censored and Truncated Data. New York, Springer, 1997.
46 Walters BAJ, Augustine B, Bander SJ: Gender does not influence medical outcomes, quality of life or patient satisfaction in a major dialysis provider in the United States. Women and Renal Disease, National Institute of Health, September 14–17, 1999 (http://niddk.nih.gov/fund/reports/womenrd/poster.htm).
47 Caplin N, Sedlacek M, Teodorescu V, Falk A, Uribarri J: Venous access: Women are equal. Am J Kidney Dis 2003;41:429–432.
48 Hakim R, Himmelfarb J: Hemodialysis access failure: A call to action. Kidney Int 1998;54: 1029–1040.
49 Schwab SJ: Improving access patency: Pre-end-stage renal disease strategies. J Am Soc Nephrol 1998;9:S124–S129.
50 Zacharias JM, Weatherston CP, Spewak CR, Vercaigne LM: Alteplase versus urokinase for occluded hemodialysis catheters. Ann Pharmacother 2003;37:27–33.

51   Northsea C: Continuous quality improvement: Improving hemodialysis catheter patency using urokinase. ANNA J 1996;23:567–571.

52   Friedman AL, Walworth C, Meehan C, Wander H, Shemin D, DeSoi W, Kitsen J, Hill C, Lambert C, Mesler D: First hemodialysis access selection varies with patient acuity. Adv Ren Replace Ther 2000;4(suppl 1):S4–S10.

53   Svara E: Vascular access monitoring evaluated from automated recirculation measurement. EDTNA ERCA J 2001;27:17–22.

54   Malik J, Slavikova M, Malikova H, Maskova J: Many clinically silent access stenoses can be identified by ultrasonography. J Nephrol 2002;15:661–665.

55   Reddan D, Klassen P, Frankeenfield DL, Szczech L, Schwab S, Coladonato J, Rocco M, Lowrie EG, Owen WF Jr: National profile of practice patterns for hemodialysis vascular access in the United States. J Am Soc Nephrol 2002;13:2117–2124.

56   Krivitski NM, Gantela S: Access flow measurement as a predictor of hemodialysis graft thrombosis: Making clinical decisions. Semin Dial 2001;14:181–185.

57   Duda CR, Spergel LM, Holland J, Tucker CT, Bander SJ, Bosch JP: Lessons learned. Implementing a vascular access quality improvement program. Part II. Nephrol News Issues 2000;14:29–32.

58   Allon M, Bailey R, Ballard R, Deierhoi MH, Hamrick K, Oser R, Rhynes VK, Robbin ML, Saddekni S, Ziegler ST: A multidisciplinary approach to hemodialysis access: Prospective evaluation. Kidney Int 1998;53:473–479.

59   Tokars JI, Miller ER, Stein G: New national surveillance system for hemodialysis-associated infections: Initial results. Am J Infect Control 2002;30:288–295.

60   Taylor G, Gravel D, Johnston L, Embil J, Holton D, Paton S: Prospective surveillance for primary bloodstream infections occurring in Canadian hemodialysis units. Infect Control Hosp Epidemiol 2003;23:716–720.

61   Tokars JI, Arduino MJ, Alter MJ: Infection control in hemodialysis units. Infect Dis Clin North Am 2001;15:797–812.

62   Dopirak M, Hill C, Oleksiw M, Dumigan D, Arvai J, English E, Carusillo E, Malo-Schlegel S, Richo J, Traficanti K, Welch B, Cooper B: Surveillance of hemodialysis-associated primary bloodstream infections: The experience of ten hospital-based centers. Infect Control Hosp Epidemiol 2002;23:721–724.

63   Price CS, Hacek D, Noskin GA, Peterson LR: An outbreak of bloodstream infections in an outpatient hemodialysis center. Infect Control Hosp Epidemiol 2003;23:725–729.

64   Berns JS, Tokars JI: Preventing bacterial infections and antimicrobial resistance in dialysis patients. Am J Kidney Dis 2002;40:886–898.

65   Tokars JI, Light P, Anderson J, Miller ER, Parrish J, Armistead N, Jarvis WR, Gehr T: A prospective study of vascular access infections in seven outpatient hemodialysis centers. Am J Kidney Dis 2001;37:1232–1240.

66   Tokars JI, Gehr T, Jarvis WR, Anderson J, Armistead N, Miller ER, Parrish J, Qaiyumi S, Arduino M, Holt SC, Tenover FC, Westbrook G, Light G: Vancomycin resistant enterococci colonization in patients at seven hemodialysis centers. Kidney Int 2001;60:1511–1516.

67   Chang S, Sievert DM, Hageman JC, Boulton ML, Tenover FC, Downes FP, Shah S, Rudrik JT, Pupp GR, Brown WJ, Cardo G, Fridkin SK: Infection with vancomycin-resistant *Staphylococcus aureus* containing the van A resistance gene. N Engl J Med 2003;348:1342–1347.

68   Baquey C: New polymer, surface treatments, bioactive materials: Value of vascular access devices. Nephrologie 2001;22:399–402.

69   Haynes BJ, Quarles AW, Vavrinchik J, White J, Pedan A: The LifeSite hemodialysis access system: Implications for the nephrology nurse. Nephrol Nurs J 2002;29:27–32.

70   O'Neill WC, Ash SR, Work J, Saad TF: American Society for Diagnostic and Interventional Nephrology. Guidelines for training, certification, and accreditation. Semin Dial 2003;16:173–176.

71   Rasmussen RL: Establishing an interventional nephrology suite. Semin Nephrol 2002;22:237–241.

72   Asif A, Byers P, Vieira CF, Preston RA, Roth D: Diagnostic and interventional nephrology. Am J Ther 2002;9:530–536.

73   Asif A, Byers P, Gadalean F, Roth D: Peritoneal dialysis underutilization: The impact of an inter-
      ventional nephrology peritoneal dialysis access program. Semin Dial 2003;16:266–271.
74   US Renal Data System: Excerpts from the USRDS 2002 Annual Data Report: Atlas of End-Stage
      Renal Disease in the United States. Am J Kidney Dis 2003;41(suppl 2):S189–S204.

Brian A.J. Walters, Phd, CLD
Scientific Affairs & Clinical Research
Gambro Healthcare
3951 SW 30th Avenue
Ft. Lauderdale, FL 33312 (USA)
E-Mail Brian.Walters@us.gambro.com

Ronco C, Levin NW (eds): Hemodialysis Vascular Access and Peritoneal Dialysis Access.
Contrib Nephrol. Basel, Karger, 2004, vol 142, pp 350–362

....

Systemic Barriers to Vascular Access Care: Implications for Clinical Outcomes

Jeffrey J. Sands[a]*, Andrea L. Montis*[b]*, Gina D. Etheredge*[b]

[a] Fresenius Medical Care NA, Celebration, Fla., and
[b] Tulane University School of Public Health and Tropical Medicine,
New Orleans, La., USA

Vascular access failure remains among the most frequent causes of hospitalization for patients with end-stage renal disease (ESRD). In fact, vascular access complications may be considered to have reached epidemic proportions in the United States. PTFE grafts remain the most commonly used vascular access, catheter use continues to increase and patients continue to have more than one access procedure per patient-year [1]. The Clinical Practice Measurement Project reported that only 28% of incident and 27% of prevalent US patients utilized arteriovenous fistulas (AV fistulas) as their primary access. In contrast, 43% of incident and 50% of prevalent US patients utilized PTFE grafts; catheter use was 30% in incident and 23% in prevalent patients [2]. This practice pattern leads directly to extensive morbidity and high costs. The United States Renal Data System (USRDS) reported that access-related expenditures by Medicare alone were greater than USD 1.5 billion in 2002 [1].

The high rate of catheter and graft placement is significantly different in the United States than in Europe. Data from the Dialysis Outcomes Practice Pattern Study (DOPPS) revealed that 67% of patients used an AV fistula for their first dialysis ever in European DOPPS centers. In contrast, only 15% of patients used an AV fistula and 59% relied on catheter access for their first dialysis in the United States. This marked difference in the type of access persists in prevalent patients. The vast majority of prevalent European patients used AV fistulas (81%); only 10% of prevalent European patients used PTFE grafts and 8% used catheters. This is in stark contrast to the US aggregate totals of 24% AV fistulas, 58% PTFE grafts and 17% catheters even after controlling for case mix variation including age, diagnosis, sex and body mass index [3].

This pattern of access use has profound implications for clinical outcomes. AV fistulas have significantly fewer complications than PTFE grafts or cuffed catheters. The relative risk of requiring a declotting procedure or revision is 7-fold greater in patients with grafts compared to patients with AV fistulas and 8-fold higher for requiring any access procedure [3]. While positive outcomes associated with PTFE graft use are fewer than for patients with AV fistulas, the increased use of cuffed catheters results in even worse outcomes [4, 5]. It has been reported that nondiabetic prevalent patients with cuffed catheters had a 70% increase in the relative risk of mortality compared to patients with AV fistulas even after adjusting for case mix [4]. The increased mortality risk is also striking in diabetics. Prevalent diabetic patients with cuffed catheters had a 54% increase and patients with PTFE grafts a 41% increase in the relative risk of death when compared to AV fistula patients. Among incident cases, catheter patients had a 91% increase in the relative risk of death and graft patients had a 64% increase in the relative risk of death compared to fistula patients. Similar data have been reported elsewhere and support these findings [Lowrie, pers. commun.]. In a sample of greater than 38,000 patients adjusted for case mix and laboratory values including KT/V and serum albumin, patients with cuffed catheters had a relative risk of death of 1.96 compared to patients with AV fistulas while graft patients had a relative risk of 1.32.

Mortality, however, is not the only concern. Patients with cuffed catheters develop frequent episodes of catheter-related septicemia, generally reported in the range of 2.3/1,000 patient-days [6–8]. A major proportion of these episodes are caused by *Staphylococcus aureus* and result in a significant incidence of major complications including epidural abscess, endocarditis and other serious metastatic infectious complications. In a US catheter population of approximately 80,000, these complications represent projected preventable deaths or major complications of up to 8,000 patients/year. Although the best approach is to avoid catheters, appropriate catheter care can make a difference. A randomized placebo-controlled trial of polysporin applied during weekly dressing changes showed that the polysporin group had a significantly lower infection rate (1.02 vs. 4.1/1,000 catheter-days), decreased catheter-related bacteremia (1.63 vs. 2.48/1,000 catheter-days) and significantly decreased hospitalization (7 vs. 24%) and mortality (4 vs. 16%) than the control group [9]. These data points signal there is significant room for improvement in catheter-related care even for patients who cannot have alternative access.

The National Kidney Foundation Dialysis Outcomes Quality Initiative (DOQI) and its recent revision K/DOQI, have established national guidelines for access-related care [10, 11]. This publication sets down strict recommendations for AV fistula placement, catheter reduction, specific catheter location, hemo-dialysis access surveillance and intervention/outcome results. These recommendations have received approval and praise throughout the ESRD community in the United States and throughout Europe. However, despite general agreement, most of these recommendations have not been put into practice in the majority of dialysis facilities in the United States. Why have practice patterns in the US not changed to reflect the K/DOQI recommendations? The dichotomy between accepted guidelines and actual practice is evidence of the systemic nature of patient care [12]. Clinical outcomes are dependent upon the structure of the health care delivery system and its inherent incentives and disincentives. Each delivery system attributes that result in differing approaches to patient care. Many of the outcome and practice pattern differences between Europe and the United States are a reflection of both cultural and learned behaviors, and incentives and disincentives which are built into the delivery system. These result in specific systemic barriers to improving care delivery.

There are many factors that contribute to the fact that vascular access outcomes have improved only marginally in the United States. One problem is that the focus has been only on dialysis facilities. The greatest opportunity for improving access outcomes is to increase AV fistula prevalence and to reduce catheter use. This is dependent upon the efforts of vascular surgeons, nephrologists and hospitals. Dialysis facilities, however, play only a small role in access choice and creation. Another concern is a general lack of accountability for patient outcomes and access choices. Hospitals, vascular surgeons and interventional radiologists often do not track a patient's vascular access outcomes or their aggregate use of AV fistulas, grafts and catheters. There is no requirement to achieve or enforce accepted standards such as the K/DOQI. Neither are they routinely involved in the dialysis facility's quality improvement process. As a result, they are often unaware and uninvolved with the implications of their decisions.

Physicians and hospitals face significant financial disincentives to providing optimal vascular access care. This has fostered an industry that reacts to complications rather than preventing them and rewards the care of failing or infected accesses instead of the prevention of complications. Some of the financial disincentives for increasing fistula placement are illustrated by the Medicare allowable payment schedule [13]. Physician reimbursement for AV fistula placement is generally in the range of USD 570–640 compared to USD 760–845 for PTFE graft placement (2001 data). Although transposed fistulas are reimbursed at a higher rate (approximately USD 815–910), transposed fistula creation requires significantly increased effort and prolonged surgery. Graft declotting pays USD 420–475 when performed without surgical revision and up to USD 725 when performed with revision. In a very real sense, PTFE grafts become an annuity, incited by quick and easy placement at a higher reimbursement, followed by the frequent need for declotting and revision with their own separate reimbursements. Although catheter placement is reimbursed at a lower amount (approximately USD 160–175 for temporary catheters and USD 350 for permanent catheters), catheter placements are short-term solutions that shift the burden to other providers. By providing the patient with a short-term fix, the problem disappears. However, as previously discussed, long-term complications increase.

Improving vascular access outcomes should begin from the patient-centered perspective. In this context, vascular access represents a cycle that goes from initial access placement, to access maintenance, to repair and finally, to access loss resulting in the placement of a secondary access. The goal of nephrologists and caregivers is to slow down the cycle by placing accesses that function every time without complications. Understanding the delivery system's impact requires a careful review of each step in the vascular access process and ascertaining which changes will have the greatest impact on patient outcomes.

First, patients need to be identified, preferably when they reach stage 3 of chronic kidney disease (CKD) (glomerular filtration rate of 30–59 ml/min) and referred to a nephrologist for CKD care. Surgical evaluation for AV fistula placement is indicated when their glomerular filtration rate is less than 25–30 ml/min. Arterial and venous mapping by duplex ultrasound to find appropriate vessels for AV fistula creation must be a routine part of surgical evaluation. Finally, careful follow-up for maturation of the AV fistula is crucial. Barriers that result in late referrals, inadequate surgical evaluations, access placement without preoperative imaging and lack of follow-up result in increased numbers of emergency access placements and an increase in the use of catheters and grafts. The resulting decrease in AV fistulas inevitably leads to poorer outcomes.

The areas that provide the best opportunities to improve access placement are early referrals and preoperative imaging. Preoperative imaging maximizes successful AV fistula placement. Early referral provides time to resolve or minimize complications before the patient requires an emergency catheter. The cooperation of primary care physicians, nephrologists and vascular surgeons is required to enact these changes. Vascular surgeons have the greatest ability to increase AV fistula creation. Holding hospitals and surgeons accountable for the type and success of accesses they place is an important component of increasing the number of fistulas and limiting the use of catheters. Unfortunately, preoperative imaging is not routinely reimbursed in the United States. The importance of preoperative imaging must be underscored; without careful planning and identification of an adequate artery and outflow vein, AV fistula creation can potentially result in more harm than good. Patients with failed fistulas often return to the hospital for emergency access usually in the form of a catheter. Thus, without the knowledge gained through preoperative imaging, AV fistula placement initiatives run the risk of increasing catheter use and catheter-related complications.

These opportunities for improving access care through early patient identification, appropriate referrals, and preoperative imaging have been highlighted [14]. It was demonstrated that patients followed by a nephrologist and with a gradual, predictable progression towards ESRD used AV fistulas as their initial access 46% of the time, while 19% used a PTFE graft and 35% a cuffed catheter. Only 21% of patients followed by a nephrologist who had an unexpected acceleration of their renal failure used fistulas as their first dialysis access while 15% used grafts and 62% utilized catheters. Patients who presented with an acute need for dialysis utilized AV fistulas only 2% of the time, grafts 10% of the time and catheters 85% of the time, illustrating the marked impact of CKD care on the type of vascular access placed.

Preoperative imaging is the standard of care for evaluating patients for all types of vascular surgery including carotid bypass and abdominal aneurysm surgery. It is also used extensively in Europe to select appropriate vessels prior to AV fistula creation [15, 16]. In the United States, however, dialysis accesses historically have been created based on physical exam alone without the benefits of preoperative imaging, even though the impact of performing arterial and venous mapping on patients prior to access creation has been demonstrated [17]. Successful AV fistula creation increased from 14% in 1992–1994 to 63% in 1994–1997. This was coupled with a decrease in catheter use from 24 to 7% during the same time frame. Most importantly, early fistula failure was decreased from 38 to 8.3%. This was accomplished by identifying and utilizing veins that met the following specific criteria: (1) a luminal diameter ≥2.5 mm for AV fistulas and ≥4 mm for grafts, (2) exhibit continuity with a deep venous system and (3) demonstrate the absence of segmental stenosis, occluded segments and have patent central veins. Arteries were required to be: (1) ≥2 mm in diameter at the wrist or ≥2.5 mm at the elbow, (2) exhibit no significant pressure differential between the two arms and (3) have a patent palmer arch [17]. Similar results were achieved by others who reported an increase in AV fistula placement from 5 to 68% using a program that included preoperative arterial/ venous mapping by duplex ultrasound to select appropriate vessels (vein diameter ≥2 mm at the wrist or ≥3 mm in the upper arm) and the use of basilic transposition where appropriate. Primary 1-year fistula patency was 85% and only 4% required revisions [18]. In the last year of the program over 95% of patients underwent AV fistula placement. Over three quarters of patients had maturation times of less than 6 weeks, defined as the ability to perform dialysis at prescribed blood flows greater than 300 ml/min with two dialysis needles. Other groups have reported marked increases in AV fistula prevalence utilizing this combination of preoperative imaging, the use of vein transpositions and a focus on maximizing AV fistula creation [19–24]. One report showed fistula placement increasing from approximately 12% in 1993 to over 75% in 1998 [24]. When transposed fistulas were included, their aggregate fistula creation rate was over 95%. Significant cost savings are observed by allowing the increased use of outpatient access placement rather than emergency inpatient procedures. In a review of Medicare payment data on 149,362 access placements, outpatient access placements were USD 9,105.00 less expensive on average than similar procedures performed in the in-patient area (1996 data) [25]. These findings have significant implications for health care policy and delivery.

Access maintenance involves access monitoring followed by imaging of accesses at high risk of developing subsequent access failure, coupled with elective intervention to correct significant areas of stenosis. Surgical evaluation with elective surgical repair is necessary for the subgroup of patients not amenable to or with poor results from angioplasty. Follow-up monitoring and planning is important to ensure successful lesion correction and to assure the most appropriate course of action if further problems develop. Barriers to provision of any of these services result in an increase in emergency access procedures leading to hospitalization, higher procedure rates, increased use of catheters and decreased AV fistula rates. Most gains can be achieved by developing monitoring programs coupled with elective revision. This facilitates the change from emergent inpatient procedures to outpatient procedures, reduces total procedure rates and the need for catheters. Although dialysis facilities play an important role, physicians, especially nephrologists, vascular surgeons, and interventional radiologists, have the greatest potential for improving patient outcomes.

The utility of access monitoring, coupled with elective intervention, has been illustrated [26]. It was reported that when monthly access flow measurement was instituted, graft thrombosis rates decreased from 0.71/patient-year in patients without access monitoring and 0.67/patient-year in grafts undergoing dynamic venous pressure monitoring to 0.16 thrombosis/patient-year. AV fistula thrombosis rates fell from an average of 0.14–0.15/patient-year before access flow monitoring to 0.07/patient-year with active access flow monitoring. The type of monitoring technique, the target population, and the speed of elective intervention are crucial to improving outcomes. Prolonged wait times of greater than 2 weeks for elective procedures can result in a significant loss of program efficacy and can create additional work without significant outcome improvements.

Recently, however, the effectiveness of access monitoring in predicting future thrombosis has become controversial. A meta-analyses and a prospective trial demonstrated that access flow measurement was only approximately 80% sensitive and 80% specific for identifying future access thrombosis [27, 28]. Others reported that neither dynamic nor static venous pressures were predictive of graft thrombosis [29]. Although access flow monitoring was the best predictor of future thrombosis, the area under the curve (ROC) was only 0.73. This is consistent with a screening test that is neither highly sensitive nor specific. (An ROC of 1.0 denotes a perfect test with 100% sensitivity and 100% specificity, while an ROC of 0.5 describes a test that is no more sensitive or specific than random sampling.) How can we interpret this conflicting data that on the one hand shows significant decreases in thrombosis using access surveillance programs and yet, on the other, poor sensitivity and specificity of these monitoring techniques?

The impact of prevalence on positive and negative predictive value is well understood among epidemiologists and has a profound influence on the utility of monitoring studies. For a given test, positive predictive values increase and negative predictive values decrease with increasing prevalence of a condition in a population. For example, if a test has an 80% sensitivity and an 80% specificity (similar to those observed for access flow monitoring) and if disease prevalence is 80% (current PTFE thrombosis rates), the positive predictive value of the test would be 94.1% with a negative predictive value of 50%. This is good for a monitoring study because over 94% of patients referred for intervention would have demonstrable disease. However, if the prevalence falls to 20% (similar to the thrombosis rate in AV fistulas), the positive predictive value of the same test would be only 50%, with a negative predictive value of 94%. This means that half the patients would be referred unnecessarily for intervention. This clearly illustrates that the effectiveness of a monitoring program is dependent on both the nature of the test (procedure) and the prevalence of disease in the target population.

Numerous authors previously have demonstrated the impact of access monitoring [26, 30–35]. Thrombosis rates in access flow monitoring programs have been demonstrated to be 0.1–0.3/patient-year in AV fistulas and 0.2–0.5/patient-year in AV grafts. This compares to baseline thrombosis rates of 0.25–0.40/patient-year in AV fistulas and 0.8–1.2/patient-year in grafts without monitoring [26, 32–35]. Procedure rates can be decreased to less than one per patient-year in PTFE grafts and the 75/25% thrombectomy/angioplasty ratio can be reversed, resulting in the replacement of emergent procedures with elective procedures [26, 30–35]. For these reasons, K/DOQI continues to recommend monthly access monitoring for all patients with grafts and fistulas (guideline 10) [11].

Unfortunately, access failure and the need for access repair is a common event. Repair requires identification and correction of the pathologic lesions and a confirmation of physiologic improvement after the procedure. Often patients have more than one lesion and unless there is a confirmation of physiologic improvement, for example, an increase in access flow, it is possible that the lesion corrected was not in fact the underlying source of the patient's problem. Additionally, all patients who undergo access repair should be evaluated for a secondary AV fistula and an access plan should be incorporated into the patient record to guide future interventions. This results in fewer procedures, more fistulas and fewer catheters. Central to facilitating these outcomes are the roles of nephrologist, vascular surgeon and interventionalist. Dialysis facilities play a part by documenting the access plan as elaborated by the treating physician. Recently, with the introduction of outpatient percutaneous access intervention centers, it has become much easier to perform emergent procedures. They provide excellent service and care for patients. Unless used appropriately, this ease of use can lead to decreased planning and result in a procedure epidemic. Their availability must be coupled with careful planning to ensure that the appropriate procedure is performed at each juncture.

In reality, most patients have adequate sites for AV fistula placement. Our group performed arterial and venous mapping by Doppler ultrasound on prevalent patients with catheters or grafts. Using Silva's criteria, over 65% of catheter patients and over 73% of graft patients were identified as having suitable arteries and veins for subsequent AV fistula creation. Over 85% of patients with forearm loop grafts have adequate vasculature for fistula creation in the upper arm [36, 37]. This is not surprising because one has to have adequate inflow and venous outflow to have a functioning forearm graft. The strategy of creating secondary fistulas has been demonstrated. A program dictating the replacement of failing PTFE grafts with secondary fistulas successfully increased in AV fistula prevalence from less than 45 to 71% [38]. This strategy has high impact and poses little risk for patient complications.

In reviewing the vascular access cycle from creation to maintenance, loss and replacement, we have identified a number of potential targets for intervention. Those with the highest impact include, but are not limited to, early referral to nephrologists prior to their need for dialysis (CKD program), preoperative imaging and mapping to increase successful AV fistula placement, and the creation of secondary AV fistulas in patients with failing grafts. These are also the most cost-effective interventions. This combination of high impact on improving patient outcomes and the potential for significant cost savings emphasizes that these interventions (early nephrologic referral, pre-ESRD care, preoperative imaging and secondary AV fistula creation) should be the improvement targets for our care delivery system.

Understanding clinical process dynamics is necessary when considering the role of a care delivery system on patient outcome. Clinical effectiveness is defined by the impact of a program on patient outcomes. In the vascular access setting this is the result of a series of interventions rather than one simple procedure. For any intervention to be effective, one must first identify the group of patients at high risk, i.e. the target population. These patients must then be enrolled in the program. Once this has occurred, each therapy has a particular efficacy. It is only by multiplying the effects of each of these steps that one can ascertain the cumulative impact. The interaction of these factors is defined by the system of care. For example, 80% of patients are known to be candidates for fistula creation. This represents the identification of the target group. If only 50% of these patients are referred for AV fistula creation, as is currently the practice in the United States, and if fistula creation is successful in 67% of the patients in whom it is attempted (current success rate without preoperative monitoring), then multiplying these numbers ($0.8 \times 0.5 \times 0.67$) results in a 26.8% impact (i.e. the current 27% AV fistula rate in the United States). This is the real explanation of why we have only 27% AV fistulas. Improvements will come from making changes in the most fruitful places: by both increasing AV fistula creation from its current 50% and by increasing the efficacy of each fistula creation through the use of preoperative imaging. A similar calculation can be made with vascular access monitoring. If access monitoring identifies 80–90% of the patients at high risk of developing thrombosis and if 80–90% of these patients are referred for imaging and undergo angioplasty with an 80% efficacy, the impact will be approximately 50–65%. This is exactly the outcome improvement seen in access monitoring programs, which reduces thrombosis rates to approximately 50–75% of the rates in programs without monitoring.

Another significant factor in the efficacy of access care delivery systems are the incentives provided. Each reimbursement system creates its own particular set of incentives and disincentives. High-cost or high-work patients are constantly shifted to other locations for care. For example, if the patient is admitted for acute dialysis in a hospital, frequently a catheter is placed and the patient is transferred to the outpatient dialysis center with plans to place a permanent access at a later date. The transfer of a potentially high-cost patient results in a cost shift from the hospital to the outpatient center. In reality, it represents a care tax on the outpatient dialysis facility because caring for catheter patients results in an increased financial burden. Unfortunately, many of these patients never undergo fistula creation. This results in both an increase and a shift in the overall cost of care to the society as a whole to the benefit for the hospital or insurance company. Solutions to these issues will require a better alignment of incentives. The system gets the behaviors it encourages. Financial barriers, although unpleasant to discuss, are central to this argument.

Mandating particular behaviors without providing the financial resources to cover the added cost are often futile and at best misguided. This is not to say that solutions cannot be financially neutral. However, resources must be provided to compensate for the cost of additional services required, either as shared savings, or with some incentive to provide additional outpatient care to prevent future complications. Additionally, options need to be available for localities where services are not available.

Improving vascular access outcomes requires extending the focus outside the dialysis facilities to involve hospitals, physicians, surgeons, and interventional radiologists, and providing the required additional resources needed to ensure service delivery. A multidisciplinary team utilized to address all access issues including access creation, maintenance, loss and repair can be achieved by involving hospitals, physicians and dialysis providers. This type of coordinated effort will strengthen interactions, and maximize the efficiency of all parties in order to reduce the potential for poor outcomes. Additionally, all parties including physicians and hospitals, in addition to dialysis facilities, must be held accountable for their outcomes. Internationally, different countries have had varying success at aligning incentives and creating coordinated care teams, often centered on the use of an access coordinator. From the United States perspective, there are multiple potential opportunities for improvement. Minor adjustments in reimbursement including coverage for preoperative imaging, increased payment for AV fistulas and payment for access monitoring would improve outcomes. Furthermore, accountability at the source of fistula creation and catheter placement, involving hospitals and surgeons, is necessary.

Another opportunity for improving care is to consider what measurements or indicators should be used to evaluate the effectiveness of a care delivery system. Following indicators such as the inability to provide adequate blood flow to reach the adequacy target, access-related missed treatments, access-related hospitalizations and access-related mortality instead of using only the current measures of access placement type and thrombosis rate to improve care may be more appropriate. This is necessary because what is important is not whether a fistula or catheter is placed, but rather does the patient have an access that provides adequate blood flow to achieve a particular dialysis adequacy target and that can function for prolonged periods of time without complications. These other indicators also take into account changes in process and technology. One of the hallmarks of quality improvement is the choice of appropriate metrics. From a quality improvement perspective, operations and quality are tied together by metrics that are financial and also are equivalent to quality metrics. In this setting the role of operations is to drive quality outcomes and the role of quality teams is to streamline operations. The metrics described above have both financial and quality components and are examples of the types of metrics that may need to be developed to help spur outcome improvement.

The final issues to address regarding barriers to providing effective vascular access care involve overall structural change. In the United States, regionalization of access care and the possibility of limited capitation or performance-based payments are currently under discussion. Disease management programs such as those through Optimal, Kaiser, Renaissance, and RMS have demonstrated significant improvement in access outcomes. These types of programs can be used to facilitate overall outcome improvement.

In conclusion, systemic variables have a significant impact on vascular access outcomes. These factors provide a road map to improving access care by decreasing morbidity and mortality and decreasing the costs associated with access failure. Sustainable improvements, however, require addressing the systemic barriers that limit the potential improvements. This can best be accomplished by aligning incentives to reward desired behaviors and to drive outcomes improvement. Stressing the areas that have the maximum potential to provide benefits, including pre-ESRD (CKD care) with early referral to nephrology and surgery for access creation, preoperative imaging by duplex ultrasound to identify the most appropriate site for AV fistula creation, and secondary fistula creation in patients with failing PTFE grafts or cuffed catheters can result in significant improvement in patient outcomes at a lower global cost. The overall system of care must include reasonable reimbursement that rewards excellence and penalizes cost shifting. Lastly, all parties must be held accountable for their outcomes. Vascular access care can be improved only by involvement and cooperation of all parties including payers, providers, patients, industry, and hospitals in a multidisciplinary team. This is our opportunity and challenge.

References

1   US Renal Data System: USRDS 2002 Annual Data Report. The National Institutes of Health, National Institute of Diabetes and Digestive and Kidney Diseases, Bethesda, 2002.
2   Centers for Medicare and Medicaid Services: 2001 Annual Report: ESRD Clinical Performance Measures Project. Am J Kidney Dis 2002;39(suppl 2):S1–S98.
3   Pisoni RL, Young EW, Dykstra DW, Greenwood RN, Hecking E, Gillespie B, Wolfe RA, Goodkin DA, Held PJ: Vascular access use in Europe and the United States: Results from the DOPPS. Kidney Int 2002;61:305–316.
4   Dhingra RK, Young EW, Hulbert-Shearon TE, Leavey S, Port FK: Type of vascular access and mortality in US hemodialysis patients. Kidney Int 2001;V60:1443–1451.
5   Pastan S, Soucie JM, McClellan WM: Vascular access and increasing risk of death among vascular access patients. Kidney Int 2002;62:620–626.
6   Marr KA, Sexton D, Conlon PJ, et al: Catheter related bacteremia and the outcome of attempted catheter salvage in patients undergoing hemodialysis. Ann Intern Med 1997;127:275–280.

7   Saad TF: Bacteremia associated with cuffed hemodialysis catheters. Am J Kidney Dis 1999;34:
    1114–1124.

8   Stevenson KB, Hannah EL, Lowder CA, Adcox MJ, Davidson RL, Mallea MC, Narasimhan N,
    Wagnild JP: Epidemiology of hemodialysis vascular access infections from longitudinal
    surveillance data: Predicting the impact of the NKF-DOQI clinical practice guidelines for vascular
    access. Am J Kidney Dis 2002;V39:549–555.

9   Lok C, Stanley KE, Hux JE, Richardson R, Tobe SW, Conly J: Hemodialysis infection prevention
    with polysporin ointment. J Am Soc Nephrol 2003;14:169–179.

10 NKF DOQI clinical practice guidelines for hemodialysis vascular access. Am J Kidney Dis
    1997;30(suppl 3):S154–S196.

11 NKF-K/DOQI clinical practice guidelines for vascular access: Update 2000. Am J Kidney Dis
    2001;37(suppl 1):S137–S181.

12 Sands JJ, Ferrell LM, Perry MA: Systemic barriers to improving vascular access outcomes. Adv
    Ren Replace Ther 2002;V9/2:109–115.

13 2001 Locality Fee Schedule Report: 2001 Medicare Fee Schedule. www.cms.hhs.gov/
    esrd/default.asp

14 Friedman AL, Walworth C, Meehan C, Wander H, Shemin D, DeSoi W, Kitsen J, Hill C, Lambert C,
    Mesler D: First hemodialysis access selection varies with patient acuity. Adv Ren Replace Ther
    2000;7/4(suppl 1):S4–S10.

15 Konner K: Primary vascular access in diabetic patients: An audit. Nephrol Dial Transplant 2000;
    15:1317–1325.

16 Malovrh M: Native arteriovenous fistula: Preoperative evaluation. Am J Kidney Dis 2002;39:
    1218–1225.

17 Silva MB, Hobson RW 2nd, Pappas PJ, Jamil Z, Clifford AT, Goldberg MC, Gwertzman G,
    Padberg FT: A strategy for increasing use of autogenous hemodialysis access procedures: Impact
    of preoperative noninvasive evaluation. J Vasc Surg 1998;27:302–308.

18 Ascher E, Gade P, Hingorani A, Mazzariol F, Gunduz Y, Fodera M, Yorkivich W: Changes in the
    practice of angioaccess surgery: Impact of dialysis outcome and quality initiative recommenda-
    tions. J Vasc Surg 2000;31:84–92.

19 Glazer S, Crooks P, Shapiro M, Diesto J: Using CQI and the DOQI guidelines to improve vascular
    access outcomes: The Southern California Kaiser Permanente experience. Nephrology News
    Issues 2000;14:21–26.

20 Silva M, Hobson R, Pappas P, Haser P, Araki C, Goldberg M, Jamil Z, Padberg F: Vein transposi-
    tion in the forearm for autogenous hemodialysis access. Vasc Surg 1998;27:302–307.

21 Sedlacek M, Teodorescu V, Falk A, Vassalotti J, Uribarri J: Hemodialysis access placement with
    preoperative noninvasive vascular mapping: Comparison between patients with and without
    diabetes. Am J Kidney Dis 2001;38:560–564.

22 Huber TS, Ozaki CK, Flynn TC, et al: Prospective validation of an algorithm to maximize native
    arteriovenous fistulae for chronic hemodialysis access. J Vasc Surg 2002;V36:3.

23 Spuhler CL, Schwarze KD, Sands JJ: Increasing AV fistula creation: The Akron experience.
    Nephrol News Issues 2002;16/6:44–47, 50, 52.

24 Gibson K, Caps M, Kohler T, Hatsukami T, Gillen D, Aldassy M, Sherrard D, Stehman-Breen C:
    Assessment of a policy to reduce placement of prosthetic hemodialysis access. Kidney Int 2001;
    59:2335–2345.

25 Collins AJ, Ebben J, Chen S, Ma JZ: Cost-effectiveness outpatient vascular access services. ABS,
    ASN, 1999.

26 McCarley P, Wingard RL, Shyr Y, Pettus W, Hakim RM, Ikizler A: Vascular access blood flow
    monitoring reduces access morbidity and costs. Kidney Int 2001;V60:1164–1172.

27 Paulson WD, Ram SJ, Birk CG, et al: Accuracy of decrease in blood flow in predicting hemodialysis
    graft thrombosis. Am J Kidney Dis 2000;35:1089–1095.

28 Paulson WD, Ram SJ, Work J: Use of vascular access blood flow to evaluate vascular access. Am
    J Kidney Dis 2001;38:916.

29 McDougal G, Agarwal R: Clinical performance characteristics of hemodialysis graft monitoring.
    Kidney Int 2001;60:762–766.

30 Schwab SJ, Raymond JR, Saeed M, et al: Prevention of hemodialysis fistula thrombosis. Early detection of venous stenoses. Kidney Int 1989;36:707.

31 Besarab A, Sullivan LK, Ross RP, Moritz MJ: Utility of intra-access pressure monitoring in detecting and correcting venous outlet stenosis prior to thrombosis. Kidney Int 1995;47: 1364–1373.

32 Smits JH, Van Der Linden J, Hagen C, et al: Graft surveillance: Venous pressure, access flow or the combination? Kidney Int 2001;59:1551–1558.

33 Sands J, Jabyac P, Miranda C, Kapsick B: Intervention based on monthly monitoring decreases hemodialysis access thrombosis. ASAIO J 1999;45:147–150.

34 Schwab S, Oliver M, Suhocki P, McCann R: Hemodialysis arteriovenous access: Detection of stenosis and response to treatment by vascular access blood flow. Kidney Int 2001;59:358–362.

35 Sands JJ, Young SF, Miranda CL: The effect of Doppler flow screening studies and elective revisions on dialysis access failure. Trans Am Soc Artif Intern Organs 1992;38:524–527.

36 Sands J, Espada C, Ferrell L, Lazarus J: 73% of patients with prosthetic bridge grafts have suitable sites for secondary arterio-venous fistula creation (abstract). NKF Spring Clinical Meeting, 2001.

37 Sands J, Espada C, Ferrell L, Lazarus J: 65% of patients with cuffed catheters have adequate vasculature for arterio-venous fistula creation (abstract). NKF Spring Clinical Meeting, 2000.

38 Nguyen V, Tomford R, Jackson A, Griffith C: Should we stop revising thrombosed hemodialysis grafts (G). A 2-year experience at Providence St. Peter Hospital Dialysis Program. J Am Soc Nephrol 1999;10:A1085.

Jeffrey J. Sands, MD,
Fresenius Medical Care,
NA, 231 Celebration Blvd., Celebration, FL 34747 (USA)
Tel. +1 407 566 0683, Fax +1 407 566 0676, E-Mail Jeffrey.Sands@fmc-na.com

Ronco C, Levin NW (eds): Hemodialysis Vascular Access and Peritoneal Dialysis Access.
Contrib Nephrol. Basel, Karger, 2004, vol 142, pp 363–375

....

The Vascular Access: A Long-Term Patient's Considerations and Reflections

John M. Newmann

Health Policy Research & Analysis, Inc., Reston, Va., USA

Introduction

This chapter touches on nearly 18 years' experience in the US with an AV fistula, and what I've learned from a variety of professionals and patients since 1971, when I began hemodialysis. I cannot write 'the patient's perspective'. Although patients may share much in common with their vascular access experiences, there are important differences, which influence a patient's access placement, function, quality, care, and maintenance. These differences include individual patient insurance coverage and economic resources, psychological and social behavior, as well as physiology, attending nephrologists, vascular surgeons, doctor/patient relationships, and other chronic dialysis staff. I provide one patient's perspective informed and enhanced by scores of fascinating and frustrated patients' and professionals' experiences.

While patients often share the same or similar diagnoses of renal failure and comorbidities, we come to realize, perhaps when we least expect it, there are important differences in the ways our bodies, minds, and emotions respond to the many caregivers we require as they try to meet the challenges of creating, using, and monitoring our accesses. In addition, patients may be advised quite differently on appropriate access protection, cleaning, exercise, and possibly cannulation.

Aspects of critically important staff and patient communication required for successful patient education and understanding will be discussed. Thoughtful suggestions from other patients provide options readers may consider for their own practice. Reading this chapter with a clinically critical eye may provide little, if any insight. Read this to be reminded how desperately serious patients are when suggesting new and established patients may benefit from their past lessons. Readers might choose to vary some previously normative methods and behavior, to bring about constructive improvement in both vascular access function and longevity, and increased patient and professional satisfaction.

A Brief Personal Vascular Access History and Commentary

Two weeks before I began thrice weekly, 6-hour home hemodialysis at age 30 in 1971, an AV fistula was created in my nondominant left forearm. By chance, I had the double good fortune of being nondiabetic with healthy veins and arteries, and having an experienced vascular surgeon skilled at AV fistula placement. Over the first few years of consistent cannulation, four separate areas, including one above the elbow, were developed long enough to accommodate both arterial and venous needles. This AV fistula was used for 16 years prior to my receiving a cadaver transplant.

During the first few months of dialysis, while the fistula was maturing, I was infiltrated a few times, once very badly. I soon began to dread inexperienced or incompetent 'needle stickers', as we called them. It was easy for a patient, as a captive audience in a dialysis chair, to observe staff and categorize them as excellent, good, mediocre, or incompetent. It not only became painfully clear who was to be avoided, but quite apparent whom we'd prefer! As in other dialysis centers, unit policy prohibited individual patient choice of who would put in the needles. 'Staff shortages and cost' explanations have not persuaded me why medical directors, directors of nursing, and attending nephrologists don't insist each dialysis shift have one or two very skillful staff members to regularly cannulate the most problematic accesses. The costs of partial and missed treatments for outpatient or inpatient access intervention, not to mention considerable dialysis staff time for recannulation and associated problems may not be fully appreciated. Patients do understand the physiological and emotional costs they pay for inadequately skilled staff.

Differences among Vascular Surgeons and Inconsistent Medicare Physician Payment Fees for Vascular Access Options

The timing for predialysis kidney disease patient referral to a nephrologist and placement of accesses differs widely [1–3]. Some patients may be informed of the superior function and longevity of AV fistulae [4–9]. Few are likely to be aware of the serious scarcity of vascular access surgeons skilled at placing AV fistulae, the different types of surgeons involved in AV fistula and graft placement [2], and the variety of surgical approaches employed [10–12]. Most patients will have to trust the referral process, particularly when emergently referred for immediate access placement. In addition, most patients may be unaware of the greater time and skill normally required to place an AV fistula when compared to a graft. Finally, patients are unlikely to know if the practice of vascular surgeons to whom they have been referred is influenced by the Medicare physician fee schedule, which favors graft over fistula replacement, and often varies geographically.[1]

Changing the organization of care at the dialysis unit level by implementing programs which provide high levels of AV fistula use, along with training floor staff to provide the quality of care necessary to maintain and monitor AV fistulae has demonstrated excellent results [13–18]. Some companies (e.g. Fresenius Medical Care of North America, and Renal Management Systems, a new division of DaVita, Inc., recently acquired from Baxter Health Care) have undertaken serious efforts to encourage increasing the numbers and skills of vascular surgeons for dialysis patient needs. Dedicated outpatient vascular access surgical centers continue to be established and a number of vascular surgeons have begun emphasizing hemodialysis vascular access as a subspecialty in their practices.

Even though the AV fistula has become and remains the clinically superior and preferred vascular access when appropriate for hemodialysis patients, Medicare's lower physician payment schedule for AV fistula placement, when compared to fees paid for graft placement, remains an ironic and inappropriate payment policy. The differential appears to provide an incentive for surgeons to place grafts, which are relatively easy to create, and a disincentive for placing the more effective, but difficult and time-consuming AV fistulae. One would expect greater payment for fistula placement, the more technical, and time-consuming procedure, or at the very least, comparable fee schedules for grafts and fistulae. Complicating this issue is the unknown degree to which nephrologists establish effective relationships with, and persuade vascular surgeons of the clinical superiority of AV fistula function and longevity.

---

[1]For example for Washington, D.C., the current Center for Medicare & Medicaid Services participating fee schedule for creating an AV fistula autogenous graft (ICD9 code 36825) is USD 612.71; for an AV anastomosis, open, direct any site, Cimino type (ICD9 code 36821) the payment is USD 554.10. For an AV synthetic graft (ICD9 code 36830), the payment is USD 720.98; 16% greater than an AV fistula autogenous graft, and 30% greater than an AV Cimino fistula [pers. commun., Anderson]. The differences also vary up to 33% in North East Philadelphia and Florida (pers. commun., Sands, coauthor of another chapter in this volume [20]). These differences can be greater or smaller, depending upon the billing codes used.

Self-Cannulation

I traveled frequently, arranging dialysis treatments at first throughout the USA; later (related to my work) in Asia, South America, and North Africa. I disliked the worry and tension when meeting a nurse or patient care technician assigned to cannulate my fistula. How experienced were they? Would they listen to the informed description I would provide about the characteristics of the part of the fistula I knew was appropriate for cannulation for that treatment? Obviously the answers were quite variable. Once, after a few years of hemodialysis, I dialyzed next to a rather small woman who inserted her own needles, a talent I had heard about, but had never seen before. She asked if I put in my needles. I said I didn't, and asked how she decided to learn. She explained she used to sit next to a large truck driver who took a very dim view of being infiltrated. He finally asked his nurse, 'Can you teach me to put in those needles?' She had never been asked this before, and had to check with the charge nurse, who decided the man could be taught. After a short time, he was able to stick himself quite well. My new dialysis friend told me she thought, 'If he can do it, I can do it.' And my reaction to this was the same, 'If she can do it, so can I.'

A skilled 'sticker' with patience can teach self-cannulation, once the access has matured. After I learned, occasionally some assistance from a nurse or technician to steady a rolling vein was helpful. The feelings of accomplishment and relief, which accompany self-cannulation, are wonderful! At first, I was nervous about my ability. With experience, I began to know my fistula better and gain more confidence. Though it's not for everyone, my and other patients' successful years of self-cannulation confirm it is worth an honest try. The benefits include:

(1) Personal stress is markedly reduced because there is no more fear or uncertainty about who will be doing the cannulation, whether at the local dialysis unit or when traveling.

(2) One seldom feels the stick, since concentration is so complete to cannulate smoothly. No more waiting for the pain!

(3) It's usually clear if the needle is in the middle, along the side, or caught in the side or top of the vein. Nerves sense when the needle is not sliding though the middle of the vein. The fingers holding the needle being inserted can feel a smooth insertion, or a slight resistance or stick if the needle is caught on the vein. A motivated self-cannulating patient may be more likely to sense these subtleties than the nurse or patient care technician with limited dialysis experience and cannulation training. Certainly an unknown proportion of the limited number of highly motivated and skilled nurses and technicians may have excellent cannulaton skills and sensitivities.

(4) A new sense of independence and satisfaction accompanies the added control of this critically important step in dialysis treatment initiation.

Aseptic Preparation

I don't like the inevitable increased risk of infection, which accompanies every dialysis treatment. The risk is likely to be higher in a dialysis unit or hospital setting when compared to the risk in my home. I favor competent, unhurried protection against infection. Too often, I've seen other patients' bandaged, reddened and tender access sites, and caregivers who appear rushed and less than focused. I do hope it is reasonable to assume each dialysis unit has adequate space and proper facilities for patients to wash the access area with soap and water prior to going to their assigned dialysis stations. While traveling, I witnessed many methods for preparing the access for cannulation. Seldom have I seen used the method I was taught and told was preferred. Frequently alcohol wipes and stronger disinfectants have been used on gauze, which is wiped back and forth a few times over the intended insertion site. This may reduce contaminants, but repeatedly rubs the materials to be cleaned over the site. Disinfectants stronger than alcohol were always recommended to me. I was taught to use a circular motion beginning directly over the intended site of insertion, and moving clockwise in slightly larger circles, away from the intended point of puncture. This increases the chances of effectively clearing the needle site of potentially infectious material. Unfortunately, this method may unintentionally remain a well-kept secret from patients and dialysis staff. I would not be surprised if this method, or a variation of it, is known to nursing staff leadership, but has not been given priority in training and monitoring of dialysis floor staff.

Other Patients' Comments and Suggestions

I have neither been dialyzed, nor been in a dialysis center on a regular basis for 10 years. As one way to learn what other hemodialysis patients currently consider important about vascular access, I used a dialysis patient listserv:dialysis_support-owner@yahoogroups.com, to post this request: 'I've been asked to write a chapter, "A Patient's Comments on Vascular Access" in a book for ESRD professionals on vascular access. Very simply, I'd like to know what you think are the three most important points you would make if writing the chapter for hemodialysis staff. For practical reasons, I limit this to three, knowing there are more. All names and email addresses will be kept confidential.'

Eleven submissions were chosen and provide an interesting composite of views, though all with the common thread of using patients' experiences as examples. Emphasis appeared to be concentrated around effective patient-to-staff and staff-to-patient communication. Respondents wanted to increase staff awareness of the patients' educational, medical and emotional needs, and encourage staff to use their knowledge for increased patient understanding of the important issues in successful access use, care, and maintenance. Mention was also made, though less frequently, of appreciation for staff competence and compassion. Several discussed needle insertion, choice of who does it and how, with a number favoring self-cannulation. Preferences among patients and staff for type of access, not surprisingly, mirrored well-understood problems of convenience versus access functionality and longevity. Topics are categorized and italicized. When available, short descriptions of the author's dialysis experience are provided.

These comments/suggestions come from a married couple brought together through kidney failure, each with over 15 years of dialysis and transplantation experience:

Vascular access surgeon choice: 'Too often nephrologists refer only to one surgeon, when others are available. Several options for surgeons could be made available to the patients by their nephrologists.'

Information about vascular access surgeons: 'Technicians are the folks who do most of the cannulating and see the accesses on a frequent basis. They may be in a position to provide substantive comments about which surgeon's accesses tend to be superior and have higher success rates. Patients and nephrologists ought to have information from experienced technicians available to them when considering referral to vascular access surgeons.'

Temporary catheters: 'When poor surgery does occur, patients are all too willing to give into the allure of temporary catheters, without being made aware of their inferiority. Some of these patients understandably conclude the temporary catheters do not require needle sticks and in addition, the put-on and take-off times are decreased, reducing the overall time spent at the unit.'

Standardized access care information: 'I have received wildly varied information on how to take care of my access. In terms of post-surgery care, I've experienced everything from 'you don't have to do anything', to a clear plan of exercise and wound care. I've also experienced great variation in how to take care of my access over the long term, and how to prepare for treatment. I'd like to see standardized care information for post-surgery and daily access care.'

Self-cannulation: 'I would like to see more discussion by staff with patients of self-cannulation. I don't believe patients even know this is an option. I realize many patients will not be interested, but every patient should be made aware of the option, its pros and cons.'

Patient care technician preference for grafts: 'Since the NKF/DOQI Vascular Access Guidelines have been published, almost everyone would tell a patient a fistula is preferred over a graft. It seems technicians too often express their preferences for sticking grafts, since they are easier, more uniform in shape, and not as "tough". We hope there would be extensive technician training on how to stick the two different types of vascular access and, most importantly, how to discuss the differences with patients.'

The importance of saving an access: 'Staff should be as aggressive in saving an access as they are in saving a transplant. For us, they are equally important. I have had nine accesses and believe that number would be considerably less, if early on, problems had been dealt with more aggressively. The attitude seemed to be: a new access could always be placed. Now that many patients are living longer on dialysis, each and every access is of the utmost importance!'

A registered nurse, who has been a renal patient for over 35 years, on dialysis four times, and currently enjoying her fourth transplant described her most important issues:

(1) 'Careful *sterile technique to prevent infections.*'

(2) 'Always *do your own needle placements.* At the very least, have the same person, who knows your access, do them. A skilled, competent person is needed. When cared for properly, an AV fistula can last a lifetime. This is not so with a graft… Actually, the people I have known who do their own punctures do not want anyone else doing it, if they have had bad experiences in the past.'

(3) '*Protecting all the veins is a constant and necessary task for renal patients.* The last thing you want is to run out of veins to use!'

This was submitted by a near octogenarian from England: *Trusting and comfortable with cannulation staff* – He began by partially quoting an earlier posting from a US patient: '…understand our natural protectiveness of what is to you an arm, but to us is our LIFE LINE'. He added: 'I say, I say, isn't that laying it on a bit too thick?…I certainly don't feel any sense of apprehension when the nurses (always, without fail, gentle and caring and efficient) approach with the twin needles. They don't lunge, act unsteady, get distracted, use too much pressure or work roughly. It is, I hope, the same everywhere. I just lie back, offer my arm to them as a sacrifice and gently murmur, 'into thy hands I commend my arm' and then return to my Walkman and the delights of Classic FM…'

Differences in patient age and responsibilities may influence attitudes and priorities: A young woman's respectful disagreement in response to the Englishman: 'Perhaps it is because of your age that you are able to, in your words, sacrifice your arm to the dialysis needles. If you were in my shoes, when I started dialysis I had a four year old in tow, and was not willing to just look the other way as my longevity truly was in the hands of people who had little medical training. I have, on a few occasions, had a technician talking to the next patient or to another technician just as I was about to be stuck. I have no problem saying, "Hold the conversation when you're sticking a needle the size of a nail in my arm, please".'

A 31-year veteran of hemodialysis (15 at home, 16 in center) provides *counsel to staff for cannulation, education, and encouragement to patients*:

(1) 'Be gentle, those needles hurt more than you know. Don't be a tech/nurse with an ego, be man or woman enough to admit when you have failed making a good cannulation and let someone else try.'

(2) 'Encourage the person on dialysis to learn to stick themselves…and encourage rotation of sites.'

(3) 'Encourage regular exercising of the arms to keep the access from clotting and to keep the non-access arm's veins and arteries in good shape, you never know when you might need them!'

A home hemodialysis patient of 4 years picks up on another's observation: *when a hemodialysis treatment begins, there should be solemn respect for the moment.* 'I like this a lot. It is a significant moment. Even as a self-cannulator, I tense up when in center, and the staff seem too cavalier when hooking the lines to the needles or taping the needles to the arm.'

Suggestions of a patient with over 3 years of hemodialysis experience:

'*Needle removal is just as important as insertion.* Do not apply too much pressure to the needle when removing. Enlist the help of the patient if necessary. I have had more pain inflicted by needle removal than insertion.'

'*Do not swab only with alcohol*; use Betadine after. Alcohol is used for cleaning, not killing germs/bacteria. It will burn the patient's access if it is not followed by the Betadine swab (which does kill germs/bacteria and allows for pain-free needle insertion).'

Another patient (of 21 years, diagnosed at age 8; with peritoneal dialysis, hemodialysis, and transplant experience) emphasizes *access as a lifeline, and the importance of staff getting cannulation help sooner than later*: 'I hope staff understand and care that our access is our lifeline and treat it as such. I have a two stick rule: if a nurse cannot get a needle in with two sticks, they have to quit and get someone who can, or let me go home and come back after my arm has gotten over the trauma. I have seen nurses stick patients over and over again, with no care as to what damage they might be doing to a patient. However, I have also seen other staff telling patients how important their access is when it is an issue with the patient, like not exercising their arm or something.'

Some straight talk for staff from a first year patient: *The importance of empathy and knowing patients are also people:* 'First of all, when it hurts so bad, believe me; don't tell me to calm down and be still – it HURTS!!! I'll gladly trade you places or you let me stick YOU just once. Don't complain about your job – you have a job and some of us would like to escape that chair and go to work. When you're in front of us, don't talk about food when we cannot eat.'

Sticking grafts doesn't hurt much and certain staff may be unacceptable stickers for some patients: 'When I first started on dialysis (almost four years ago), YES the sticks hurt, but I had a fistula then. Now I have a graft, they do not hurt. It can also depend on who is doing the sticking. Some techs are better than others, and there are certain people in my unit I will not let stick me…I know this may offend some of the techs, but it is my arm and if I do not feel comfortable with someone, I will not let them stick me. I tell them it has nothing to do with them, that I am just more comfortable with other people. Most understand, but some of the newer people may feel a bit offended. I have never used Emla cream, I just make a fist, turn my head, and close my eyes.'

Self-cannulation: 'I've been sticking myself for over twenty-three years. I do recommend you go this route when you feel up to it. I find it does reduce pain based on one basic point; I know where the nerves are in my arm and can stay away from them. I have found that even fractions of an inch can make a huge difference.'

Communication: 'Tain't What You Do' (It's the Way That Cha Do It) [19]

This tune, often performed by Louis Armstrong, reflects an important suggestion for improving communication among patients and staff, and can be applied to vascular access issues. The manner in which something is said and done has an important impact on patients' attitudes and their ability to cope with thrice-weekly dialysis treatments, which could compromise their health status, quality of life and longevity.

There Is No Substitute for Listening to Patients
Has self-cannulation received disproportionate attention in this chapter? For the minority who swear by it, most recognize the majority of patients are unlikely to want or be able to do it. Perhaps most centers have one or two patients who may self-cannulate, but it's doubtful every shift has such a patient. Interestingly, the patients' comments never referred to being asked by staff to learn self-cannulation, though I imagine some staff suggested it. Patients directly experience access problems due to inadequate staff skills. They also observed other patients benefiting from self-cannulation and some staff promoting it. Why is this not something commonly discussed as an option, and promoted for those interested and suitable? Some possible reasons and responses include:

(1) Individual staff members may neither want to self-cannulate if they required dialysis, nor the responsibility of teaching it. Therefore, they may not encourage it. Many patients are likely to have heard at least one hemodialysis

staff member opine, 'I don't know what I'd do if my kidneys failed. Perhaps I'd want a transplant or try PD.' Though a speculative comment, a staff member's personal judgments may influence patients, but should not interfere with the professional obligation to clearly communicate patient information and self-care options, and engage patients in these conversations.

(2) So few patients are interested, training a patient is time consuming, and valuable staff time cannot be wasted consistently helping those who may have been poor prospects for self-cannulation in the first place. The same can be said concerning adherence to dietary guidelines for hemodialysis patients: few patients are interested, training takes time, and valuable staff time may be wasted consistently reminding patients who may be poor prospects for dietary adherence. Both topics are very important, although there is a substantive distinction between increasing the number who successfully self-cannulate, and those who improve dietary compliance. The more competent, suitable patients are informed about, and trained to self-cannulate, the less time staff will be spending with them, and the more experienced staff and time will be available to patients with problematic accesses. The more patients adhere to the dialysis dietary guidelines, the more successful their dialysis, the less staff time spent dealing with hypotension and cramping, and the more staff time available for self-cannulation training and other educational issues!

Patients Helping Patients

It is not uncommon to take an interest in the experiences of other patients facing similar, serious health problems and challenges. Patient support groups are plentiful among the population with chronic, life-threatening illnesses. Patients listen to each other, and learn from each other. Just as some health professionals may be misinformed, pass on inappropriate or dated information, the same can occur among patients. Each dialysis unit may have a few patients exemplary in their care and understanding of AV fistulae and grafts. Staff at all dialysis units can easily identify patients with whom they have had difficulty communicating about understanding vascular access care and protection. Encouraging nonthreatening, constructive communication between these two types of patients may resolve some previously troublesome staff/patient vascular access problems. Some units may develop training programs for patient 'peer counselors' who can serve in this capacity.

Information for Patients Is Widely Available

The growing video, internet, and print literature for patients with chronic kidney disease and kidney failure includes numerous examples of reader-friendly definitions, explanations, and suggestions for understanding hemodialysis vascular access.[2] Patient groups consistently have medical advisors who review the information prior to publication. In addition, corporate partnerships with patient organizations have provided funding and medical expertise for producing educational materials. References are often made to the NKF-K/DOQI Vascular Access Guidelines. If nephrologists and staff direct patients to reliable vascular access information, and respond to patient questions related to the information patients bring to the unit, serious confusion may be reduced and understanding increased.

Concluding Remarks

This book adds to the available resources professionals can use to improve vascular access care. Understanding the nature and depth of patient needs for clear and empathetic (not sympathetic) communication remains an important objective and challenge for hemodialysis staff. Those directly and indirectly responsible for appropriate vascular access referral, choice of access, placement, cannulation, protection, care, and monitoring are likely to increase their success when providing care which is sensitive to patient vascular access and hemodialysis experience. Patient perceptions of staff competence and respect for vascular access lifelines deserve serious staff attention.

[2]The following organizations with websites provide a variety of patient information, along with links to other informative patient sites:

The American Association of Kidney Patients (AAKP) has several publications, among them, *Understanding Your Hemodialysis Access Options* on line at: www.aakp.org. In addition *Care of Your Hemodialysis Access* by William J. Plaus, MD, FACS is free, available by calling AAKP at (800) 749-AAKP.

IKidney has a website, www.iKidney.com with useful links and includes: *Just the Facts: Vascular Access* by the Life Options Rehabilitation Advisory Council, and *Caring for Your Vascular Access* by Lori Hartwell, a renal patient and advocate.

The Life Options Rehabilitation Advisory Council has a fact sheet on vascular access at: www.lifeoptions.org, and a patient interactive teaching module, Vascular Access – A Lifeline for Dialysis at: www.kidneyschool.org.

The National Kidney Foundation (NKF) at: www.kidney.org has materials on the K/DOQI Vascular Access Clinical Practice Guidelines and a patient and family section with excerpts from *Your Hemodialysis Access* brochure. A free brochure, *Getting the Most from Your Treatment: What You Need to Know about Hemodialysis Access*, is available by calling the National Kidney Foundation at (800) 622-9010.

The National Kidney and Urologic Diseases Cleaning House (of the National Institutes of Health) has a publication *Vascular Access for Hemodialysis* available on line: http://www.niddk.nih.gov/health/kidney/nkudic.htm

Staff behavior might be modified based upon lessons from patient/staff interaction and listening to patients' suggestions, even when they are in the throws of difficulty with access placement, use, or reliability. Educational efforts, which encourage patient understanding and participation in vascular access care, and constructive patient role model support may reduce staff and patient stress, and contribute to improved access function and longevity.

References

1   Pisoni RL, Young EW, Dykstra DM, Greenwood RN, Hecking E, Gillespie B, Wolfe RA, Goodkin DA, Held PJ: Vascular access use in Europe and the United States: Results from the DOPPS. Kidney Int 2002;61:305–316.
2   Pisoni RL, Young EW, Mapes DL, Keen ML, Port FK: Vascular access use and outcomes in the U.S., Europe, and Japan: Results from the Dialysis Outcomes and Practice Patterns Study. Nephrol News Issues 2003;17/6:38–43.
3   Rayner HC, Pisoni RL, Gillespie BW, Goodkin DA, Akiba T, Akizawa T, Saito A, Young EW, Port FK: Creation, cannulation and survival of arteriovenous fistulae: Data from the Dialysis Outcomes and Practice Patterns Study. Kidney Int 2003;63:323–330.
4   Woods JD, Port FK: The impact of vascular access for haemodialysis on patient morbidity and mortality. Nephrol Dial Transplant 1997;12:657–659.
5   Hakim R, Himmelfarb J: Hemodialysis access failure: A call to action. Kidney Int 1998;54: 1029–1040.
6   Culp K, Flanigan M, Taylor L, Rothstein M: Vascular access thrombosis in new hemodialysis patients. Am J Kidney Dis 1995;26:341–346.
7   Woods JD, Turenne MN, Strawderman RL, et al: Vascular access survival among incident hemodialysis patients in the United States. Am J Kidney Dis 1997;30:50–57.
8   Schwab SJ, Harrington JT, Singh A, et al: Vascular access for hemodialysis. Kidney Int 1999;55: 2078–2090.
9   Dhingra RK, Young EW, Hulbert-Shearon TE, Leavey SF, Port FK: Type of vascular access and mortality in U.S. hemodialysis patients. Kidney Int 2001;60:1443–1451.
10 Konner K: A primer on the av fistula-Achilles' heel, but also Cinderella of haemodialysis. Nephrol Dial Transplant 1999;14:2094–2098.
11 Coburn MC, Carney WI Jr: Comparison of basilic vein and polytetrafluoroethylene for brachial arteriovenous fistula. J Vasc Surg 1994;20:896–904.
12 Humphries AL Jr, Colborn GL, Wynn JJ: Elevated basilic vein arteriovenous fistula. Am J Surg 1999;177:489–491.
13 Bonucchi D, D'Amelio A, Capelli G, et al: Management of vascular access for dialysis: An Italian survey. Nephrol Dial Transplant 1999;14:2116–2118.
14 Allon M, Bailey R, Ballard R, Deierhoi MH, Hamrick K, Oser R, Rhynes VK, Robbin ML, Saddekni S, Zeigler ST: A multidisciplinary approach to hemodialysis access: Prospective evaluation. Kidney Int 1998;53:473–479.
15 Kalman PG, Pope M, Bhola C, et al: A practical approach to vascular access for hemodialysis and predictors of success. J Vasc Surg 1999;30:727–733.
16 Miller A, Hölzenbein TJ, Gottlieb MN, et al: Strategies to increase the use of autogenous arteriovenous fistula in end-stage renal disease. Ann Vasc Surg 1997;11:397–405.
17 Ascher E, Gade P, Hingorani A, et al: Changes in the practice of angioaccess surgery: Impact of dialysis outcome and quality initiative recommendations. J Vasc Surg 2000;31:84–92.
18 Silva MB Jr, Hobson RW 2nd, Pappas PJ, et al: A strategy for increasing use of autogenous hemodialysis access procedures: Impact of preoperative noninvasive evaluation. J Vasc Surg 1998; 27:302–307.

19   Oliver S, Young J: The Original Decca Recordings, 'Louis Armstrong – The California Concerts'
      (MCA, Inc., Warock Corp./ASCAP), performed at the Crescendo Club, January 21, 1955; reissue
      1992 MCA Records and 1992 GRP Records, Inc.
20   Sands JJ, Montis AL, Etheredge GD: Systemic barriers to vascular access care: Implications for
      clinical outcomes. Contrib Nephrol. Basel, Karger, 2003, vol 142, pp 350–362.

John M. Newmann, PhD, MPH,
Health Policy Research & Analysis, Inc.,
1698 Chimney House Road, Reston, VA 20910 (USA)
Tel. +1 703 709 9335, Fax +1 703 709 9696, E-Mail JohnNewm@aol.com

Ronco C, Levin NW (eds): Hemodialysis Vascular Access and Peritoneal Dialysis Access.
Contrib Nephrol. Basel, Karger, 2004, vol 142, pp 376–386

....

An Experimental Temporary Vascular Access Catheter for Intracorporeal Plasma Separation

Harold. H. Handley Jr.[a], Rey Gorsuch[a], Harold Peters[a], Lutgardo Punzalan[a], Thomas G. Cooper[b], Nathan W. Levin[c], Claudio Ronco[d]

[a]Transvivo, Inc., Napa, Calif., [b]Cooper Consulting Services, Friendswood, Tex., and [c]Renal Research Institute, New York, N.Y., USA; [d]St. Bortolo Hospital, Department of Nephrology, Vicenza, Italy

Introduction

Access to whole blood for hemodialysis requires high blood flow rates (BFR) necessitating one of three predominant vascular access techniques. These include (1) surgical anastomosis of an artery and vein to create a shunt or native (arteriovenous, AV) fistula in the arm, (2) creation of an autologous or synthetic AV graft, or (3) placement of a temporary vascular access catheter in the internal jugular or femoral vein [1–3]. The Dialysis Outcomes and Practice Patterns Study (DOPPS) found that AV fistulas were preferred in Europe and Japan with fistulas present in 81 and 93%, respectively, of established hemodialysis patients [4, 5]. In contrast, only 24% of current US patients possessed AV fistulas. Instead, 58% of US patients possessed AV grafts and 18% utilized temporary catheters. Further, the use of catheters amongst new ESRD patients in the US was over 60% as opposed to 22 and 32% of new European or Japanese patients, respectively. Just over half of all temporary catheters placed in the US were tunneled (cuffed) catheters. Despite the susceptibility of temporary catheters to infection, tunneled catheters have been shown to last over 9 months in 60% of recipients whereas nontunneled catheters failed to last more than 2 months [5, 6]. The large differences between the US and other countries may be attributed to reimbursement issues, clinical site preferences and the use of inadequately prepared surgical staff trainees at dialysis centers [5].

Amongst congestive heart failure (CHF) patients suffering from acute fluid overload, however, permanent vascular access is much less common. These patients typically receive diuretic drug therapy and temporary catheters are placed only as a secondary resort, despite the suggestion of outcomes superior to those on diuretics [7]. Although chronic fluid accumulation is characteristic of these patients, diuretic drug therapy can fail. In such cases, immediate device-based intervention to alleviate fluid overload is appropriate. Temporary vascular access catheters require high BFR of 100–400 ml/min through their extracorporeal circuit to minimize clotting and formation of fibrin sheaths within the external circuit. The use of anticoagulants, heparin or its derivatives with or without protamine reversal, regional citrate, or thrombolytic enzymes can increase the longevity of these catheters and the hemofiltration cartridge. The major drawback to the longevity of externally communicating catheters, however, is their greater susceptibility to bacterial infection when compared to fistulas [5, 8].

We have previously described an experimental temporary vascular access catheter which performs plasmapheresis as an in vivo prefiltration step for second stage extracorporeal ultrafiltration of the plasma, rather than whole blood, of Yorkshire pigs [9–12]. Slow continous ultrafiltration (SCUF) of plasma is physiologically similar to whole blood SCUF. A slow continuous intravenous plasma filtration (SCIP™) system performs plasma SCUF after SCIP™ catheters are placed in the inferior vena cava of pigs by percutaneous (Seldinger) insertion through either the femoral or internal jugular veins [11]. A Fluid Control Module (FCM) automates fluid removal as well as catheter patency during continuous therapy protocols in excess of 72 h without significant requirements for heparin, labor, or the septic potential from frequent changes of the hemofiltration cartridge or tubing sets [11]. The catheter has been shown to be free of leachable toxins and capable of removing over 2 net liters of plasma water per day with only nominal changes in blood chemistry, gross or histopathology [12]. In this paper, we describe an in vitro test apparatus designed to explore the theoretical limitations and vascular plasma access flow rate potential of varied experimental SCIP™ catheter designs and a method by which to assess the potential performance of SCIP™ catheters designed for humans.

Equivalence of SCIP™ to Slow Continuous Ultrafiltration

Plasma SCUF therapy with the SCIP™ system is effectively comparable to slow continuous ultrafiltration (SCUF) as outlined in table 1. The slow continuous methods used by either therapy have been shown to enhance the hemodynamic stability of the patient over that of short, intermittent therapy [13]. Both technologies require a temporary vascular access catheter for

Table 1. Operational similarities between SCUF and SCIP™ therapy

Characteristics	SCUF	SCIP™
Indication for use	Continuous solute and/or fluid removal in patients with acute renal failure or fluid overload	Continuous solute and/or fluid removal in patients with acute renal failure or fluid overload
Fluid process	SCUF	SCUF
Benefit	Hemodynamic stability	Hemodynamic stability
Method	Convective transport of plasma water to waste bag	Convective transport of plasma water to waste bag
Catheter	Intravascular double lumen (whole blood)	Intravascular triple lumen (plasmapheresis)
Catheter placement	Internal jugular/femoral vein	Internal jugular/femoral vein
Extracorporeal fluid	Whole blood	Plasma
Whole BFR	100–400 ml/min (access pump)	2–5 liters/min (BFR in vivo)
Access fluid flow rates	100–400 ml/min (access)	2–10 ml/min (access pump)
Access pressure	~200 mm Hg (hemofilter)	~5–35 mm Hg (prefilter)
Extracorporeal red cells	100% of whole blood count	~0.0% of whole blood count
Extracorporeal platelets	100% of whole blood count	~0.2% of whole blood count
Plasma water removal	~10–15%	50–65%
Hemofilter longevity	6–12 h	>72 h

The therapeutic principles of SCUF are effectively identical in both techniques except for the absence of cells in the extracorporeal circuit and lower relative operational flow rates and pressures with SCIP™.

removal of either whole blood or plasma to an extracorporeal circuit for fluid removal by convective transport of solutes across an ultrafiltration cartridge. SCIP™ employs a vascular access catheter which excludes cells from the external circuit. Both systems require a vascular access pump and an effluent removal pump; however, the operational speeds and transmembrane pressures (TMP) are significantly lower with SCIP™. The absence of whole cells, particularly platelets, in the external hemofilter of the SCIP™ system has allowed continuous therapy for more than 3 days without changing the hemofilter or associated tubing. Elimination of red cells from the extracorporeal circuit should alleviate red cell lysis and anemia in the patient. In the absence of cells, SCIP™ allows the removal of 60% of the plasma water volume through an HF-400 (Minntech, Inc.) hemofilter ($0.3 m^2$) without coagulation of the extracorporeal circuit or complications to the animal.

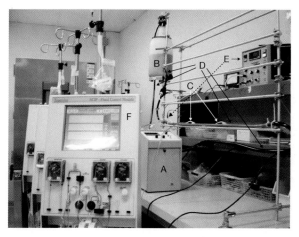

Fig. 1. In vitro whole blood test apparatus. Whole bovine blood was heparinized upon collection at an abattoir. Blood was centrifuged to remove limited flocculants/coagulants and plasma and whole cells slurry were reconstituted to a packed cell volume of 33%. The system consists of a variable speed blood pump (A), a collection reservoir (B), a continuous loop of 1/2 in (diameter) silicone tubing (D), into which test catheters (C) are introduced and the entrance sealed with silicone 24 h prior to the test. BFR is monitored with a flow meter (E) and the BFR adjusted with the blood pump (A). Plasma access, effluent removal rate and backflush cycles are controlled by the pumps on the fluid control module (F), SCIP™-FCM.

In vitro Test Results

Each SCIP™ catheter, tested in vivo, rests in the inferior vena cava of experimental pigs, but its length and surface area was anatomically restricted in these animals to ~11 cm, whereas in the human anatomy, the theoretical length of a catheter could exceed 20 cm. To determine the theoretical performance of human-sized catheters, an in vitro testing apparatus was developed (fig. 1) and validated for housing larger catheters. A variety of catheter sizes, as seen in figure 2, are tested in this apparatus, including functional catheters recovered from experimental animals. The typical range of test catheters (fig. 2) include small 20 fiber units, called SCIP™-20 mini-modules, developed for investigation of varied design configurations, porcine SCIP™-60 catheters, and catheters containing 80, 100, or 120 fibers.

Whole bovine blood was obtained from a local abattoir in 5-gallon buckets thoroughly coated with concentrated heparin to a final blood volume of 10 IU/ml whole blood. The blood was prepared by centrifugation to create a loose cellular slurry pellet from which plasma was decanted. Activated platelet aggregates and extraneous tissues were also carefully decanted following

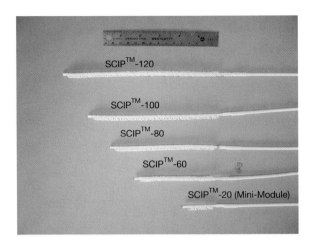

Fig. 2. SCIP™ plasmapheresis catheters are made in a variety of sizes and labeled by filtration fiber count. The human prototype catheter is the SCIP™-120, the porcine catheter used in all animal studies is the SCIP™-60, while catheter design changes are typically measured with mini-modules (SCIP™-20) containing only 20 plasma filtration fibers.

centrifugation. The bovine blood was then reconstituted to a final hematocrit of ~33% before use. Reconstituted blood was placed in a water-jacketed reservoir warmed to 37°C. During each study, reconstituted blood was continuously passed through a 37-μm arterial filter (Gish Medical, Inc.) within the test apparatus circuit to remove any cellular aggregates. The resultant bovine blood possessed normal blood chemistry levels except for elevated creatine kinase levels and a substantial thrombocytopenia introduced by the preparation process (data not shown). The experimental in vitro bench test apparatus is illustrated in figure 1. A variable speed blood pump (A) removed heparinized blood from a 10-liter lower reservoir and pumped it into a 3-liter upper reservoir (B). Blood drained from the upper reservoir past each test catheter (C) sealed within a 1/2-ft silicone tube (D) into the lower reservoir by gravity. The BFR was determined by the adjustable column height difference between upper and lower reservoir and measured with a flow meter (E). The access flow rate and TMP of the catheter and the TMP of the hemofilter were recorded every 10 s by the SCIP™-FCM.

To validate the in vitro test apparatus, two SCIP™-60 catheters were recovered from necropsy following two animal studies and their performance was evaluated in vitro. Experimental catheter XMD-017 had removed over 2 liters of plasma water from a pig during 22 h of operation at an average flow rate of 3.8 ml/min and had attained a peak performance of 4.5 ml/min in vivo. In contrast, catheter XMD-020 failed to perform satisfactorily in vivo, attaining a

Table 2. Comparative performance of two SCIP™-60 catheters tested in vitro following their experimental use in vivo in Yorkshire pigs

Catheter performance (in vivo) h	In vivo ml/min	In vitro ml/min
XMD-017 (22 h)	4.5	4.2
XMD-020 (6 h)	1.2	1.6

peak flow rate of only 1.2 ml/min in vivo. Each catheter was mounted in the test apparatus and found to provide comparable plasma access flow rates in vitro with a BFR of 6 liters/min (table 2). In vitro BFR lower than 6 liters/min failed to provide access flow rates as high as those obtained in vivo. Thus, under proper conditions, the in vitro test system was capable of estimating access flow rates comparable to those observed in vivo.

To assess varied aspects of the catheter design, SCIP™-20 mini-modules were designed which differed in only one design parameter. For example, to determine the effect of a SCIP™ catheter's filter surface area upon the plasma access flow rate at constant BFR and TMP, four sets of triplicate catheters were built. These catheters had either (1) all fibers open (7.6 cm²), (2) every third fiber blocked with polyurethane (5.7 cm²), (3) every other fiber blocked (3.8 cm²), or (4) three out of four fibers blocked (1.9 cm²). Each set of varied surface area catheters was tested in a single tube against the same blood at the same BFR. The data, presented in figure 3a, demonstrate as expected that catheters with a larger surface area performed more effectively than catheters of a lower surface area. The relationship did not appear to be linear in these tests, however. In a second series, the effect of catheter diameter was tested. Again, four sets of triplicate catheters were produced. In these catheters, surface area was held constant within evenly spaced fibers of varied length, producing catheter diameters of 31, 26, 21 and 18 french. Figure 3b demonstrates that catheters of larger diameter allow greater access flow at a constant BFR and TMP. Significant loss of access flow capacity was observed with the 18-french catheter when compared to either the 26- or 31-french catheter. We are currently uncertain as to the specific cause of this phenomenon, but consider restricted flow to the inner surfaces of the filters to be one potential limiting factor.

Insertion of catheters larger than 18 french, however, will not likely be well tolerated by patient or physician, particularly in patients with poor blood

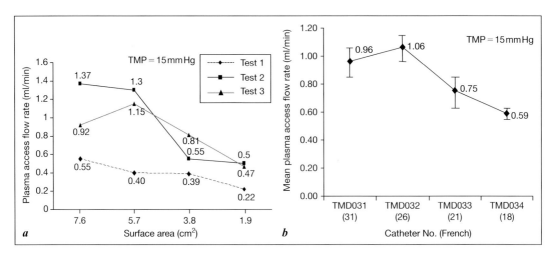

Fig. 3. a Plasma access fluid flow rates at constant TMP were a direct function of the filtration surface area. Mini-modules were constructed having the same number of fibers with the same catheter diameter, spacing and length, but with either 3 of 4 (1.9 cm²), 2 of 4 (3.8 cm²), 1 of 4 (5.6 cm²), or no fibers (7.6 cm²) occluded with polyurethane adhesive. A section of silicone tubing contained one mini-module of each surface area type allowing all catheters to be tested in the same blood sample at the same BFR. Three independent tests were conducted. **b** Plasma access fluid flow rates at constant TMP were directly proportional to the diameter of the mini-module. Catheter diameter (french) is a function of the filtration fiber length. Mini-modules were constructed having the same surface area, fiber number, and spacing, but with some fibers occluded with polyurethane adhesive to equalize surface area. Three sections of silicone tubing each contained four mini-modules representing one of each catheter diameter. All catheters were tested in the same blood sample at the same BFR.

pressure, bleeding complications or organ perfusion. Further, many patients are likely to have poor BFR in the inferior vena cava. Therefore, design features which maximize SCIP™ access flow rates must be emphasized to attain satisfactory clinical performance from the SCIP™-FCM system.

To determine the functional capacity of an 18-french SCIP™-120 catheter in vitro, several experimental catheters were constructed and inserted into the in vitro test apparatus. These catheters had a functional surface area exceeding ~32 cm². For reference, 18-french porcine SCIP™-60 catheters possess a surface area of ~15 cm². Additionally, SCIP™-120 catheters were tested at in vitro BFR which were more comparable to those expected in humans, in this case BFR = 3.1 liters/min. Access flow rate data collected from four 18-french SCIP™-120 catheters over 8 h of operation at incrementally increased TMPs are shown in figure 4. The data indicated that all

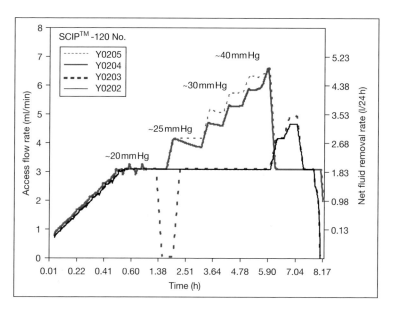

Fig. 4. Plasma access flow rates in vitro for four SCIP™-120 catheters, human catheter prototypes. All SCIP™ catheters undergo a ~30-min conditioning phase of slowly increasing access flow, with a TMP limit of 25 mm Hg, until the prescribed fluid removal rates (2 net liters/day) were attained. Two catheters (Y0202 and Y0203) were operated at 2 net liters per 24 h over 6 continuous hours before access flow was increased stepwise to determine peak plasma access flow rate potential and TMP. Two other catheters were subjected to a stepwise increase in access flow rate without restricting the TMP, which commensurately increased until the desired flow rate was achieved. Flow rates achieved the maximum rate allowed by the access tubing (diameter). Net fluid removal rates (clearance minus backflush) approached 5 liters/day. The data suggest that experimental prototype SCIP™-120 catheters may remove clinically significant quantities of plasma water from humans.

SCIP™-120 catheters were capable of sustained operation at net fluid removal rates in excess of 2 net liters plasma water per day with a 20 mm Hg TMP. Two catheters (Y0204, Y0205) were operated for >4 hours with incremental increases in TMP, allowing access flow rates to rise. These catheters maintained a constant access flow rate >6.5 ml/min with a stable TMP of 40 mm Hg. The stability of TMP at higher access flow rates suggested these catheters remained patent and functional even at the net fluid removal rate of ~5 liters/day. Maximum access flow in these two catheters was ultimately limited only by tubing set diameter used in the test. While these data are promising, SCIP™ catheter performance in humans cannot be accurately predicted until clinical studies are conducted.

Discussion

Plasma SCUF with the SCIP™ system represents a novel, yet logical approach to temporary vascular access for fluid management of the CHF or renal failure patient. Although initial use of SCIP™ is intended only for temporary vascular access in critical care cases, longer-term applications can be envisioned. Since tunneled or cuffed catheters have been shown to last 9 months or more in 60% of recipient patients [6] and infectious incidents may be significantly reduced with antibiotic bonding [14], the use of tunneled SCIP™ catheters for longer-term use in ambulatory or daily ultrafiltration is not an unreasonable proposition for prolonged use.

Rationally, there is no logical reason for processing whole blood within an extracorporeal blood purification circuit. Numerous hemodynamic complications arise directly from removing blood cells from the body, particularly with intermittent hemofiltration therapies. First, during extracorporeal treatment blood is necessarily removed at access fluid flow rates as high as 10% or more of the endogenous BFR to minimize stagnation and platelet aggregation within the external circuit. This also necessitates warming the processed blood before it reenters the body and raises concerns for access recirculation of purified blood. Second, hemofiltration necessarily processes an access fluid volume of 25–80% or greater than the solute-containing volume (plasma) depending upon the packed cell volume of the patient. Third, patients typically suffer therapy-induced anemia, to a varying degree, induced through oxidative stress and thrombocytopenia. Anemia may be improved by treatment with vitamin E and antioxidant therapy [15]. Extracellular processing of blood cells may induce the elevation of proinflammatory cytokines [16] although the degree, profile and impact of such is still unclear. Fourth, hemofiltration therapy is limited in time as the filtration cartridge clogs with activated platelets and fibrin sheaths. Fifth, pre- or postfiltration dilution of the whole blood is often employed to enhance the efficiency of fluid removal and extend filter cartridge operational life. Additionally, slow continuous renal replacement therapies minimize the potential for device-induced dry weight syndrome [17]. The elimination of cells from the extracorporeal circuit allows the hypothesis that all or some of the above-mentioned complications should be eliminated or minimized by extracorporeal plasma processing. In fact, stable hematocrits, plasma-free hemoglobin and blood chemistry values have been consistently observed in vitro (data not shown). Further, we have demonstrated the removal of up to 60% water from thrombocyte-free extracorporeal plasma removed by the porcine SCIP™-60 catheter for ultrafiltration through $0.4\text{-}m^2$ hemofilter cartridges for over 72 h.

While these in vitro studies suggest that clinically beneficial fluid removal will be observed in human trials, numerous other physiologic factors may influence in vivo plasma access flow rates and pressures. These include, but are not limited to postsurgical or postanesthetic thrombocytopenia, diminished BFR, hematocrit, dry weight, sepsis, thrombus formation, fibrin sheath formation or inflammation.

The patient population most likely to benefit from SCIP™ will present with CHF and resulting acute respiratory distress from accumulation of as much as 20 liters of excess fluid. Typically, these patients are prescribed high-dose, intravenous diuretic drugs that can effectively induce the elimination of up to 2 liters/day, necessitating hospitalization of up to or exceeding 10 days. However, significant numbers of these fluid overload patients eventually fail diuretic drugs. Such patients will require device-assisted fluid removal to avoid death. Yet, only infrequently do these patients receive ultrafiltration or dialytic therapy. Key impediments to replacement of devices with diuretics are reimbursement policies, interdisciplinary experience between cardiology and nephrology departments and certainly the extra labor required to regularly monitor the patient and device as well as to replace clogged hemofiltration cartridges and tubing sets.

Conclusions

The current experimental SCIP™-FCM prototypes are designed for ease of use by hospital staff familiar with central venous catheter insertions and provide a safe, labor-free, continuous 3-day fluid removal therapy for use in the intensive or critical care unit. SCIP™-120 catheters may provide net fluid removal rates up to 5 liters/day, a rate sufficient to remove clinically relevant amounts of fluid from diuretic refractory patients. It is expected that this therapy will provide the same clinical benefits already attributed to SCUF [7] and may reduce hospitalization stays, incidence of comorbidities and, quite possibly, the dosage of intravenous diuretics and recombinant human erythropoietin. We are currently planning clinical trials for early 2004 to investigate the safety and efficacy of SCIP™ therapy for such patients.

References

1   Bonello M, Levin NW, Ronco C: History and evolution of the vascular access for hemodialysis; in Ronco C, Levin NW (eds): Hemodialysis Vascular Access and Peritoneal Dialysis Access. Contrib Nephrol. Basel, Karger, 2004, vol 142, pp 1–13.
2   Ronco C, Ghezzi PM, La Greca G: The role of technology in hemodialysis. J Nephrol 1999;12: S68–S81.
3   Khosla N, Ahya SN: Improving dialysis access management. Semin Nephrol 2002;22:507–514.

4   Pisoni RL, Young EW, Dykstra DM, Greenwood RN, Hecking E, Gillespie B, Wolfe RA, Goodkin DA, Held PJ: Vascular access use in Europe and the United States: Results from the DOPPS. Kidney Int 2002;61:305–316.

5   Pisoni RL, Young EW, Mapes DL, Keen ML, Port FK: Vascular access use and outcomes in the US, Europe and Japan: Results from the Dialysis Outcomes and Practice patterns Study. Nephrol News Issues 2003;17:38–47.

6   Combe C, et al: Dialysis Outcomes and Practice Patterns Study: Données sur l'utilisation des cathéters veineux centraux en hémodialyse chronique. Néphrologie 2001;22:379–384.

7   Agostoni P, Marenzi G, Lauri G, Perego G, Schianni M, Sganzerla P: Sustained improvement in functional capacity after removal of body fluid with isolated ultrafiltration in chronic cardiac insufficiency: Failure of furosemide to provide the same result. Am J Med 1994;96:191–199.

8   Oliver MJ, Callery SM, Thorpe KE, Schwab SJ, Churchill DN: Risk of bacteremia from temporary hemodialysis catheters by site of insertion and duration of use: A prospective study. Kidney Int 2000;58:2543–2545.

9   Ronco C, Ricci Z, Bellomo R, Bedogni F, Handley H, Gorsuch R, Levin N: A novel approach to the treatment of chronic fluid overload with a new plasma separation device. Cardiology 2001;96: 202–208.

10   Ronco C: Extracorporeal therapies: Can we use plasma instead of blood? Int J Artif Organs 1999; 22:342–346.

11   Handley HH, Gorsuch R, Levin NW, Ronco C: I.V. catheter for intracorporeal plasma filtration. Blood Purif 2002;20:61–69.

12   Handley HH, Gorsuch R, Levin NW, Ronco C: Slow continuous intracorporeal plasmapheresis for acute fluid overload. Blood Purif 2003;21:72–78.

13   Swartz RD, Messana JM, Orzol S, Port FK: Comparing continuous hemofiltration with hemodialysis in patients with severe acute renal failure. Am J Kidney Dis 1999;34:424–432.

14   Kamal GD, Pfaller MA, Rempe LE, Jebson PJ: Reduced intravascular catheter infection by antibiotic bonding. A prospective, randomized, controlled trial. JAMA 1991;265:2364–2368.

15   Usberti M, Gerardi G, Micheli A, Tira P, Bufano G, Gaggia P, Movilli E, Cancarini GC, De Marinis S, D'Avolio G, Broccoli R, Manganoni A, Albertin A, Di Lorenzo D: Effects of a vitamin E-bonded membrane and of glutathione on anemia and erythropoietin requirements in hemodialysis patients. J Nephrol 2002;15:558–564.

16   Malaponte G, Bevelacqua V, Fatuzzo P, Rapisarda F, Emmanuele G, Travali S, Mazzarino MC: IL-1beta, TNF-alpha and IL-6 release from monocytes in haemodialysis patients in relation to dialytic age. Nephrol Dial Transplant 2002;17:1964–1970.

17   Levin NW, Zhu F, Keen M: Interdialytic weight gain and dry weight. Blood Purif 2001;19: 217–221.

H.H. Handley, Jr., PhD
Transvivo, Inc.,
1100 Lincoln Ave., suite 108, Napa, CA 94558 (USA)
Tel. +1 707 254 9597, Fax +1 707 254 9599, E-Mail hhandley@transvivo.com

Ronco C, Levin NW (eds): Hemodialysis Vascular Access and Peritoneal Dialysis Access.
Contrib Nephrol. Basel, Karger, 2004, vol 142, pp 387–401

....

History and Development of the Access for Peritoneal Dialysis

Zbylut J. Twardowski

University of Missouri, Columbia, Mo., USA

Introduction

One of the most important components of the peritoneal dialysis system is a permanent and trouble-free access to the peritoneal cavity. Although in the development of peritoneal access various ideas have been tried, nowadays only catheters penetrating the abdominal integument are in use. Unfortunately, none of the currently used catheters is trouble free; poor dialysate drainage, peri-catheter leaks, exit site and tunnel infections, and recurrent peritonitis episodes are frequently encountered. Therefore, there is an incessant search for new technological solutions, including new shapes of intraperitoneal and intramural catheter segments and new catheter materials are tried. This chapter will present a brief history of peritoneal catheter development and describe the designs of the most commonly used catheters.

Early History of Catheter Development (1923–1968)

In the early years of peritoneal dialysis the access was not specifically designed for the peritoneal dialysis, rather the available equipment used for other purposes was adapted. Ganter [1] used a metal trocar; Rosenak and Siwon [2] adjusted a glass cannula with multiple side holes used for surgical drains. Engel and Kerkes [3] from Prague used a glass catheter with a mushroom-like opening inside the peritoneum to maximize fluid distribution and prevent obstruction. Reid et al. [4] used a Foley catheter. Major problems in these years were leakage, infection and catheter occlusion by clot or omental fat sucked into the catheter lumen. Fine et al. [5] created a subcutaneous tunnel to hamper periluminal bacterial migration into the peritoneal cavity. They adapted a stainless steel sump drain for dialysate outflow and a rubber mushroom catheter for dialysis solution inflow. Although these innovations showed some improvement in infection rate and drainage, the overall results were not satisfactory and pericatheter leaks were frequent. Some unusual problems that we do not see these days were rigidity of the tube with resulting pressure to viscera, suction of contaminated air into the peritoneal cavity, and difficulties of proper aseptic fixation of the tube to the abdominal wall.

Stephen Rosenak, a Hungarian physician, who became interested in continuous flow peritoneal dialysis in his medical student years in the 1920s [2] while working with Oppenheimer at the Mt. Sinai Hospital in New York, for the first time developed an access specifically for peritoneal dialysis [6]. The Rosenak and Oppenheimer access consisted of a stainless steel flexible coil attached to a rubber drain. The outer portion of the steel tube was attached to an adjustable tie plate for fixation and prevention of leakage. The access was suitable for continuous flow dialysis with inflow through the outer tube and outflow through the inner tube. This device did not gain popularity because major problems were not solved: the rigid tube irritated viscera; dialysate leakage and peritoneal contamination were not eliminated.

A major advance was the introduction of less rigid materials by French physicians. Derot et al. [7] and Marcel Legrain, while working with John Merril [8] in New York used polyvinyl tube for peritoneal dialysis in acute renal failure. The next major progress was made in late 1950s when Maxwell et al. [9] from the University of California in Los Angeles introduced a polyamide (nylon) catheter with multiple tiny distal perforations. The small diameter of perforations prevented particles of omentum from entering the catheter. At the same time, Doolan et al. [10] developed a polyvinyl catheter with multiple ridges to prevent omental wrapping. Both catheters were inserted into the peritoneal cavity with the help of a paracentesis trocar. Smooth, plastic materials were much less irritating to the peritoneum than previously used glass, rubber or steel, thereby omental occlusion became less frequent. The drainage of fluid from the peritoneal cavity was markedly improved, but leakage and pericatheter infections continued to plague the access.

In the early 1960s, Dr. Belding Scribner from Seattle invited Dr. Boen from the Netherlands to continue his peritoneal dialysis research. With limited capacity for hemodialysis, Scribner expected that peritoneal dialysis would be a good alternative for treating a larger number of patients. Boen implanted a Teflon® button in the abdominal wall. Through this button a long catheter was inserted into the peritoneal cavity. After each dialysis the catheter was removed and the button was capped; thus, periodic peritoneal dialysis for chronic renal failure was introduced [11]. Because the method was plagued by frequent peritonitis episodes, Boen et al. [12] in 1963 developed the repeated puncture method. The available catheters, which were semirigid and poorly secured with a short pericatheter path, were not suitable for permanent implantation. For each dialysis, a new catheter had to be inserted. The insertion procedure required penetration of the abdominal wall with a paracentesis trocar. The resulting abdominal opening was of greater diameter than the catheter and pericatheter leaks were frequent.

To circumvent the dialysate leakage problem, Weston and Roberts [13] invented a stylet catheter, which was inserted without a trocar. A sharp stainless steel stylet inserted through the catheter was used to penetrate the abdominal wall. As a result, the abdominal opening fitted snugly around the catheter, thereby preventing leakage. This type of catheter is still being used for acute renal failure.

In another approach to facilitate repeated puncture, Mallette et al. [14] implanted a subcutaneous button. Only skin and subcutaneous tissue had to be penetrated for each catheter insertion. Jacob and Deane [15] used a Teflon® rod to replace the catheter between dialyses. No puncture was necessary. To decrease the possibility of leakage around the catheter, Barry et al. [16] revived the Rosenak and Oppenheimer idea for providing an external seal. They used a Plexiglas disc and a polyvinyl balloon instead of a metal plate for the trans-abdominal cannula. A polyvinyl catheter was inserted through the cannula for each dialysis. The necessity of repeated puncture or catheter insertion through the permanent opening has not gained popularity because this was impractical, especially for the home peritoneal dialysis. These catheters were also plagued with infections, dialysate leaks, and obstructions.

A major step forward in creating a permanent peritoneal access was made in 1964. Gutch [17] noticed lower protein losses with silicone rubber catheters as compared to polyvinyl ones, which suggested less irritation of the peritoneum with a new material. About the same time, Russell Palmer, a physician at the Canadian Army Medical Corps, was developing a peritoneal access made of polyethylene, polypropylene, and nylon [18]. These catheters were relatively rigid and not better than the others available at that time. He was looking for a better material, softer, and more biocompatible. With the help of Wayne Quinton, already successful in manufacturing silicone rubber shunts for hemodialysis, they developed a catheter, which is a prototype of currently used coiled catheters [19]. The catheter was made of silicone rubber; the intraperitoneal end was coiled and had numerous perforations extending 23 cm from the tip; a long subcutaneous tunnel was supposed to hinder periluminal infection. To impede further infection and leakage, a triflanged step was created for securing the catheter in the deep abdominal fascia.

In 1965, Henry Tenckhoff, at the University of Washington, was beginning to treat patients on chronic peritoneal dialysis [20]. After an initial few dialyses in the hospital, the patients would be trained for home dialysis. On the weekends, Tenckhoff would go to the patient's home, insert a temporary catheter and begin dialysis. After the appropriate time on dialysis, the patient would remove the catheter and cover the exit wound with a dressing. Although the method was successful in Tenckhoff's hands, the technique was cumbersome, and Tenckhoff recognized its limitations. He was thinking of a more practical solution.

In 1968, McDonald et al. [21] developed an external seal composed of a polyester (Dacron®) sleeve and a polytetrafluoroethylene (Teflon®) skirt. Tissue ingrowth into these elements created a firm external seal to prevent leakage and microorganism migration. No subcutaneous tunnel was created; the catheter was inserted straight through the abdominal wall.

In the same year, Tenckhoff and Schechter [22] published the results of their studies on a new catheter. Their catheter was an improved version of the Palmer catheter. An intra-abdominal flange was replaced by a Dacron® cuff, a subcutaneous tunnel was shortened and a second, external cuff was used to decrease the length of the catheter sinus tract. Ultimately, the coiled intraperitoneal portion was replaced by a straight segment resembling the Gutch catheter. The intraperitoneal segment was kept open ended and the size of the side holes was optimized to 0.5 mm to prevent tissue suction. A shorter subcutaneous tunnel and a straight intraperitoneal segment facilitated catheter implantation at the bedside with the aid of a specially designed trocar. To avoid excessive bleeding the catheter was inserted through the midline. The Tenckhoff catheter has become the gold standard of peritoneal access. Some of the original recommendations for catheter insertion such as an arcuate subcutaneous tunnel with downward directions of both intraperitoneal and external exits are still considered very important elements of catheter implantation. Few complications were reported in patients treated by periodic peritoneal dialysis in the supine position. However, in patients treated with continuous ambulatory peritoneal dialysis, complications became more frequent, due to high intra-abdominal pressure in the upright position and numerous daily manipulations. Nevertheless, even today, 35 years later, the Tenckhoff catheter in its original form is one of the most widely used catheter types.

Modifications to Mitigate Complications of the Tenckhoff Catheter

The most common complications of the Tenckhoff catheter included exit/tunnel infection, external cuff extrusion, obstruction (which was usually a sequela of catheter tip migration out of the true pelvis with subsequent omental wrapping or tip entrapment in peritoneal adhesions), dialysate leaks, recurrent peritonitis, and infusion or pressure pain.

Exit Infection

To prevent exit infection, a subcutaneous catheter was developed by Stephen et al. [23]. The catheter had two tubes in the peritoneal cavity, and a subcutaneous container. The container was to be punctured for each dialysis. Another subcutaneous catheter was developed by Gotloib et al. [24]. Yet another approach to decrease exit site infection rates was to position the subcutaneous cuff at the skin level [25]. Unfortunately, contrary to expectations, such a position tends to increase infection rates [26].

Catheter Obstruction

To decrease catheter migration and omental wrapping the intraperitoneal segment of the catheter was provided with a saline inflatable balloon [27] or discs [28]. Valli et al. [29, 30] revived an idea of Goldberg and Hill [27] and made a silicone rubber catheter with a balloon-shaped intraperitoneal segment surrounding the catheter tip. Ash et al. [31] replaced the intraperitoneal tubing with a disc located immediately beneath the abdominal wall. Recently Ash et al. [32, 33] changed the intraperitoneal segment of the catheter from the column disc to a longitudinal tube with 1-mm wide 'flutes' or grooves on the surface. The intraperitoneal segment lies against the parietal peritoneum and is connected perpendicularly to a transabdominal tube, thus creating a 'T'-shaped catheter. Both catheters cannot migrate, but still may be obstructed by bowels, adhesions, or omentum.

Another approach was undertaken by Chiaramonte et al. [34–36] from Vicenza. Because the best position of the catheter tip is the true pelvis, the Vicenza group decided to shorten the catheter and implant it very low, just a few centimeters above the symphysis pubis. Such a catheter has a limited capability to migrate outside of the true pelvis and the omental wrapping was less likely as in the majority of people the omentum does not reach below the pelvic brim. According to the authors, the long-term experience with Vicenza catheter was very positive [36]: the catheter obstruction rate was very low, and other complications were not worse than with the Tenckhoff catheter, with the exception of pericatheter leaks, which were significantly higher. This was related to the low, near the pubis, insertion site of the catheter, where intra-abdominal pressure in the upright position is higher compared to that of the insertion site of Tenckhoff catheter near the navel.

As mentioned above, the omentum rarely reaches below the pelvic brim, so keeping the catheter tip in the true pelvis should prevent catheter migration with subsequent obstruction. To keep the catheter tip in the true pelvis,

Di Paolo et al. [37] decided to incorporate a tungsten weight at the catheter tip. In the upright position, such a catheter tip tends to remain in the true pelvis due to gravity. In the original study, 32 'self-locating' catheters were followed for 468 patient-months and compared to 26 Tenckhoff catheters followed for 415 patient-months. No translocations of the self-locating catheter were observed, whereas nine dislocations occurred with Tenckhoff catheters. The rate of Tenckhoff catheter dislocations was unusually high in this study. The other complications were similar with both types of catheters. The lower dislocation rates of the self-locating catheter compared to Tenckhoff catheter were confirmed by other groups [38, 39]. No bowel or bladder perforations were observed with self-locating catheters [39].

Pericatheter Leak

As pericatheter leakage was frequently observed in ambulatory peritoneal dialysis patients, a design to prevent this complication was introduced in Toronto in 1979 [40], shortly after continuous ambulatory peritoneal dialysis was introduced into the treatment of chronic renal failure. The catheter, dubbed the Toronto Western Hospital Type 2 (TWH-2), was made of silicone rubber tubing and was provided with two cuffs, similar to the Tenckhoff catheter and two silicone rubber discs to curtail catheter migration [28]; however, it had new features. The catheter was provided with a polyester flange at the base of the deep cuff and a silicone rubber ring (or bead) situated close to the flange that provided a groove in which a purse string could tie the peritoneum tightly [40]. These innovations by themselves did not decrease leakages until the implantation technique was modified. Instead of implantation through the linea alba, the catheter was inserted though the rectus muscle [40]. After implantation the flange was situated on the posterior rectus sheath, the deep cuff in the rectus muscle and the purse string was placed through the posterior rectus sheath, transversalis fascia, and the peritoneum.

Infusion or Pressure Pain

Some patients experience pain at the tip of the catheter with the straight intraperitoneal segment. This pain is partly related to a 'jet effect' of the rapidly flowing dialysis solution and to the pressure of the straight catheter tip. Catheters with a coiled intraperitoneal segment, as in the Palmer catheter [19], are less likely to induce abdominal pain because more of the solution flows shower-like through side holes with only part of it through the main lumen that is not in direct contact with the peritoneal membrane. Moreover, the poking force of the coiled catheter is smaller than that of the straight one because the coiled intraperitoneal segment is more flexible. Finally, the larger contact area of the coiled catheter with the parietal peritoneum further reduces the pressure compared to the straight catheter tip. Many of the currently used catheters include this feature.

External Cuff Extrusion

The simplest way to avoid external cuff extrusion is not to use it; however, a single cuff catheter is associated with more exit/tunnel infections, higher peritonitis rates, and shorter survival [41–44]. Another remedy would be to locate the external cuff far away from the exit so it would be impossible to have it extruded; however, a long sinus tract (from the exit to the cuff) creates a situation similar to the single cuff catheter predisposing to exit/tunnel infections. A localization of the cuff close to the exit predisposes to its extrusion. There are at least two forces favoring cuff extrusion: (1) the pushing force of catheter resilience and (2) pulling and tugging on the catheter. The resilience (shape memory) of the straight catheter implanted in an arcuate tunnel plays the most important role in cuff extrusion.

As a compromise between the requirements of a short sinus tract to prevent infections but not so short to favor cuff extrusions the cuff should be implanted approximately 2–3 cm beneath the skin. Moreover, resilience forces should be eliminated by designing the catheter in a shape similar to the shape of the tunnel. To follow original Tenckhoff recommendations that the catheter should be implanted with an arcuate subcutaneous tunnel with downward directions of both intraperitoneal and external exits, the catheter should have a permanent bend between the cuffs. The catheters with such a bend are called swan-neck catheters [45]. Similar principles were applied by Cruz to polyurethane catheters [46].

Double-Lumen Catheters for Continuous Flow Peritoneal Dialysis

Continuous flow peritoneal dialysis, introduced in 1925 by Rosenak and Siwon [2], was used concomitantly with intermittent flow peritoneal dialysis until the late 1960s. High fluid flows were used with either two catheters [47] or double-lumen catheters [48]. The method was abandoned in the 1970s as associated with technical difficulties due to catheter obstruction, abdominal pain related to high flow, and less than expected dialysis efficiency because of fluid channeling [49].

There is a renewed interest in continuous flow peritoneal dialysis, as it is believed that new peritoneal accesses may make this modality successful. One of these catheters, a fluted double-lumen catheter, has been recently described by Diaz-Buxo [50]. Within the abdominal wall, this catheter consists of two tubes using a novel configuration, where one slightly oval-shaped tube embeds within the other crescent-shaped tube. Externally, the tubes are separate. Internally the tubes are also separated, with each tube terminating with a fluted section. The internal part of this double-lumen catheter is similar to the T-fluted catheter with the exception that the latter is a single-lumen catheter. Another catheter, a double-lumen catheter with diffuser, has been recently developed by Ronco et al. [51]. The intraperitoneal segment of the outflow tubing has a coiled design. The intraperitoneal segment of the inflow tubing is a short, thin-walled, silicone rubber, round tapered diffuser with multiple side holes, which allow the inflowing dialysis solution to be dispersed just below the parietal peritoneum, far away from the outflow tubing tip. In vitro studies showed excellent flow characteristics and very low recirculation [51].

Clinical trials are needed to determine whether continuous flow peritoneal dialysis can be revived after more than a quarter century hiatus.

Most Commonly Used Chronic Peritoneal Catheters

Straight and Coiled Tenckhoff Catheters

The catheters consist of the silicone rubber tubing with a 2.6-mm internal diameter and 5-mm external diameter. The catheter is provided with one or two polyester (Dacron®), 1-cm-long cuffs. The overall length of the adult straight double cuff catheter is about 40 cm. The lengths of segments are: intraperitoneal about 15 cm, intercuff 5–7 cm, and external 16 cm. The intraperitoneal segment has an open end and multiple 0.5-mm perforations on a distance of 11 cm from the tip. The coiled Tenckhoff catheter differs from the straight in having a coiled, 18.5-cm-long perforated distal end. As mentioned above, the coiled catheter reduces inflow infusion 'jet effect' and pressure discomfort. All Tenckhoff catheters are provided with a barium-impregnated radiopaque stripe to assist in radiological visualization of the catheter. The catheters are manufactured by numerous companies.

Swan-Neck Catheters

The design of the swan-neck catheters is based on a retrospective analysis of complication rates with Tenckhoff and Toronto Western Hospital catheters. The analysis showed that the lowest complication rates were with double cuff catheters implanted through the belly of the rectus muscle and with both internal and skin exits of the tunnel directed downward; however, the resulting arcuate tunnel led to frequent external cuff extrusion [45]. All swan-neck catheters feature a permanent bend between cuffs [45]. The catheter was dubbed 'swan neck' because of its shape. Because of this design, catheters can be placed in an arcuate tunnel in an unstressed condition with both external and internal

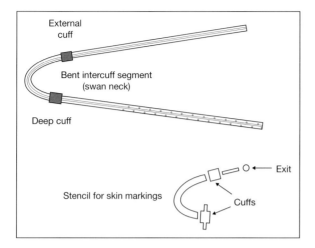

Fig. 1. Swan-neck Tenckhoff catheter with straight intraperitoneal segment and stencil for skin markings.

segments of the tunnel directed downward. The downward directed exit, two cuffs, and optimal sinus length reduce exit/tunnel infection rates. A permanent bend between cuffs eliminates the silicone rubber resilience force or the 'shape memory' which tends to extrude the external cuff. Downward peritoneal entrance tends to keep the tip in the true pelvis reducing its migration. Insertion through the rectus muscle decreases pericatheter leaks. Lower exit/tunnel infection rates curtail peritonitis episodes. Finally, swan-neck catheters with a coiled intraperitoneal segment minimize infusion and pressure pain. Several types of swan-neck catheters are available [52]. Swan-neck catheters are designed to have an exit in the abdominal integument (swan-neck abdominal catheters, fig. 1, 2) or in the chest (swan-neck presternal catheter, fig. 3). Stencils have been developed for skin markings to facilitate creation of proper tunnels for swan-neck catheters (fig. 1, 2). The stencils follow exactly the shape of the intra-mural segments of the catheters and the catheter tunnels must follow the shape of the catheters exactly as designed to maximize the advantages of this design.

Swan-Neck Abdominal Catheters

Swan-neck abdominal catheters are one of the most commonly used catheters at present. According to the manufacturer (Kendal Healthcare, Mansfield, Mass., USA), over 17,000 swan-neck abdominal catheters were sold worldwide in 2002. Long-term studies from a number of peritoneal dialysis programs reported lower complications and better survival of swan-neck catheters compared to other catheters [53–57].

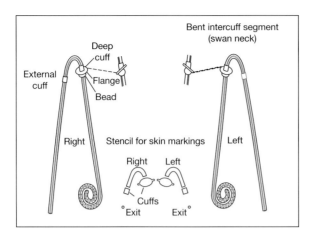

Fig. 2. Swan-neck Missouri catheters and stencils for right and left tunnels. The flange and bead are slanted 45°; once the catheter is properly implanted, the intraperitoneal tubing is directed downward to keep the tip in the true pelvis.

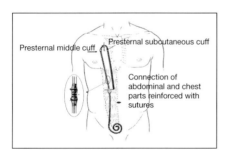

Fig. 3. Implanted swan-neck prester-nal peritoneal catheter in relation to torso.

Swan-Neck Tenckhoff Straight and Coiled. The Tenckhoff type of the swan-neck peritoneal dialysis catheter (fig. 1) is provided with two Dacron cuffs. It differs from the double cuff Tenckhoff catheter only by being perma-nently bent between cuffs. This type of catheter may be inserted at the bedside; however, a subcutaneous tunnel has to be created in the same way as for other swan-neck catheters. The intraperitoneal segment of the swan-neck coiled catheter is identical to that of the Tenckhoff coiled catheter.

Swan-Neck Missouri Straight and Coiled. The swan-neck Missouri catheter has a flange and bead circumferentially surrounding the catheter just below the internal cuff, similar to the TWH-2 catheter [40]; however, the flange and bead are not perpendicular but slanted approximately 45° relative to the axis of the catheter (fig. 2). The slanted flange and bead, and bent tunnel segment require that the swan-neck Missouri catheters for right and left tunnels be mirror images of each other. To facilitate recognition of right and left Missouri catheters, the tubings have a radiopaque stripe in front of the catheter. It is imperative to implant the catheter with an appropriate tunnel direction, otherwise the catheter will not provide any advantages, and rather worse results may be encountered. The intraperitoneal segment may be straight or coiled.

Moncrief-Popovich Catheter. This catheter is a modified swan-neck Tenckhoff coiled catheter with a longer subcutaneous cuff (2.5 cm instead of 1 cm). It is most commonly used in conjunction with the Moncrief-Popovich implantation technique, whereby the external part is kept under the skin until the ingrowth of the tissue into the cuff is strong. Only after several weeks (3–6 or more), is the external part exteriorized [58].

Swan-Neck Presternal Catheter

The idea of a presternal exit location stemmed from several observations indicating that this location may decrease exit infections [59]. The chest is a sturdy structure with minimal wall motion; the catheter exit located on the chest wall is subjected to minimal movements decreasing chances of trauma and contamination. Also, in patients with abdominal ostomies and in children with diapers, a chest exit location decreases chances of contamination. Moreover, a loose garment is usually worn on the chest and there is less pressure on the exit. Clinical surgical experience indicates that wounds heal better after thoracic surgery than after abdominal surgery; this may be related to less chest mobility or some other reasons. Obese patients have higher exit site infection rates and a tendency to poor wound healing, particularly after abdominal surgery. The subcutaneous fat layer is several times thinner on the chest than on the abdomen. If fat thickness per se is responsible for quality of healing and susceptibility to infection then chest location may be preferred for obese patients. The catheter is particularly useful in obese patients (body mass index > 35), patients with ostomies, children with diapers and fecal incontinence, and patients who want to take tub bath without the risk of exit contamination. Many patients prefer presternal catheter because of better body image.

To accommodate these principles, we modified the swan-neck peritoneal catheter to have an exit on the chest but preserving all advantages of the swan-neck Missouri coiled catheters, minimizing catheter obstruction, cuff extrusion, pericatheter dialysate leak and infusion pain. A major difference from the swan-neck Missouri catheter is in the length of the subcutaneous tunnel.

The presternal peritoneal dialysis catheter is composed of two flexible (silicon rubber) tubes, which are connected end to end at the time of implantation (fig. 3). The implanted lower (abdominal) tube constitutes the intraperitoneal catheter segment and a part of the intramural segment. The upper or chest tube constitutes the remaining part of the intramural segment and the external catheter segment. The lower tube is identical to the swan-neck Missouri catheter, with the exception that it is not bent and does not have a second cuff. The proximal end of the lower tube is straight and with a redundant length to be trimmed to the patient's size at the time of implantation. A titanium connector, provided in a package, is to be coupled with the distal part of the upper or chest part at the time of implantation. The connection is reinforced with sutures placed over the connector grooves on both the abdominal and thoracic tubes. Details of the catheter implantation technique have been recently published [59].

Ten years of experience with this catheter confirmed theoretical predictions. The results regarding infectious complication and catheter survival were superior to other catheters, including swan-neck abdominal catheters [59]. Their use has gradually been increasing in recent years; according to the manufacturer (Kendal Healthcare, Mansfield, Mass., USA), 217 catheters were sold worldwide in 2000, 386 in 2001, and 371 in 2002.

Disadvantages of the presternal catheter are minimal. Compared to abdominal catheters, dialysis solution flow is slightly slower due to the increased catheter length; however, the slower flow is insignificant clinically. There is a possibility of catheter disconnection in the tunnel but this complication is extremely rare in adults and easily corrected. Finally, the implantation technique is more challenging compared to that of single-piece, abdominal catheters. This may be one of the reasons of limited use. A video showing the implantation technique in detail is available from the manufacturer.

Concluding Remarks

The Tenckhoff catheter, developed in 1968, continues to be widely used for chronic peritoneal dialysis, although its use is decreasing in favor of swan-neck catheters. Soft, silicone rubber instead of rigid tubing virtually eliminated early complications such as bowel perforation or massive bleeding. Other complications, such as obstruction, pericatheter leaks, and superficial cuff extrusions, have been markedly reduced in recent years, particularly with the use of swan-neck catheters and insertion through the rectus muscle instead of the midline. However, complications still occur so new designs are being tried. A renewed interest in continuous flow peritoneal dialysis stimulated inventions of imaginative, double-lumen catheters.

References

1   Ganter G: Ueber die Beseitigung giftiger Stoffe aus dem Blute durch Dialyse. Munch Med Wochenschr 1923;70:1478–1480.

2   Rosenak S, Siwon P: Experimentelle Untersuchungen über die peritoneale Ausscheidung harnpflichtiger Substanzen aus dem Blute. Mitt Grenzgeb Med Chir 1925;39:391–408.

3   Engel D, Kerkes A: Beiträge zum Permeabilitätsproblem: Entgiftungsstudien mittels des lebenden Peritoneums als 'Dialysator'. Z Ges Exp Med 1927;55:574–601.

4   Reid R, Penfold JB, Jones RN: Anuria treated by renal decapsulation and peritoneal dialysis. Lancet 1946;ii:749–753.

5   Fine J, Frank HA, Seligman AM: The treatment of acute renal failure by peritoneal irrigation. Ann Surg 1946;124:857–878.

6   Rosenak SS, Oppenheimer GD: An improved drain for peritoneal lavage. Surgery 1948;23:832–833.

7   Derot M, Tanzet P, Roussilon J, Bernier JJ: La dialyse péritonéale dans le traitement de l'urémie aiguë. J Urol 1949;55:113–121.

8   Legrain M, Merril JP: Short term continuous peritoneal dialysis. N Engl J Med 1953;248: 125–129.

9   Maxwell MH, Rockney RE, Kleeman CR, Twiss MR: Peritoneal dialysis. JAMA 1959;170:917–924.

10 Doolan PD, Murphy WP, Wiggins RA, Carter NW, Cooper WC, Watten RH, Alpen EL: An evaluation of intermittent peritoneal lavage. Am J Med 1959;26:831–844.

11 Boen ST, Mulinari AS, Dillard DH, Scribner BH: Periodic peritoneal dialysis in the management of chronic uremia. Trans Am Soc Artif Intern Organs 1962;8:256–265.

12 Boen ST, Mion CM, Curtis FK, Shilipetar G: Periodic peritoneal dialysis using the repeated puncture technique and an automated cycling machine. Trans Am Soc Artif Intern Organs 1964; 10:409–413.

13 Weston RE, Roberts M: Clinical use of stylet catheter for peritoneal dialysis. Arch Intern Med 1965;115:659–662.

14 Mallette WG, McPhaul JJ, Bledsoe F, McIntosh DA, Koegel E: A clinically successful subcutaneous peritoneal access button for repeated peritoneal dialysis. Trans Am Soc Artif Intern Organs 1964;10:396–398.

15 Jacob GB, Deane N: Repeated peritoneal dialysis by the catheter replacement method: Description of technique and a replaceable prosthesis for chronic access to the peritoneal cavity. Proc Eur Dial Transplant Assoc 1967;4:136–140.

16 Barry KG, Shambaugh GE, Goler D: A new flexible cannula and seal to provide prolonged access for peritoneal drainage and other procedures. J Urol 1963;90:125–128.

17 Gutch CF: Peritoneal dialysis. Trans Am Soc Artif Intern Organs 1964;10:406–407.

18 Palmer RA, Maybee TK, Henry EW, Eden J: Peritoneal dialysis in acute and chronic renal failure. Can Med Assoc J 1963;88:920–927.

19 Palmer RA, Quinton WE, Gray JE: Prolonged peritoneal dialysis for chronic renal failure. Lancet 1964;i:700–702.

20 Tenckhoff H, Schechter H, Boen ST: One year experience with home peritoneal dialysis. Trans Am Soc Artif Intern Organs 1965;11:11–14.

21 McDonald HP Jr, Gerber N, Mischra D, Wolm L, Peng B, Waterhouse K: Subcutaneous Dacron and Teflon cloth adjuncts for silastic arteriovenous shunts and peritoneal dialysis catheters. Trans Am Soc Artif Intern Organs 1968;14:176–180.

22 Tenckhoff J, Schechter H: A bacteriologically safe peritoneal access device. Trans Am Soc Artif Intern Organs 1968;14:181–187.

23 Stephen RI, Atkin-Thor E, Kolff WJ: Recirculating peritoneal dialysis with subcutaneous catheter. Trans Am Soc Artif Intern Organs 1976;22:575–584.

24 Gotloib L, Nisencorn I, Garmizo AL, Galili N, Servadio C, Sudarsky M: Subcutaneous intraperitoneal prosthesis for maintenance of peritoneal dialysis. Lancet 1975;i/7920:1318–1320.

25 Daly BDT, Dasse KA, Haudenschild CC, Clay W, Szycher M, Ober NS, Cleveland RJ: Percutaneous energy transmission systems: Long-term survival. Trans Am Soc Artif Intern Organs 1983;29: 526–530.

26 Ogden DA, Benavente G, Wheeler D, Zukoski CF: Experience with the right angle Gore-Tex® peritoneal dialysis catheter; in Khanna R, Nolph KD, Prowant BF, Twardowski ZJ, Oreopoulos GD (eds): Advances in Continuous Ambulatory Peritoneal Dialysis. Selected Papers from the Sixth Annual CAPD Conference, Kansas City, Missouri, February 1986. Toronto, Peritoneal Dialysis Bulletin, 1986, pp 155–159.

27   Goldberg EM, Hill W: A new peritoneal access prosthesis. Proc Clin Dial Transplant Forum 1973;3:122–125.

28   Oreopoulos DG, Izatt S, Zellerman G, Karanicolas S, Mathews RE: A prospective study of the effectiveness of three permanent peritoneal catheters. Proc Clin Dial Transplant Forum 1976;6: 96–100.

29   Valli A, Comotti C, Torelli D, Crescimanno U, Valentini A, Riegler P, Huber W, Borghi M, Gruttadauria C, Scavoranat P, Pecchini F: A new catheter for peritoneal dialysis. Trans Am Soc Am Intern Organs 1983;29:629–632.

30   Valli A, Andreotti C, Degetto P, Midiri R, Mazzon M, Rovati C, Valentini A, Crescimanno U, Depaoli Vitali E, Manili L, Camerini C: 48-months' experience with Valli-2 catheter; in Khanna R, Nolph KD, Prowant BF, Twardowski ZJ, Oreopoulos DG (eds): Advances in Continuous Ambulatory Peritoneal Dialysis. Selected Papers from the Eight Annual CAPD Conference, Kansas City, Missouri, February 1988. Toronto, Peritoneal Dialysis Bulletin,1988, pp 292–297.

31   Ash SR, Johnson H, Hartman J, Granger J, Koszuta J, Sell L, Dhein C, Blevins W, Thornhill JA: The column disc peritoneal catheter. A peritoneal access device with improved drainage. ASAIO J 1980;3:109–115.

32   Ash SR, Janle EM: T-fluted peritoneal catheter. Adv Perit Dial 1993;9:223–226.

33   Ash SR, Sutton JM, Mankus RA, Rossman J, de Ridder V, Nassivi MS, Ross J: Clinical trials of the T-fluted (Ash Advantage) peritoneal dialysis catheter. Adv Ren Replace Ther 2002;9/2: 133–143.

34   Chiaramonte S, Feriani M, Biasoli S, Bragantini L, Brendolan A, Dell'Aquilla R, Fabris A, Ronco C, La Greca G: Clinical experience with short peritoneal dialysis catheters. Proc Eur Dial Transplant Assoc Eur Ren Assoc 1985;22:426–430.

35   Chiaramonte S, Feriani M, Biasoli S, Fabris A, Ronco C, Borin D, Bragantini L, Brendolan A, Dell'Aquilla R, Milan M, La Greca G: Clinical experience with short peritoneal dialysis catheters; in Peritoneal Dialysis – Proc 2nd International Course. Milano, Wichtig, 1986, pp 161–164.

36   Chiaramonte S, Bragantini L, Brendolan A, Conz P, Crepaldi C, Dell'Aquilla R, Feriani M, Milan M, Ronco C, La Greca G: Long-term experience with the Vicenza catheter; in Ota K, et al (eds): Current Concepts in Peritoneal Dialysis. Amsterdam, Elsevier Science, 1992, pp 160–163.

37   Di Paolo N, Petrini G, Garosi G, Buoncristiani U, Brardi S, Monaci G: A new self-locating catheter. Perit Dial Int 1996;16/6:623–627.

38   Cavagna R, Tessrin C, Tarroni G, Casol D, De Silvestro L, Fabbian F: The self-locating catheter: Clinical evaluation and comparison with the Tenckhoff catheter. Perit Dial Int 1999;19:540–543.

39   Minguela I, Lanuza M, Ruiz de Gauna R, Rodado R, Alegria S, Andreu AJ, Gonzalez MJ, Rodriguez B, Vitores JM, Castellanos T, Martinez C, Aurrekoetxea B, Chena A: Lower malfunction rate with self-locating catheters. Perit Dial Int 2001;21(suppl 3):S209–S212.

40   Ponce SP, Pierratos A, Izatt S, Nathews R, Khanna R, Zellerman G, Oreopoulos DG: Comparison of the survival and complications of three permanent peritoneal dialysis catheters. Perit Dial Bull 1982;2/2:82–86.

41   US Renal Data System, USRDS 1992 Annual Data Report, VI: Catheter-related factors and peritonitis risk in CAPD patients. Am J Kidney Dis 1992;5(suppl 2):48–54.

42   Honda M, Iitaka K, Kawaguchi H, Hoshii S, Akashi S, Kohsaka T, Tuzuki K, Yamaoka K, Yoshikawa N, Karashima S, Itoh Y, Hatae K: The Japanese National Registry data on pediatric CAPD patients: A ten-year experience. A report of the Study Group of Pediatric PD Conference. Perit Dial Int 1996;16/3:269–275.

43   Lindblad AS, Hamilton RW, Nolph KD, Novak JW: A retrospective analysis of catheter configuration and cuff type: A National CAPD Registry report. Perit Dial Int 1988;8/2:129–133.

44   Gokal R, Alexander S, Ash S, Chen TW, Danielson A, Holmes C, Joffe P, Moncrief J, Nichols K, Piraino B, Prowant B, Slingeneyer A, Stegmayr B, Twardowski Z, Vas S: Peritoneal catheters and exit-site practices toward optimum peritoneal access: 1998 update (Official report from the International Society for Peritoneal Dialysis). Perit Dial Int 1998;18/1:11–33.

45   Twardowski ZJ, Nolph KD, Khanna R, Prowant BF, Ryan LP: The need for a 'swan neck' permanently bent, arcuate peritoneal dialysis catheter. Perit Dial Bull 1985;5/6:219–223.

46   Cruz C: Clinical experience with a new peritoneal access device (the Cruz® catheter); in Ota K, Maher J, Winchester J, Hirszel P, Ito K, Suzuki T (eds): Current Concepts in Peritoneal Dialysis:

Proceedings of the Fifth Congress of the International Society for Peritoneal Dialysis, Kyoto, July 21–24, 1990. Amsterdam, Excerpta Medica, 1992, pp 164–169.

47 Miller JH, Gipstein R, Margules R, Swartz M, Rubini ME: Automated peritoneal dialysis: Analysis of several methods of peritoneal dialysis. Trans Am Soc Artif Intern Organs 1966;12:98–105.

48 Lange K, Treser G, Mangalat J: Automatic continuous high flow rate peritoneal dialysis. Arch Klin Med 1968;214/3:201–206.

49 Twardowski ZJ: New approaches to intermittent peritoneal dialysis therapies; in Nolph KD (ed): Peritoneal Dialysis, ed 3. Dordrecht, Kluwer Academic Publishers, 1989, chap 8, pp 133–151.

50 Diaz-Buxo JA: Streaming, mixing, and recirculation: Role of the peritoneal access in continuous flow peritoneal dialysis (clinical considerations). Adv Perit Dial 2002;18:87–90.

51 Ronco C, Gloukhoff A, Dell'Aquila R, Levin NW: Catheter design for continuous flow peritoneal dialysis. Blood Purif 2002;20/1:40–44.

52 Twardowski ZJ, Nichols WK: Peritoneal dialysis access and exit site care including surgical aspects; in Gokal R, Khanna R, Krediet RT, Nolph KD (eds): Peritoneal Dialysis, ed 2. Dordrecht, Kluwer Academic Publishers, 2000, chap 9, pp 307–361.

53 Twardowski ZJ, Prowant BF, Nichols WK, Nolph KD, Khanna R: Six year experience with swan neck catheter. Perit Dial Int 1992;12/4:384–389.

54 Gadallah MF, Mignone J, Torres C, Garfield R, Pervez A: The role of peritoneal dialysis catheter configuration in preventing catheter tip migration. Adv Perit Dial 2000;16:47–50.

55 Plaza MM, Rivas MC, Dominguez-Viguera L: Fluoroscopic manipulation is also useful for malfunctioning swan-neck peritoneal catheters. Perit Dial Int 2001;21/2:193–196.

56 Neu AM, Ho PL, McDonald RA, Warady BA: Chronic dialysis in children and adolescents. The 2001 NAPRTCS Annual Report. Pediatr Nephrol 2002;17:656–663.

57 Harvey EA: Peritoneal access in children. Perit Dial Int 2001;21(suppl 3):S218–S222.

58 Moncrief JW, Popovich RP, Broadrick LJ, He ZZ, Simmons EE, Tate RA: Moncrief-Popovich catheter: A new peritoneal access technique for patients on peritoneal dialysis. ASAIO J 1993; 39/1:62–65.

59 Twardowski ZJ: Pre-sternal peritoneal access. Adv Ren Replace Ther 2002;9/2:125–132.

Zbylut J. Twardowski, MD, PhD,
Professor Emeritus of Medicine,
University of Missouri, Dialysis Clinic, Inc.,
3300 LeMone Industrial Blvd., Columbia, MO 65201 (USA)
Tel. +1 573 443 1531, ext. 256, Fax +1 573 884 5506,
E-Mail twardowskiz@health.missouri.edu

Ronco C, Levin NW (eds): Hemodialysis Vascular Access and Peritoneal Dialysis Access.
Contrib Nephrol. Basel, Karger, 2004, vol 142, pp 402–409

....

Techniques of Peritoneal Catheter Insertion

A. Rodrigues[a], *A. Cabrita*[a], *C. Nogueira*[b]

Departments of [a]Nephrology and [b]Surgery, Hospital Geral Santo Antonio,
Porto, Portugal

Introduction

Peritoneal dialysis needs an access to the peritoneal cavity for instillation of
dialysis fluid. Different devices and implantation methodologies have been used
to access the peritoneal cavity for either acute or chronic peritoneal dialysis.

In the early times of peritoneal dialysis semirigid catheters have been used
for acute peritoneal dialysis [1] with blind bedside percutaneous implantation.
Initially a small trocar was used for insertion of a commercially available small-
bore nylon catheter. By the end of 1964, a stylet catheter was used. A high rate
of leaks, poor drainage and peritonitis made it necessary to develop new methods.
In 1968, Tenckhoff described a two-cuffed silicone rubber catheter implanted
through a special trocar. Increased experience with these catheters made the
maintenance of a reliable and long-standing access for chronic peritoneal dialysis
possible. A key factor to the technical success of chronic peritoneal dialysis is
a correctly positioned and functioning catheter with long-term survival.
Different methods of catheter implantation have been used aiming for a low rate
of access-related complications such as pericatheter leaks, exit site/tunnel
infections, peritonitis, mechanical dysfunction due to luminal obstruction,
epiploon entrapment or intraperitoneal tip migration, infusion/pressure-related
pain, bleeding, and rarely, visceral perforation.

Preimplantation Care

Before the description and critical review of placement techniques some
general preimplantation rules should be considered. During the predialysis visits

the patient should be fully informed about the modality and an integrated plan of chronic renal replacement therapies. A careful examination of the abdominal wall should be done, looking for hernias and scars. An adequate choice of the exit site, avoiding the belt line and fat folds, is also essential. Constipation should be treated before surgery to allow adequate postimplantation catheter function. It is recommended that nasal swabs are used to identify *Staphylococcus aureus* carriers and treat them with mupirocin before catheter implantation [2].

General Guidelines for Peritoneal Catheter Insertion

Regardless the implantation technique, the placement of the catheter calls for strict asepsis. Either a surgeon or a nephrologist can do it, since the results are mainly related to the skills of the operator. The role of preoperative vancomycin or cephalosporins in preventing early infection in newly placed peritoneal catheters has been controversial, but enough evidence-based data clearly support this antibiotic prophylaxis [3–5]. Cefazolin is a good option, leaving the use of vancomycin for the treatment of allergic patients and specific therapies.

The patients should be instructed to empty their bladder before catheter insertion. Local anesthesia, with some intravenous sedation, usually allows most of the catheter implantations, either in an outpatient procedure room and in a surgical theater. Admission is only necessary for some patients. Catheter implantation can preferably be safely managed as an outpatient procedure, reducing the costs involved.

Considering Some Historical General Rules [6–10]

The incision for catheter insertion, as it is classically described, can be infraumbilical midline (3 cm below the umbilicus), paramedian (at the medial edge of the rectus muscle) or lateral to the border of the rectus muscle. The midline incision has the advantage of avoiding epigastric vessels but is associated with a higher risk of subsequent leaks or hernia. It was the common place of implantation of acute catheters, but is no longer widely used. The left side is recommended because the cecum can be avoided. Nowadays, a paramedian incision at the left side with a transrectus dissection of the muscle is the most frequently used place. The catheter is soaked and flushed with sterile saline prior to insertion. The cuffs are squeezed in saline to expel air, promoting good tissue ingrowth. The intraperitoneal portion should be directed toward the lower peritoneal cavity.

The deep cuff should be placed within the abdominal wall under the rectus muscle providing better vascularization and stronger fibrous tissue ingrowth

Table 1. Techniques of peritoneal catheter placement

Implantation methodology	Technique
Blind	Trocar
	Seldinger
Surgical	Minilaparotomy

compared to a cuff placed in the subcutaneous tissue. After closing the aponeurosis, an arcuate subcutaneous tunnel is made with a tunneler and a downward-facing exit site is recommended. If a double-cuffed catheter is used, the external cuff should be 2 cm from the exit site. In some patients, such as in children [11], the experience with double-cuffed catheters brought the risk of external cuff extrusion due to external pulling and catheter resilience forces.

Fluid (either peritoneal solution or preferably saline) is infused and drained through the catheter to check for adequate function.

Techniques of Peritoneal Catheter Insertion

Catheter insertion may be done with a blind abdominal puncture (commonly labeled blind percutaneous), surgically (with minilaparotomy) or peritoneoscopically (table 1). Peritoneoscopy is also a surgical technique but nephrologists usually list it separately due to its specific characteristics. Besides, since the use of acute catheters has been abandoned, literally abdominal blind percutaneous implantation is no longer done. Chronic catheters always make a small dissection incision through the skin and abdominal structures towards the peritoneum necessary. At this stage the insertion may be blind (with a trocar or Seldinger technique), a dissection with minilaparotomy, or peritoneoscopic.

Blind Insertion

Acute catheters were usually placed by a blind percutaneous puncture in the midline, under local anesthesia, over a stylet or with a guidewire, into a pre-filled abdomen. They should no longer be used.

For blind insertion of chronic catheters an incision through the skin and the subcutaneous tissue, and then separation of the rectus muscle fibers is done. The parietal peritoneum is punctured with a trocar or a needle and guidewire (Seldinger technique) through which the catheter is passed. The rectus aponeurosis is closed over the deeper cuff, left among the fibers of the muscle, and the subcutaneous tunnel is then created. The patient should preferably be alert to cooperate in tensing the abdominal wall.

Viscera perforation is an ever-present complication of blind implantation. Patients with ileus or previous abdominal surgeries and adhesions are poor candidates for this technique.

Surgical Insertion

Few centers are at present using blind catheter implantation [12], mainly because of the risk of organ perforation and catheter dysfunction. Therefore, surgical minilaparotomy is the rule. Catheters are inserted in an operating theater using an open surgical technique, preferably under local anesthesia. Local anesthesia makes possible an outpatient procedure and patient collaboration during the procedure.

The important difference is that the dissection of the abdominal wall and peritoneum is made under direct vision. After an incision through the skin, subcutaneous fat, anterior rectus aponeurosis, and dissection of the rectus muscle, the transversalis fascia and parietal peritoneum is lifted to create an air space between it and the abdominal contents. Then a small incision in the deep fascia and in the peritoneum allows the introduction of the catheter under direct vision, avoiding organs, epiploon and adhesions. The catheter, stiffened with a stylet or simply guided with a long forceps, is guided through the peritoneal cavity into the pelvic cavity, at the Douglas pouch if possible. At that time, the patient feels a voiding sensation if the tip is in good position. It is important to use a purse-string suture in the peritoneum/deep fascia through witch the catheter is passed. In this way, the peritoneum, transversalis fascia and posterior rectus sheet are closed tightly below the inner cuff to avoid early leakage.

This technique also allows to perform partial omentectomy, but there is no evidence to recommend it as a routine.

Peritoneoscopic Implantation

Peritoneoscopic implantation as described by Ash et al. [13] allows inspection of the abdominal cavity in a minimally invasive procedure with a control of the placement of the catheter tip. Using a 2-mm Y-TEC trocar there is a reduced risk of leakage and catheter survival may prove to be superior to surgical implantation. Gadallah et al. [14] showed that peritoneoscopically placed catheters had significantly better survival (77.5% at 12 months, 63% at 24 months and 51.3% at 36 months) than those placed by minilaparotomy (62.5% at 24 months, 41.5% at 24 months and 36% at 36 months). Local anesthesia has been used in this study. However, if wider laparoscopic trocars are used it is necessary to suture the ports to prevent early leakage. Wright et al. [15] also published a randomized controlled study comparing surgical and laparoscopic techniques: the latter presented a similar rate of complications with the disadvantage of being more time-consuming. But in this study general anesthesia and a 10-mm port were used. Efficacy is probably mainly dependent on the experience of the operator and on methodological skills, therefore conflicting experiences may be reported [16–18]. Laparoscopy has the advantage of reducing the incidence of catheter flow dysfunction and permit simultaneous identification and correction of other problems such as hernias, adhesions or even cholecystectomy [19–21]. Safe immediate peritoneal dialysis induction is reported. The procedure can be performed safely under local anesthesia and on an ambulatory basis [22].

On the other hand, laparoscopic catheter replacement or revision is the preferable and cost-effective method for dysfunctional access [21, 23, 24]. In order to elect a specific method of catheter insertion, advantages and disadvantages must be considered (table 2).

Moncrief-Popovich Technique

Moncrief et al. [25] described a new peritoneal access technique in 1993 in which the external segment of the catheter is left in a subcutaneous tunnel for an extended period of time until exteriorization and peritoneal dialysis are initiated. The Moncrief catheter itself was not popular but the technique described has gained acceptance [26–28]. Common Tenckhoff or swan-neck catheters may be left buried until dialysis is needed. This procedure would theoretically allow healing and tissue ingrowth into the Dacron cuff in a sterile environment, therefore minimizing the risk of early bacterial colonization and exit site/tunnel infection, and presumably also eliminating the risk of peritonitis via the periluminal route.

Park et al. [27] compared prospectively double-cuffed swan-neck catheters implanted either with the conventional or Moncrief technique showing a significant reduction of peritonitis and exit site infections with the new technique. Although catheter survival did not differ between the two groups, these data suggest that the periluminal route of bacterial spread may be far more important than the intraluminal route already satisfactorily diminished with flush before fill connection.

A recent prospective randomized study by Danielsson et al. [29] was unable to confirm such advantages, with a similar rate of infectious complications. Besides, a higher exit site infection rate occurred with buried catheters possibly because, after exteriorization, a fresh wound is more vulnerable to pulling

Table 2. Advantages and disadvantages of implantation methods

Method	Blind	Surgical	Peritoneoscopic

Advantages	Inexpensive
	Bedside implantation
	Easily performed by
	  a nephrologist
		Dissection under
		  direct visual control
		Reduced risk of bowel
		  or vessel perforation
		Correct placement of
		  deep cuff within the
		  abdominal
		  musculature
			Wide visualization of
			  intraperitoneal cavity
			Lower rate of leak
			Immediate PD
			Role for simultaneous
			  correction of hernias or
			  adhesions (with wider
			  laparoscopic trocars)
			Outpatient procedure

Disadvantages	Need for prefilling
	  the abdomen
	Higher rate of leak
	  with trocar
	More frequent outflow
	  obstruction due to
	  misplacement
	Risk of bowel
	  perforation
	Difficult to perform
	  in uncooperative
	  patients
		Higher cost
		Need of an operating
		  room
		Some use general
		  anesthesia
		Larger incision than
		  blind Seldinger
		  technique
			Expensive
			Need to use a 2-mm
			  Y-TEC peritoneoscop
			If wider laparoscopic
			  trocars used, immediate
			  PD can be performed
			  only if side ports sutured
			Wider trocars do not
			  assure deep placement
			  of deep cuff in the
			  musculature
			Need for training in
			  laparoscopic procedures

PD = Peritoneal dialysis.

forces while nonburied catheters start peritoneal dialysis after a break-in and with a well-healed exit site. However, logistic advantages and patient comfort are clinically relevant and this new technique, therefore, is being increasingly accepted as a simple, safe, and cost-effective procedure for quality care of peritoneal dialysis patients [30].

Certain designs of catheters may influence the method of implantation. For example, Toronto Western and Missouri catheters are usually placed in a paramedian site and must be implanted surgically. Tenckhoff, swan-neck and T-fluted catheters may be implanted either by blind insertion, surgically or peritoneoscopically.

The implantation technique of presternal peritoneal dialysis catheters is more challenging with an added subcutaneous extension and tunneling of the catheter under the skin towards the upper chest but it can also be inserted laparoscopically as recently reported [31].

Conclusion

To optimize the peritoneal dialysis technique major efforts have been made with new catheter designs and connecting devices. But the operative technique is probably a stronger determinant of successful catheter function.

A center effect is a remarkable confounding factor when analyzing different implantation protocols. Blind percutaneous catheter placement in some centers [12] has a similar catheter survival when compared to surgical procedures but it implies a higher risk of bowel perforation. Minilaparotomy is a safer method and if performed with experience and skill has a low rate of leaks and infectious complications. It should be performed under local anesthesia as an out-patient procedure, unless the patient is a candidate for a simultaneous correction of adhesions or hernias or unable to cooperate with local anesthesia. Peritoneoscopy using a 2-mm Y-TEC assures excellent results in experienced hands, but it is not consistently superior to minilaparotomy. Selected patients with suspected adhesions might preferably be managed with peritoneoscopic catheter implantation. Laparoscopy, however, has a definite advantage if a simultaneous correction of intra-abdominal complications is needed or in case of the replacement of dysfunctional catheters.

Whichever method is used, the success of catheter management mainly depends on the commitment and skill of the operator and team care (surgeon, nephrologist, peritoneal dialysis nurse) [2, 11]. Monitoring and control of the complication rate are mandatory in order to optimize peritoneal catheter implantation.

References

1 Ash SR: Peritoneal access devices and placement techniques; in Nissenson AR, Fine RN (eds): Dialysis Therapy, ed 2. St Louis, Mosby-Year Book, 1993.
2 Rodrigues A, Verger C: Peritoneal access; in Ronco C, Dell'Aquila R, Rodighiero MP (eds): Peritoneal Dialysis Today. Contrib Nephrol. Basel, Karger, 2003, vol 140, pp 195–201.
3 Sardegna KM, Beck AM, Strife CF: Evaluation of perioperative antibiotics at the time of dialysis catheter placement. Pediatr Nephrol 1998;12:149–152.
4 Pecoits-Filho RF, Twardowski ZJ, Khanna R, et al: The effect of antibiotic prophylaxis on the healing of exit sites of peritoneal dialysis catheters in rats. Perit Dial Int 1998;18:60–63.
5 Gadallah MF, Ramdeen G, Mignone J, Patel D, Mitchell L, Tatro S: Role of preoperative antibiotic prophylaxis in preventing post-operative peritonitis in newly placed peritoneal dialysis catheters. Am J Kidney Dis 2000;36:1014–1019.
6 Ejlersen E, Steven K, Lokkegaard H: Paramedian versus midline incision for the insertion of permanent peritoneal dialysis catheters. A randomised clinical trial. Scand J Urol Nephrol 1990;24/2: 151–154.
7 Ash SR: Bedside peritoneoscopic peritoneal catheter placement of Tenckhoff and newer peritoneal catheters. Adv Perit Dial 1998;14:75–79.
8 Piraino B: Peritoneal dialysis access/placement/connectors; in Drukker W, Parsons FM, Maher JF (eds): Replacement of Renal Function by Dialysis, ed 4. Dordrecht, Kluwer Academic, 1996.
9 Official Report from the International Society for Peritoneal Dialysis: Peritoneal catheters and exit site practices toward optimum peritoneal access: 1998 update. Perit Dial Int 1998;18:11–33.

10   Vas SR, Daugirdas JT: Peritoneal access devices; in Daugirdas JT, Blake PG, Ing TS (eds): Handbook of Dialysis, ed 3. Philadelphia, Lippincott Williams & Wilkins, 2001, pp 309–332.

11   Harvey EA: Peritoneal access in children. Perit Dial Int 2001;21(suppl 3):S218–S222.

12   Özener C, Bihorac A, Akoglu E: Technical survival of CAPD catheters: Comparison between percutaneous and conventional surgical placement techniques. Nephrol Dial Transplant 2001;16: 1893–1899.

13   Ash SR, Handt AE, Bloch R: Peritoneoscopic placement of the Tenckhoff catheter: Further clinical experience. Perit Dial Bull 1993;3:8.

14   Gadallah MF, Pervez A, el-Shahawy MA, Sorrels D, et al: Peritoneoscopic versus surgical placement of peritoneal dialysis catheters: A prospective randomised study on outcome. Am J Kidney Dis 1999;33:118–122.

15   Wright MJ, Beleed K, Johnson BF, et al: Randomised prospective comparison of laparoscopic and operative peritoneal dialysis catheter insertion. Perit Dial Int 1999;19:372–375.

16   Tsimoyanis EC, Siakas P, Glantzounis G, et al: Laparoscopic placement of the Tenckhoff catheters for peritoneal dialysis. Surg Laparosc Endosc Percutan Tech 2000;10:218–221.

17   Eklund B, Groop PH, Halme L, et al: Peritoneal dialysis access: A comparison of peritoneoscopic and surgical insertion techniques. Scand J Urol Nephrol 1998;32:557–573.

18   Daschner M, Gfrorer S, Zachariou Z, Mehls O, Schaefer F: Laparoscopic Tenckhoff catheter implantation in children. Perit Dial Int 2002;22/1:22–26.

19   Crabtree JH, Fishman A: Videolaparoscopic implantation of long-term peritoneal dialysis catheters. Surg Endosc 1999;13/2:186–190.

20   Cabtree JH, Fishman A, Huen IT: Videolaparoscopic peritoneal dialysis catheter implantation and rescue procedures under local anesthesia with nitrous oxide pneumoperitoneum. Adv Perit Dial 1998;14:83–86.

21   Giannattasio M, La Rosa R, Balestrazzi A: How can videolaparoscopy be used in a peritoneal dialysis programme? Nephrol Dial Transplant 1999;14:409–411.

22   Crabtree JH, Fishman A: A laparoscopic approach under local anesthesia for peritoneal dialysis access. Perit Dial Int 2000;20:757–765.

23   Yilmazlar T, Yavuz M, Ceylan H: Laparoscopic management of malfunctioning peritoneal dialysis catheters. Surg Endosc 2001;15:820–822.

24   Crabtree JH, Kaiser KE, Huen IT, Fishman A: Cost-effectiveness of peritoneal dialysis catheter implantation by laparoscopy versus by open dissection. Adv Perit Dial 2001;17:88–92.

25   Moncrief JW, Popovich RP, Broadrick LJ, He ZZ, Simmons EE, Tate RA: The Moncrief-Popovich catheter. A new peritoneal access technique for patients on peritoneal dialysis. ASAIO J. 1993;39:62–65.

26   Caruso DM, Gray DL, Kohr JM, et al: Reduction of infectious complications and costs using temporary subcutaneous implantation of PD catheters. Adv Perit Dial 1997;13:183–189.

27   Park MS, Yim AS, Chung SH, et al: Effect of prolonged subcutaneous implantation of peritoneal catheter on peritonitis rate during CAPD: A prospective randomised study. Blood Purif 1998;16: 171–178.

28   Dasgupta MK, Fox S, Card J, Maitland C, Perry D: Catheter survival is improved by the use of Moncrief-Popovich catheters. J Am Soc Nephrol 1998;9:190A.

29   Danielsson A, Blohme L, Tranaeus A, et al: A prospective randomised study of the effect of a subcutaneously 'buried' peritoneal dialysis catheter technique versus standard technique on the incidence of peritonitis and exit-site infection. Perit Dial Int 2002;22/2:211–219.

30   Dasgupta MK: Moncrief-Popovich catheter and implantation technique: The AV fistula of peritoneal dialysis. Adv Ren Replace Ther 2002;9/2:116–124.

31   Crabtree JH, Fishman A: Laparoscopic implantation of swan neck presternal peritoneal dialysis catheters. J Laparoendosc Adv Surg Tech A 2003;13:131–137.

Anabela Rodrigues,
Department of Nephrology, Hospital Geral Santo Antonio,
Largo Abel Salazar, PT–4100 Porto (Portugal)
Tel. +351 22 2074881, Fax +351 22 20774880, E-Mail ar.cbs@mail.telepac.pt

Ronco C, Levin NW (eds): Hemodialysis Vascular Access and Peritoneal Dialysis Access.
Contrib Nephrol. Basel, Karger, 2004, vol 142, pp 410–421

....
Maintenance of Functioning PD Access and Management of Complications

Christian Verger

Service de Dialyse, Hôpital R. Dubos, Pontoise, France

A perfectly functioning peritoneal catheter is essential both for the adequacy of dialysis and for the accuracy of peritoneal tests and clearance assessment. The maintenance of a functional catheter includes adequate placement, normal inflow and outflow rates, preservation of its integrity, and absence of infection. We will not discuss the different types of catheters and the different techniques of insertion in this chapter; this has been done in previous or following chapters.

The maintenance of a functioning access, however, starts in the operating room. Catheter patency should always be assured before the patient leaves the operating room by infusing several small volumes of dialysate or by instilling and aspirating saline solution [1].

Break-In Period after Catheter Implantation

For many years it has been stated that during the days following catheter placement, daily small-volume lavages should be performed to avoid catheter obstruction. There is no prospective randomized study demonstrating that this may be useful. However, it is of particular interest to point out that, by definition, no postoperative lavage is performed when a catheter is implanted using the Moncrief technique [2]. In this case the external part of the catheter is left unused under the skin and may be exteriorized sometimes more than 2 years later without being obstructed. We performed these lavages for several years with dialysate; due to a shortage of nursing staff during the weekend, the lavage was usually interrupted for 2 days and we often observed a displacement of the catheter on the next Monday. Displacement was usually due to catheter wrapping by epiploic fringes or omentum. We then postulated that the dialysate might be irritating, especially during the postoperative period inducing an inflammatory response and tissue proliferation of the omentum which tended to colonize some of the lateral holes of the intraperitoneal section of the catheter. In addition to the partial obstruction of the catheter and alteration of the flow rate, this often provokes displacements due to movements of the omentum. We then changed our technique: in the operating room the patency of the catheter was checked by the introduction of 60 ml of saline solution instead of dialysate, then pure heparin was introduced into the lumen and the catheter was closed. No lavage was performed before 10–15 days and we did not observe obstructions or displacements any more. Other groups have had the same experience and practice and have left the catheter undisturbed under the dressing for several days before using it [1]. The usefulness of heparin may be argued as follows: it is very hypothetical that it has a real effect, without substrate and during a long period of time, in preventing catheter clotting and some teams do not use it. But basically there is now some consensus that rinsing the catheter with saline instead of dialysate during its placement is less irritating and postoperative lavage does not have any advantage, but might theoretically increase the risk of infection due to manipulations without flushing before the fill procedure.

In summary, it seems that better chances to have a functional catheter are obtained by using saline solution in the operating room and by keeping the catheter unused for at least 10 days. It may be kept functional without any postoperative lavage even for several weeks or months as proven by the practice with the Moncrief technique.

Basic Rules for Preserving the Catheter Integrity

Although a catheter may be kept for many years (normally a silicone catheter can be maintained for many years), the actuarial survival of a catheter should be around 90–95% at 2 years [3, 4]. In the French Language PD Registry (RDPLF) catheter survival is 81% at 2 years and 74% at 5 years in a recent retrospective analysis of 1,146 catheters implanted in 31 different centers (fig. 1). Such a result may be obtained only by taking care and applying some basic rules:

- If for some reason the catheter needs to be clamped, to change the adapter or the extension line for example, one must take care of using a nontraumatic clamp and putting a compress between the clamp and the catheter to protect it.

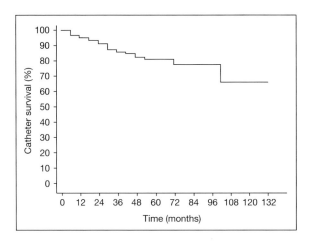

Fig. 1. Catheter survival in the RDPLF: 1,146 catheters from 31 different centers have been included since 1998 [24; full text available on http://www.rdplf.org/bdpsom/somfrdec02.html].

- Disinfectant such as povidone-iodine may interfere with the catheter; ether must never be used as the silicone is soluble in it. Alcohol and mupirocin ointment can damage a polyurethane catheter such as the Cruz catheter [5].
- The patient must be trained to keep the external part of the catheter wound regularly under the dressing to avoid any kinking.
- Prevent exit site infection: in the RDPLF quoted above, 74% of catheter loss were due to infection. Prevention and treatment of tunnel and exit site infection are discussed in another chapter.

Catheter Obstruction

Once the catheter has been placed, filling with two liters should not take more than 10 min, drainage not more than 15 min. Two different types of slowing of the dialysate flow may be observed: two-way obstructions and one-way obstructions.

In case of catheter obstruction the first absolute rule is never try to aspirate liquid out of the catheter with a syringe: most of the time this would just result in aspirating adjoining tissue digitations inside the lumen of the catheter and definitely obstruct it. The dialysate should drain spontaneously or, when a

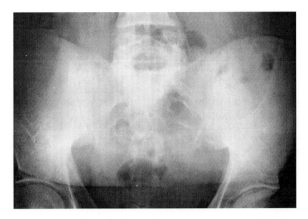

Fig. 2. Displacement of the tip of a swan neck catheter towards the left hypochondria.

syringe is attached to the catheter, just a very gentle aspiration can be performed and immediately stopped if any resistance is felt.

The second rule is to perform an abdominal x-ray to visualize the catheter position to see whether it is displaced upward in direction of the left or right hypochondria (fig. 2).

Two-way obstruction: Inflow as well as outflow are very slow. This is usually due to partial obstruction of the catheter by fibrin or tissue ingrowth inside the lateral holes. If fibrin clotting is responsible for the obstruction, it may often be fixed by introducing 10–20 ml of dialysate or saline solution several times into the catheter at high pressure. In practice, use a 20-ml syringe filled with 20 ml of solution, adapt it to the catheter and firmly hold both catheter and syringe in the same hand, use the other hand to press the piston of the syringe as vigorously as possible; there is absolutely no risk in doing that. The aim is to detach the fibrin from the lumen and the lateral holes of the catheter. After several fast and violent flushes, try to drain or aspirate very carefully as described at the beginning of this paragraph; once again, never aspirate under high pressure, otherwise the catheter would definitely be lost. If this mechanical maneuver does not work, a fibrinolytic agent may be used. Urokinase as well as streptokinase have been proposed, but urokinase is not available in all countries; 5,000 units are introduced into the peritoneal cavity and left for 2 h, then the dialysate is drained. However, we must admit that in our clinical experience this treatment has very seldom been effective. In children it has been demonstrated that it was effective when catheter obstruction was related to fibrin production during peritonitis, but less so when clotting was independent of peritonitis [6]. In addition, some cases of candida peritonitis have been described following the use of urokinase. The explanation is not clear, but it is likely that in patients who have an asymptomatic colonization of the intraluminal part of the catheter by candida imbedded in glycocalyx and fibrin coating, the use of fibrinolytic agents may reveal their presence. An association with urokinase followed by an intraperitoneal loading dose of an antifungal agent might be evaluated or recommended. Alteplase which is recombinant tissue-type plasminogen activator or tPA, a recombinant protease specific for fibrin, has been utilized in clotted peritoneal dialysis (PD) catheters, with some anecdotal success [7]. The dose is between 1 and 2 mg, depending on the volume of the catheter lumen and transfer set.

One-way obstruction: The dialysate is rapidly introduced into the peritoneal cavity, but no drainage or very slow drainage is observed. Most of the time this is the sign of a catheter displacement which is confirmed by abdominal x-ray. The dialysate is easily introduced because there is no catheter obstruction, but as its intraperitoneal tip is not in the declining position, the dialysate cannot be drained. Sometimes by asking the patients to adopt different positions (upright, supine, lateral, declining, sitting) it can be attached better to permit a normal outflow. Another possibility may be an obstruction of lateral holes of the catheter so that only the distal hole is permeable; during the drainage phase, due to the slight depression, it may come into contact with the parietal wall or an intestinal loop. The techniques described previously associated with vigorous pressures and mobilization of the abdomen may be attempted by hand. When the catheter is displaced, the use of a laxative such as sorbitol or lactulose [8] has been recommended with varying success. Another approach may be, under radioscopy, to introduce a semirigid metallic leader into the lumen of the catheter and to try to mobilize the catheter [9]. However, this is possible only with straight catheters, not with swan neck ones. In addition, even with a high rate of immediate success, there is often recurrent displacement.

As most of the above procedures may be the source of contamination, we would recommend to systematically perform a dialysate culture and then add an antibiotic, such as cefazolin, into the peritoneum. If there is an associated exit site infection, use the same antibiotic active on the organism present at the exit site.

Whatever the type of obstruction, if all the above procedures fail the catheter must be surgically replaced or unblocked. If possible, keeping the same catheter may be useful if there is no tunnel or exit site infection, as the catheter cuffs are already colonized by conjunctive tissue, encouraging rapid postoperative healing and having the possibility to resume PD within the next 3 days. Unblocking or replacement under celioscopy may be very convenient and effective compared to conventional surgery [10].

Finally, we would like to add that occasionally a catheter is displaced but works perfectly; obviously, in this case, there is no need to apply the above procedures.

Catheter Rupture

Whatever precautions are taken, catheters are occasionally spontaneously or accidentally cut; if the rupture is close to the adaptor, sectioning the damaged segment of the catheter and inserting another adaptor is simple. However, sometimes the rest of the catheter may be too short as the rupture is close to the exit site. In this case there is a kit (Peri-Patch Repair Kit, Quinton Instrument, Bothwell, Wash., USA) which makes it possible to perform a splicing procedure on the catheter and to reestablish its normal length [11]. The procedure is described in detail in the kit. To summarize, after sectioning the damaged part of the catheter a catheter extension with a double-barbed Teflon connector is attached to the indwelling catheter (fig. 3a) and a mold is wrapped around the barbed connector (fig. 3b). Then a tube of silicone glue is attached to the mold and the glue is pressed out (fig. 3c). The mold is left for 72 h, then it is removed (fig. 3d). Prophylactic antibiotics are recommended to avoid contamination.

Removal of the Catheter

In addition to mechanical causes described above, the removal of the catheter may be indicated for reasons of infection such as yeast colonization, *Pseudomonas aeruginosa* infection, or recurrent peritonitis. These different causes are described in another chapter.

Prevention of Transcutaneous Trauma during Abdominal Medication Injection

It is evident for the nephrologist that no medication should be injected into the abdominal wall of PD patients. However, these patients may sometimes be hospitalized in other units, not trained for PD. The staff of these units should be advised of the risk of injecting medications through the abdominal wall around the catheter as it could be accidentally perforated. The patient should also be taught that he should not have substances such as heparin or insulin injected subcutaneously into the abdominal wall by untrained nurses. Besides the risk of catheter trauma, abdominal subcutaneous heparin seems to have a high risk of inducing parietal hematoma. We recently had 2 patients (pers. data) who

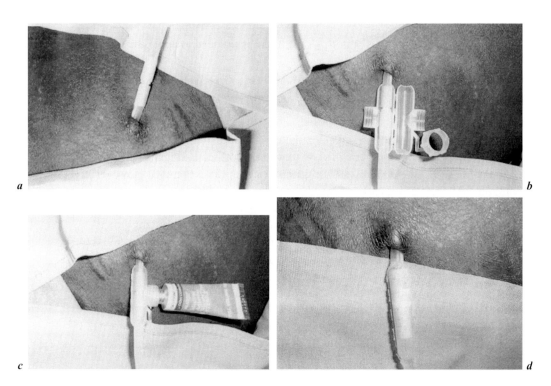

Fig. 3. *a* The extension tube with the double-barbed Teflon adaptor is connected to the indwelling catheter. *b* The mold is wrapped around the extension, the Teflon and the catheter, and then closed. *c* Glue is introduced into the mold to envelope the entire connection. *d* 72 h later, the mold is removed, the silicone glue fixes the indwelling catheter and its new extension completely.

subcutaneously received heparin into the abdominal wall in a cardiology department and who developed severe hematoma which needed surgery in one case. The presence of the catheter as well as the variations of peritoneal volume with rapid tension on the abdominal muscle facilitated microtraumatisms that may be aggravated by a high local concentration of anticoagulant. The management in such a case, besides obviously stopping abdominal perforations, is to stop PD for several weeks in order to minimize the parietal variation of the tension, until the hematoma is reabsorbed.

Catheter Cuff Extrusion

Although conflicting reports discuss the advantages and disadvantages of using double cuff or single cuff catheters, most are double cuff nowadays.

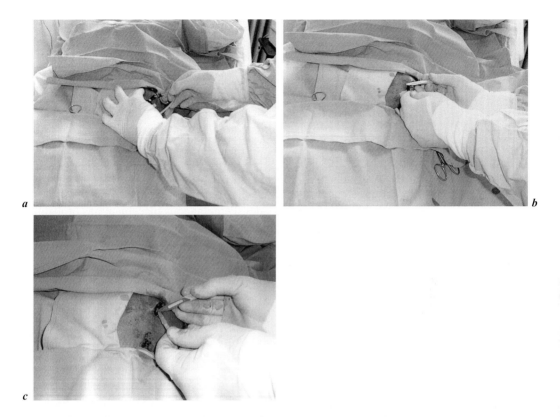

Fig. 4. a Extrusion of the subcutaneous cuff. *b* Careful shaving of the cuff with a scalpel. *c* End of shaving of the cuff.

It seems in addition that double cuff catheters have less infections and a longer survival [12]. To prevent spontaneous extrusion of the external cuff, it should be left 2 cm deep from the exit site at the time of placement. However, sometimes due to infection or to an excessively superficial placement, the subcutaneous cuff may erode the skin through the outer abdominal wall [13, 14]. Tissue in contact with the extruding cuff becomes ischemic and is prone to become infected or to maintain a quiescent local infection. It is therefore advisable to extrude the cuff completely under sterile conditions and local anesthesia. Usually at an advanced state, just gently pulling the catheter is enough to extrude the superficial eroding cuff, but most of the time it is better to remove the contaminated or necrotic tissue around the exit site. After extrusion, the Dacron must be shaved carefully with as scalpel avoiding any traumatism of the catheter underneath (fig. 4a–c). Our protocol for the following days is to inject a local antibiotic along the catheter tunnel twice a day for 3 days, then once a day for 5 days. Rapid healing is usually observed; if not and if some signs of the infection are still present, the catheter must be replaced.

Pericatheter Leakage

Pericatheter leakage usually occurs early after catheter placement at the level of the exit site. The technique of the placement plays a role and it seems that peritoneoscopically placed catheters have a lower incidence of leakage [15, 16] than surgically implanted ones. Percutaneous placement has probably the highest incidence, and a report on the technique of initial subcutaneous embedding of peritoneal catheters demonstrated no leakage at all. Intraperitoneal hyperpressure may play a role too. The nutritional status of the patient is probably important as well as the previous duration and amount of cortisone: this is why, in our practice, we recommend to wait for up to 4 or 6 weeks before starting PD in a patient who starts after a renal transplantation failure.

Clinically the diagnosis is made on the basis of dialysate at the exit site; sometimes it appears slightly rose colored due to having been mixed with some residual subcutaneous blood. It must, therefore, be differentiated from serosanguineous fluid extruding from the subcutaneous tissue. Dextrostick testing will demonstrate a very high level of glucose in case of dialysate leakage compared to serosanguineous fluid from the subcutaneous tissue. The leakage may be demonstrated by CT scanning after intraperitoneal addition of contrast material [17]. However, in case of minimal leakage the difference in contrast may be difficult to appreciate and peritoneal scintigraphy may be indicated as it is more sensitive. It has also been suggested that magnetic resonance imaging using dialysate as the contrast material may be useful [18].

The management of this leakage consists primarily of decreasing intraperitoneal pressure by reducing the volume of each exchange and switching the patient to nocturnal automatic PD with a empty peritoneum during the day. However, a slight invisible leakage may persist and induce an inflammatory response and fibrosis around the preperitoneal cuff, therefore preventing healing around the preperitoneal cuff and tissue at the point of penetration of the catheter in the peritoneum. A complete interruption of PD and a temporary switch to hemodialysis [19] for 1 or 2 weeks is probably more efficient. If this conservative management does not work, surgical repair of the tissue around the preperitoneal cuff is the best solution. Usually the catheter does not have to be completely replaced.

Peritoneal Catheter Drainage Time

We finish the chapter with one of the most useful evaluation of catheter function: the peritoneal cavity drainage time and the breakpoint determination [20–23]. During drainage two phases are observed: during the first initial phase the outflow rate is around 150–250 ml/min with a conventional catheter with an internal diameter of 2.7 mm and may be up to 300 ml/min, and even more with those with a diameter of 3 mm or more. Usually 80% of the peritoneal cavity is drained during this initial phase. The second phase has a rate of about 500 ml/min and usually drains less than 20% of the peritoneal cavity or even only a few milliliters The moment at which the outflow rate drops at the end of the first phase is called the breakpoint (or turning point in some publications).

The assessment of this breakpoint is essential with automated PD, particularly during tidal PD. As the residual volume is usually low and the drainage rate very slow after the breakpoint, the time on dialysis during the second phase is usually ineffective. So, on automated PD and/or tidal PD, the different times (infusion, dwell, drainage) may be optimized according to this breakpoint. In addition this makes it possible to reduce the number of drainage alarms during the night. On CAPD, the determination of the drainage breakpoint is also very important for the patient's quality of life. Normally, a bag exchange should not take more than 30 min including drainage and infusion. It is not uncommon to get complaints from patients on CAPD spending sometimes up to 45 min on drainage, 4 times a day. In these patients the measurement of the breakpoint demonstrates that usually the volume drained after 15 min is negligible and could be bypassed without risk, allowing a more rapid bag exchange procedure and therefore a better quality of life.

Various methods have been described to determine the dialysate outflow rate and the breakpoint. This breakpoint is variable with the type of catheter, the position, sitting or supine and gravity. Usually, in the supine position, the measurement is done with a bed 60 cm above the level of the floor. Basically, a fixed volume is infused during the previous exchange and during the test in order to make the different measurements comparable from one patient to another. Then the time of the initiation of drainage is carefully recorded in hours, minutes and seconds. During the drainage the outflow rate is monitored either by continuous weighing of the drainage or by continuous measurement of its volume. The duration of drainage during the test is 30 min. This may be done manually or automatically. The change in the drainage rate is recorded (this is the breakpoint) and the volume drained before the breakpoint is noted. It will then permit to calculate, at the end of the test, the percentage of the total volume drained before the breakpoint.

On the basis of the results obtained, the prescription of automated PD as well as CAPD may be adapted. In addition any abnormality should initiate further investigations such as abdominal x-ray to determine abnormalities of the catheter position, kinking or obstruction as described at the beginning of this chapter.

References

1   Gokal R, Alexander S, Ash S, et al: Peritoneal catheters and exit-site practices toward optimum peritoneal access: 1998 update. Perit Dial Int 1998;18:11.
2   Moncrief JW, Popovich RP, Seare W, et al: Peritoneal dialysis access technology: The Austin Diagnostic Clinic experience. Perit Dial Int 1996;16(suppl 1):S327.
3   Eklund BH, Honkanen EO, Kala AR, Kyllonen LE: Peritoneal dialysis access: Prospective comparison of the swan neck and Tenckhoff catheters. Perit Dial Int 1995;15:353–356.
4   Eklund BH, Honkanen EO, Kyllonen LE, Salmela KT, Kala AR: Peritoneal dialysis access: Prospective randomised comparison of single-cuff and double-cuff straight Tenckhoff catheters. Nephrol Dial Transplant 1997;12:2664–2666.
5   Riu S, Ruiz C, Martinez-Vea A, Peralta C, Oliver J: Spontaneous rupture of polyurethane peritoneal catheter. A possible deleterious effect of mupirocin ointment. Nephrol Dial Transplant 1998;13:1870–1871.
6   Stadermann MB, Rusthoven E, van de Kar NC, Hendriksen A, Monnens LA, Schroder CH: Local fibrinolytic therapy with urokinase for peritoneal dialysis catheter obstruction in children. Perit Dial Int 2002;22/1:84–86.
7   Sahani MM, Mukhtar KN, Boorgu R, et al: Tissue plasminogen activator can effectively declot peritoneal dialysis catheters. Am J Kidney Dis 2000;36:675.
8   Leehey DJ, Daugirdas JT: Complications other than peritonitis; in Daugirdas JT, Ing TS (eds): Handbook of Dialysis. Boston, Little, Brown, 1994, p 363.
9   Moss JS, Minda SA, Newman GE, Dunnick NR, Vernon WB, Schwab SJ: Malpositioned peritoneal dialysis catheters: A critical reappraisal of correction by stiff-wire manipulation. Am J Kidney Dis 1990;15:305–308.
10 Kimmelstiel FM, Miller RE, Molinelli BM, Lorch JA: Laparoscopic management of peritoneal dialysis catheters. Surg Gynecol Obstet 1993;176:565–570.
11 Usha K, Ponferrada L, Prowant BF, Twardowski ZJ: Repair of chronic peritoneal dialysis catheter. Perit Dial Int 1998;22:419–423.
12 Warady BA, Sullivan EK, Alexander SR: Lessons from the peritoneal dialysis patient database: A report of the North American Pediatric Renal Transplant Cooperative Study. Kidney Int Suppl 1996;53:S68–S71.
13 Robison RJ, Leapman SB, Wetherington GM, Hamburger RJ, Fineberg NS, Filo RS: Surgical considerations of continuous ambulatory peritoneal dialysis. Surgery 1984;96:723–730.
14 Swartz R, Messana J, Rocher L, Reynolds J, Starmann B, Lees P: The curled catheter: Dependable device for percutaneous peritoneal access. Perit Dial Int 1990;10/3:231–235.
15 Gadallah MF, Pervez A, el-Shahawy MA, Sorrells D, Zibari G, McDonald J, Work J: Peritoneoscopic versus surgical placement of peritoneal dialysis catheters: A prospective randomized study on outcome. Am J Kidney Dis 1999;33/1:118–122.
16 Prischl FC, Wallner M, Kalchmair H, Povacz F, Kramar R: Initial subcutaneous embedding of the peritoneal dialysis catheter – A critical appraisal of this new implantation technique. Nephrol Dial Transplant 1997;12:1661–1667.
17 Leblanc M, Ouimet D, Pichette V: Dialysate leaks in peritoneal dialysis. Semin Dial 2001;14/1: 50–54.
18 Prischl FC, Muhr T, Seiringer EM, Funk S, Kronabethleitner G, Wallner M, Artmann W, Kramar R: Magnetic resonance imaging of the peritoneal cavity among peritoneal dialysis patients, using the dialysate as 'contrast medium'. J Am Soc Nephrol 2002;13/1:197–203.

19 Ash SR, Daugirdas JT: Peritoneal dialysis access; in Daugirdas JT, Ing TS (eds): Handbook of Dialysis. Boston, Little, Brown, 1994, p 274.
20 Durand P-Y: APD schedules and clinical results; in Ronco C, Dell'Aquila R, Rodighiero MP (eds): Peritoneal Dialysis Today. Contrib Nephrol. Basel, Karger, 2003, vol 140, pp 272–277.
21 Brandes JC, Packard WJ, Watters SK, et al: Optimization of dialysate flow and mass transfer during automated peritoneal dialysis. Am J Kidney Dis 1995;25:603–610.
22 Amici G, Thomaseth K: Role of drain and fill profile in automated peritoneal dialysis; in Ronco C, Amici G, Feriani MP, Virga G (eds): Automated Peritoneal Dialysis. Contrib Nephrol. Basel, Karger, 1999, vol 129, pp 44–53.
23 Neri L, Viglino G, Cappelletti A, Gandolfo C: Evaluation of drainage times and alarms with various automated peritoneal dialysis modalities. Adv Perit Dial 2001;17:72–74.
24 Vernier I, Duman M, Fabre E: Le suivi des cathéters de dialyse péritonéale. Bull Dial Perit 2002; 12/1:41–47.

Dr. Christian Verger
Service de Dialyse
Hôpital R. Dubos
6, avenue de l'Ile de France
F- 95301 Pontoise (France)
Tel. +33 1 30 75 42 58, Fax +33 1 30 32 99 38,
E-Mail christian.verger@ch-pontoise.fr

Ronco C, Levin NW (eds): Hemodialysis Vascular Access and Peritoneal Dialysis Access.
Contrib Nephrol. Basel, Karger, 2004, vol 142, pp 422–434

....

Catheter Exit Site Care in the Long Term

Zbylut J. Twardowski

University of Missouri, Columbia, Mo., USA

Introduction

Catheter exit site and tunnel infections are frequent in CAPD patients and lead to morbidity, prolonged treatment, recurrent peritonitis, and catheter failure. With the reduced incidence of peritonitis due to touch contamination, exit site and tunnel infections have become the primary infectious complications of peritoneal dialysis. Contrary to peritonitis where the clinical presentation is clearly different from that of normal, there is a spectrum of appearances from uninfected to infected exit sites. This chapter will review prevention, diagnosis, and treatment of catheter-related infections.

Prevention of Exit Site Problems

Prevention of long-term exit site exit infection should start at the time of catheter implantation. Surgery itself and exit site care in the immediate postimplantation period seem to be crucial for long-term results regarding infectious complications and external cuff extrusion. Among factors essential for proper healing is atraumatic surgery, perfect hemostasis, proper location of the external cuff [1], and delayed bacterial colonization of the exit site. The tunnel should not be too tight, to allow free drainage of necrotic tissue and to prevent tissue edema, which decreases local perfusion and O_2 tension, which are vital for the wound healing process [2]. On the other hand, too large an incision prolongs healing by the shear volume of needed repair. In addition, the movement of the catheter in a wide tunnel causes mechanical stress that slows the healing process [3]. Thus, the catheter should be relatively tightly anchored in the tunnel and well immobilized externally, especially during the break-in period. Constricting sutures, which can cause pressure necrosis with skin sloughing, must not be used. Perfect hemostasis during implantation is extremely important because a large hematoma interferes with healing.

Impaired nutrition, diabetes mellitus, uremia, and corticosteroids are all known factors decreasing wound healing by decreasing fibrosis [4]. Therefore, in patients with these risk factors preventive measures are particularly important.

Infection is the major cause of impaired wound healing [5]. It has been well established in the surgical literature that wound infection is the result of major disturbances in the balance between host defenses and bacteria; the number of bacteria is obviously a critical factor in wound infection [5]. Bacterial virulence is also important; *Staphylococcus aureus* or *Pseudomonas aeruginosa* are more likely to induce an inflammatory response than is *Staphylococcus epidermidis*. Maintaining sterility of the exit and sinus in the initial healing period is of utmost importance. An antibiotic should be present in sufficient concentration in blood and tissue fluids before the foreign body is implanted. This may be achieved if the antibiotic is given prior to the surgical procedure.

Our study clearly demonstrated the importance of delayed colonization for optimal healing, reduced exit infection and peritonitis rates, and catheter survival [6]. Positive cultures from either washout or periexit smears 1 week after implantation were associated with early exit infections, higher peritonitis rates, and high probabilities of catheter loss due to exit/tunnel infections [6]. The early-infected exits were more likely to have gram-negative bacteria and *S. aureus* in the first positive culture.

Exit Site Appearance Postimplantation

Unless a large hematoma in the wound is present, all exits look the same a week after implantation [6]. The exit is painless or minimally tender with a light pink color of less than 13 mm in diameter from border to border (including the width of the catheter). Blood clot or serosanguineous drainage is visible in the sinus. No epidermis is visible in the sinus and the sinus lining is white and plain. Signs of good healing include a decrease in color saturation and diameter around the exit, change of drainage to serous, decreased drainage amount, decreased tenderness, and progression of epidermis into the sinus. An increase in color diameter or saturation around the exit, change of drainage to yellow, change of granulation tissue color to mottled, pink or red, change of granulation tissue texture into slightly exuberant or exuberant are signs of poor healing.

Our exit site study [6, 7] revealed four types of healing exits: (1) the fast healing exits had no drainage or minimal moisture deep inside by the third week; epidermis started to enter into the sinus within 2–3 weeks, progressed steadily, and covered at least half the visible sinus tract 4–6 weeks after implantation; (2) in slow healing exits without infection, epidermis started to enter into the sinus after 3 weeks or progressed slowly and did not cover half the visible sinus by 5 weeks; the sinus might have had serous or serosanguineous, but never purulent, drainage persistent up to 4 weeks; (3) healing interrupted by infection initially looked identical to the fast healing exit, but within 6 weeks the epidermis did not progress or regressed, granulation tissue became soft or frankly fleshy; drainage increased and/or became purulent, and (4) in slow healing exits due to early infection, granulation tissue became soft or fleshy and/or drainage became purulent by 2–3 weeks; sinus epidermalization was delayed or progressed slowly, only after infection was appropriately treated.

Early Care

To delay bacterial colonization of the exit site and minimize trauma, the dressing should not be changed frequently [8]. It is generally agreed that postoperative dressing changes should be restricted to specially trained staff [9]. We do weekly dressing changes for the first 2 weeks post-catheter implantation if there is no excessive drainage. Once the exit is inevitably colonized, by week 3 in the majority of cases [6], more frequent dressing changes are indicated, because the major rationale for infrequent dressing changes, delay of exit colonization, no longer exists. Moreover, more frequent cleansing of the exit will decrease the number of bacteria at the exit. Aseptic techniques, including both masking and wearing sterile gloves, should be used for postoperative dressing changes. Nonionic surfactant, such as 20% poloxamer 188 (Shur-Clens®; Calgon Vestal Laboratories, St. Louis, Mo., USA), is used to help gauze removal if it is attached to the scab. If the scab is forcibly removed, the epidermal layer is broken, a new scab has to be made and the epidermalization is prolonged. Care is taken to avoid catheter pulling or twisting. The exit and skin surrounding the catheter are cleansed with nonionic surfactant, patted dry with sterile gauze, covered with several layers of gauze dressings, and secured with air-permeable tape.

The exit and visible sinus should be evaluated for quality of healing at each dressing change throughout the 6-week healing period. If healing does not progress, and if there are signs of deterioration or infection, the exit is probably already colonized [6]. A clinical culture of the exudate should be taken, and an appropriate systemic antibiotic should be given.

We recommend that our patients do not shower or take tub baths post-catheter implantation to avoid colonization with water-borne organisms, and to prevent skin maceration. Once more frequent dressing changes are started (after approximately 2 weeks) the patient may take a shower, but only before the dressing change, otherwise they must take sponge baths and avoid exit wetting.

Protecting the catheter from mechanical stress seems to be extremely important; especially during break-in, catheters should be anchored in such a way that the patient's movements are only minimally transmitted to the exit. The method of catheter immobilization is individualized, depending on exit location.

Extended Prophylactic Antibiotics

Our findings of the detrimental effect of the early exit colonization on the quality of healing and long-term infectious complications led us to postulate that exit infections and peritonitis rates might be decreased by delaying exit colonization using prophylactic antibiotics for at least 2 weeks after implantation [6]. Such an approach has not been evaluated in patients in prospective randomized studies; however, a study in rats showed that intraperitoneal antibiotic prophylaxis for 3 weeks after catheter implantation was an effective way to prevent early colonization of exit sites, providing a better healing quality and a lower incidence of catheter-related infections [10]. Based on these premises, our current approach is to use a systemic antibiotic against gram-positive bacteria (usually cephalothin or trimethoprim-sulfamethoxazole) for 2 weeks after implantation and a local antibiotic (usually mupirocin ointment or cream) for at least 6 weeks.

Morphology of the Healed Catheter Tunnel

A detailed description of healthy and infected peritoneal catheter tunnel morphology has been published elsewhere [11]. In uninfected peritoneal dialysis catheter tunnels, the epithelium covers only the external part of the sinus tract while the deeper part is covered with granulation tissue. The epithelium may reach the cuff located less than 15 mm from the exit. The outer cuff limits spreading of granulation tissue and/or epithelium beyond the cuff. In the deeper part of some sinus tracts, a fibrous sheath replaces the granulation tissue. A dense capsule surrounds the cuff. Giant multinucleated cells and mature collagen fibers surround polyester fibers of the cuff in well-healed catheters. Only islands of mononuclear infiltrates are seen in the cuff.

The intercuff tunnel segment resembles a tendon sheath with a dense fibrous capsule and the surface covered with amorphous, mucinous substance on top of a modified layer of fibroblasts forming pseudosynovium. Silicon rubber per se does not induce giant cell formation.

During the healing period, only the part of the cuff adjacent to the tissue is invaded by fibroblasts and macrophages coalescing into giant cells. Immature collagen fibers are also deposited. The part of the cuff adjacent to the tubing is filled with a clot. Gradually the clot is reabsorbed, giant cells surround polyester fibers and mature collagen fibers become intertwined with polyester fibers. Infection causes formation of granulocytic infiltration, which propagates through the tunnel along the catheter and usually is confined within the fibrous capsule.

Bacterial Colonization of the Sinus

Late colonization, after the healing process is completed, is inevitable and mostly harmless, if the defense mechanisms are intact. Almost all healed catheter sinuses are colonized by bacteria [12]. The number of bacteria entering deeper into the sinus depends on the number and species of bacteria at the exit site, exit direction, as well as sinus tract length; the latter is an important contributing factor in the amplitude of catheter movement in the sinus. Defense mechanisms, after the sinus is healed, are best in undamaged epidermis and granulation tissue; trauma to these structures may tilt the balance toward attacking microorganisms and allow their rapid multiplication.

S. aureus Nasal Carriage

The importance of S. aureus as an etiologic agent of peritoneal catheter exit site infection has been well established [13, 14]. Nasal carriage status of S. aureus is reported to be common in patients undergoing hemodialysis [15] and peritoneal dialysis [16]. A recent multicenter study found an increased incidence of exit site infections in nasal carriers of S. aureus; in 85% of these infections the strain from the nares and the strain causing the infection were similar in phage type and antibiotic profile [17]. In contrast, we found that even though S. aureus was more likely to be detected in nares of patients with exit infections, by antibiotic profile, the strain causing exit infection and the strain cultured from nares were different [6]. Judging from these data, there is an increased probability of exit infection in patients who carry S. aureus in nares, but the strain is usually different.

Whereas our patients usually showed colonization of nares and the exits by different strains, in other series the strains were uniform. Hands are probably the major means of spreading bacteria to distant parts of the integument. Variations in habits, hygiene, exit site care, and/or surgical practices are among the possible explanations why our results differ from those of others. However, because in all studies *S. aureus* nasal carriers are prone to exit infections, the practice of prophylactic antibiotics, either systemically or topically, on the exit is highly recommended [18].

Classification of Exit Site Appearance

The classification of healed exit sites into seven categories evolved from 565 evaluations of 61 healed exit sites in 56 patients [12]. Five basic categories of catheter exit appearances were identified: acute infection, chronic infection, equivocal (low grade) infection, perfect, and good exit. Two special categories were also described: cuff infection with or without exit infection, and exit trauma.

Acute catheter exit site infection. Purulent and/or bloody drainage from the exit site, spontaneous or after pressure on the sinus; and/or swelling; and/or erythema with diameter 13 mm or more from border to border; and regression of epithelium in the sinus. Acute catheter inflammation lasts less than 4 weeks and may be accompanied by pain, exuberant granulation tissue around the exit or in the sinus and the presence of a scab or crust. Exit culture may be negative in patients receiving antibiotics.

Chronic catheter exit site infection. Purulent and/or bloody drainage from the exit site, spontaneous or after pressure on the sinus; and/or exuberant granulation tissue around the exit and/or in the sinus; and regression of epithelium in the sinus. Chronic infection persists for more than 4 weeks and crust or scab is frequently present. Swelling, erythema, and/or pain indicate exacerbation, otherwise are absent. Exit culture may be negative in patients receiving antibiotics.

Equivocally infected catheter exit site. Purulent and/or bloody drainage that cannot be expressed outside the sinus, accompanied by the regression of epithelium, and occurrence of slightly exuberant granulation tissue around the exit and/or in the sinus. Erythema with a diameter less than 13 mm from border to border may be present, but pain, swelling, and external drainage are absent. Exit culture may be negative in patients receiving antibiotics.

Perfect catheter exit. At least 6 months old with its entire visible length of sinus tract covered with the keratinized (mature) epithelium. Exit color is natural or dark and there is no drainage. A small, easily detachable crust may be present in the sinus or around the exit. Positive periexit smear culture, if present, indicates colonization not infection.

Good catheter exit. Exit color is natural, pale pink, purplish or dark and there is no purulent or bloody drainage. Clear or thick exudate may be visible in the sinus. Mature epithelium covers only part of the sinus; the rest is covered by fragile epithelium or plain granulation tissue. Pain, swelling, and erythema are absent. Positive periexit smear culture, if present, indicates colonization not infection.

External cuff infection without exit infection. Intermittent or chronic, purulent, bloody or gooey drainage, spontaneous or after pressure on the cuff and induration of the tissue around the cuff. Exuberant granulation tissue may be seen deep in the sinus; sinus epithelium may be macerated chronically or intermittently. Exit site may look normal on external examination. Ultrasound may show fluid collection around the cuff, but negative ultrasound does not rule out cuff infection. Exit culture may be negative in patients receiving antibiotics.

Traumatized exit. Features of traumatized exit depend on the intensity of trauma and time interval until examination. Common features of trauma are pain, bleeding, scab and deterioration of exit appearance (e.g., perfect exit transforms to good or equivocal or acutely infected).

Long-Term Exit Site Care

Perfect and Good Exits

The results of a prospective study indicate that cleaning with soap and water is the least expensive and tends to prevent infections better than povidone-iodine painting and hydrogen peroxide cleaning [19]. If strong oxidants are used, they should not enter into the sinus, only the surrounding skin should be disinfected with them. After cleansing, the exit has to be patted dry with sterile gauze and well immobilized. Most of our patients use a dressing cover for 6–12 months after implantation. One year after implantation, patients are allowed to omit use of a cover dressing, if desired. We could not find any reason why in some patients an uncovered exit seems to do better, in others worse.

We recommend that our patients use only a shower and avoid submersion in water, particularly in a Jacuzzi, hot tub, or public pool, unless watertight exit protection can be implemented. Prolonged submersion in water containing high concentrations of bacteria frequently leads to severe infection with consequent loss of catheter. Swimming in the ocean and well-sterilized private pools is less dangerous. Exit care must be performed immediately after a shower or water submersion, with particular attention to obtaining a well-dried exit. The surrounding skin is coated with a skin protector and secured with Tegaderm. Patients with the swan-neck presternal catheter may take hot tub baths without exit site submersion. Because of this feature, this catheter was dubbed the 'bath tub' catheter [20].

Acute Exit Site Infection

A culture of exit site exudate or, if there is swelling/erythema without expressible exudate, a smear culture of the skin surrounding the exit should be taken as soon as a clinical diagnosis of an acute exit site infection is made. Systemic antibiotics should be started before culture results are available. Gram-positive organisms are frequently the cause of exit site infections. Accordingly, oral cephalosporin may be selected as the initial antibiotic, but more recently, quinolones have become the initial antibiotic of choice. The antibiotic prescription should be adjusted after the organism is identified and the antibiotic sensitivity results are available. The antibiotic is initially prescribed for a period of 7–10 days, the time required for an uncomplicated acute infection to heal (achieve a good appearance). If there is no improvement after this period, another appropriate antibiotic is substituted or a second synergistic antibiotic is added. Rifampicin is frequently used as a second antibiotic for staphylococcal infections. Antibiotic therapy is continued for 7 days after achieving a healthy appearance of an exit.

Conditions that delay healing or make therapy ineffective are cuff and/or tunnel infection, infection due to a resistant organism or virulent pathogens (such as *S. aureus*, *Pseudomonas* sp., *Candida*), and patient noncompliance.

Exuberant granulation tissue (proud flesh) is cauterized with a silver nitrate stick, a procedure widely used in surgical practice, veterinary and human [21, 22]. No more than one or two applications may be necessary in acute infection. This procedure speeds up the healing process and facilitates epithelialization. Cauterization should be restricted to granulation tissue only and accidental touching of the adjacent epithelium should be avoided. Use of a magnifying glass aids in precise cauterization. This can be done safely by a physician or nurse.

Recommendations for the care of infected exit sites are based on sound surgical practices, and anecdotal experiences. Increasing the frequency of dressing changes to 1 or 2 times a day helps the healing process, especially in those with copious drainage. Nonirritating solution (e.g., nonionic surfactant) is our preferred cleanser to remove drainage and reduce the number of micro-organisms. An infected exit should be covered with a sterile dressing to absorb drainage, protect against trauma, and shield against superinfection.

Topical treatments include application of soaks to the exit 2–4 times daily as well as the application of dry heat [23, 24]. Soaking solutions include normal saline, hypertonic saline, sodium hypochlorite, dilute hydrogen peroxide, povidone-iodine and 70% alcohol. Local application of povidone-iodine ointment, mupirocin, and Neosporin® cream, ointment or ophthalmic solutions have been recommended [9].

In our opinion, strong oxidants and other irritating solutions should not be used. It is our belief that topical antibiotics are of limited value in treating acute or chronic infection with copious drainage because of the inability to achieve high enough local concentrations, but they are recommended after drainage abates [22].

Catheter immobilization is a sound practice. Immobilizing a catheter protects it from accidental trauma. Trauma leads to bleeding, and blood is a good medium for microorganisms to multiply in. Catheter immobilization should be continued during the acute infection stage or implemented (if not already in practice).

Most acute infections respond favorably to therapy [12]. An exit site with an acute infection in association with proud flesh and bleeding requires prolonged antibiotic therapy. Association with a positive nasal culture had no influence on the outcome. Recurrent infections that progress to chronic infection and/or cuff infection are associated with a poor prognosis. Catheter removal is indicated when acute exit site infection leads to tunnel infection and peritonitis.

Chronically Infected Exit Site

The workup leading to the proper diagnosis of a chronically infected exit site is similar to that performed to diagnose acute infection. As outlined for acute infection, an antibiotic is started immediately after diagnosis. Once the culture and antibiotic sensitivity results are available, an appropriate antibiotic is chosen. A combination of synergistic antibiotics is preferred to a single agent to avoid emergence of resistant organisms, since the therapy is given over a prolonged period. In chronic infection, the bacterial flora or the antibiotic sensitivity may change during the course of treatment. Therefore, an unresponsive exit site may have to be cultured repeatedly for timely diagnosis. The response to treatment is usually slow. The features of the chronic infection change very slowly to those of an equivocal exit and then eventually to those of a good exit site.

The antibiotic therapy and local care of the exit site are continued until the desired features of a good exit are achieved. In some cases, exit features change to equivocal and remain as such for a long time. In such cases, the systemic antibiotic may be discontinued and replaced with a topical antibiotic. Chronic infection requires repeated cauterization of exuberant granulation tissue. Typically, weekly cauterization for several weeks is necessary. The cauterization is continued as long as the proud flesh persists. The cauterization will discolor the proud flesh from red to gray. Some cases of chronic infection may require long-term (6 months to several years) suppressive doses of a systemic antibiotic. Typically, these cases show reinfection on discontinuing the systemic antibiotic. It is likely that such cases represent undiagnosed cuff infection.

Local care is similar to that used in treating acute infection. After achieving the features of an equivocal exit, the frequency of local care may be reduced to once a day.

Equivocal Exit

The equivocal exit site is a subclinical form of infection. If left untreated, most equivocal exits will progress to acute infection. Therefore, aggressive management of equivocal exits assumes great importance. Aggressive local care with a topical antibiotic may cure most equivocal exit sites. Exits with external, slightly exuberant granulation tissue, which usually progress to acute infection, require systemic antibiotics.

Cauterization of the slightly exuberant granulation tissue in the sinus may be necessary. An acute infection may acquire equivocal features during the recovery phase. Such an exit site warrants less aggressive therapy compared to one with acute infection; discontinuation of the systemic antibiotic and daily local care is continued in such a situation.

Local therapy with topical antibiotics is the mainstay of treatment for such an equivocal exit site. A topical antibiotic is chosen based on the exit swab culture results. The topical antibiotics that we have successfully used include mupirocin, Neosporin, gentamicin, and tobramycin. This effectiveness is due to the absence of copious drainage from the sinus tract. Free-flowing drainage in both acute and chronic infections washes away the topical antibiotic. Systemic antibiotic may be used in cases unresponsive to topical therapy. Response to therapy is excellent with cure occurring in almost all instances.

External Cuff Infection with or without Exit Infection

Ultrasound examination of the tunnel is a valuable tool in the diagnosis of cuff infection. While positive findings with ultrasound examination help to establish a diagnosis of tunnel infection, a negative examination does not rule out the existence of an infection. Cuff infection responds to therapy slowly, if at all, and a complete cure is unlikely. As mentioned above, ultrasound may show fluid collection around the cuff, but a negative ultrasound result does not rule out cuff infection. Local care has to be given aggressively. Deroofing the sinus tract and cuff shaving have been practiced with some success [25]. Others find these measures ineffective [26]. In our experience, cuff shaving prolonged catheter life for approximately 6–12 months [12]. These temporary measures may be suitable for patients who are expected to stay on therapy for a short period, e.g. patients awaiting transplant; however, cuff infection is a strong indicator for catheter removal in long-term PD patients. Lately, catheter replacement and removal have been done in one procedure if there is no active peritonitis. The preliminary experience of combining the two procedures is promising.

Anecdotal reports suggest that cuff shaving may provide better results in presternal catheters [27, 28]. This may be related to the presence of three cuffs and a long tunnel in the presternal catheter. Shaving of the subcutaneous cuff leaves two cuffs as a double barrier against periluminal bacterial penetration.

Traumatized Exit

Bleeding is a common sequela of trauma. Extravasated blood is a good medium for bacterial growth. Bacteria that have colonized the exit multiply rapidly in the presence of decomposing blood and infect the disrupted tissue. Infection may occur as early as 24–48 h after trauma. The prompt administration of an antibiotic, chosen based on the history of skin colonization, may prevent acute infection. In the absence of the information about previous skin colonies, an antimicrobial agent sensitive to gram-positive organisms, such as a cephalosporin or a quinolone, may be chosen. Therapy may have to be continued for about 7 days after achieving a good appearance. Aggressive treatment is necessary in every instance of trauma reported by the patient. Local care requires gentle cleansing of all blood from the exit site.

Emerging Approach of Long Exit Care

Excellent results observed with mupirocin ointment in healing exits, in the prevention of infections in *S. aureus* nasal carriers, and in the treatment of equivocal exits and recurrent exit site infections inclined us to extend indefinitely the use of mupirocin ointment on the exit with excellent results [29]. Patients report that the epidermis around the exit is less dry and chafed as the catheter 'glides' better over the sinus epidermis. The moisturizing/lubricating action of the ointment base may contribute to the good results of mupirocin and other ointments applied on the exits. However, there is no question that the decrease of bacterial load through the application of antibiotic is mostly responsible for these good results. Because ointment base may damage polyurethane tubing, it is advisable to avoid long-term ointment use with polyurethane or glycol-based catheters. The use of ointments on silicone rubber has not been associated with changes in its physical properties.

A recently published study [30] on the use of Polysporin ointment at the hemodialysis catheter exit for prevention of catheter-related bacteremia clearly indicates that the method is effective. In this prospective, randomized study, where topical Polysporin application was compared to the topical ointment base, Polysporin reduced 4-fold the number of infections. Although the study was carried out on hemodialysis catheters, there is no reason to doubt that similar results might be obtained with peritoneal catheters.

Concluding Remarks

Catheter exit site and tunnel infections continue to be a serious problem in peritoneal dialysis patients. Prevention of long-term exit site infection problems starts at the time of catheter implantation. Surgery itself and exit-site care in the immediate postimplantation period seem to be crucial for long-term results. Among factors essential for proper healing are atraumatic surgery, perfect hemostasis, proper location of the external cuff, and delayed bacterial colonization of the exit site.

Chronic use of topical ointments on the exit, especially in patients with *S. aureus* nasal carrier status and those with equivocal appearance of the exit site, is emerging as a very valuable method of long-term exit site care.

References

1   Twardowski ZJ: History and development of the access for peritoneal dialysis; in Ronco C, Levin NW (eds): Hemodialysis Vascular Access and Peritoneal Dialysis Access. Contrib Nephrol. Basel, Karger, 2004, vol 142, pp 387–401.
2   Heppenstall RB, Littooy FN, Fuchs R, Sheldon GF, Hunt TK: Gas tensions in healing tissues of traumatized patients. Surgery 1974;75/6:874–880.
3   Kantrowitz A, Freed PS, Ciarkowski AA, Hayashi I, Vaughan FL, VeShancey JI, Gray RH, Brabec RK, Bernstein IA: Development of a percutaneous access device. Trans Am Soc Artif Intern Organs 1980;26:444–449.
4   Orgill D, Demling RH: Current concepts and approaches to wound healing. Crit Care Med 1988; 16/9:899–908.
5   Krizek TJ, Robson MC: Biology of surgical infection. Surg Clin North Am 1975;55/6:1261–1267.
6   Twardowski ZJ, Prowant BF: Exit-site healing post-catheter implantation. Perit Dial Int 1996; 16(suppl 3):S51–S70.
7   Twardowski ZJ, Prowant BF: Appearance and classification of healing peritoneal catheter exit sites. Perit Dial Int 1996;16(suppl 3):S71–S93.
8   Prowant BF, Twardowski ZJ: Recommendations for exit care. Perit Dial Int 1996;16(suppl 3): S94–S99.
9   Prowant BF, Warady BA, Nolph KD: Peritoneal dialysis catheter exit-site care: Results of an international survey. Perit Dial Int 1993;13/2:149–154.
10 Pecoits-Filho RFS, Twardowski ZJ, Khanna R, Kim YL, Goel S, Moore H: The effect of antibiotic prophylaxis on the healing of exit-sites of peritoneal dialysis catheters in rats. Perit Dial Int 1998; 18/1:60–63.
11 Twardowski ZJ, Dobbie JW, Moore HL, Nichols WK, DeSpain JD, Anderson PC, Khanna R, Nolph KD, Loy TS: Morphology of peritoneal dialysis catheter tunnel: Macroscopy and light microscopy. Perit Dial Int 1991;11/3:237–251.
12 Twardowski ZJ, Prowant BF: Exit-site study methods and results. Perit Dial Int 1996;16(suppl 3) S6–S31.
13 Zimmerman SW, O'Brien M, Wiedenhoeft FA, Johnson CA: *Staphylococcus aureus* peritoneal catheter-related infections: A cause of catheter loss and peritonitis. Perit Dial Int 1988;8/3:191–194.
14 Abraham G, Savin E, Ayiomamitis A, Izatt S, Vas SI, Mathews RE, Oreopoulos DG: Natural history of exit-site infection (ESI) in patients on continuous ambulatory peritoneal dialysis (CAPD). Perit Dial Int 1988;8/3:211–216.
15 Yu VL, Goetz A, Wagener M, Smith PB, Rihs JD, Hanchett J, Zuravleff JJ: *Staphylococcus aureus* nasal carriage and infection in patients on hemodialysis. Efficacy of antibiotic prophylaxis. N Engl J Med 1986;315/2:91–96.
16 Davies SJ, Ogg CS, Cameron JS, Poston S, Noble WC: *Staphylococcus aureus* nasal carriage, exit-site infection and catheter loss in patients treated with continuous ambulatory peritoneal dialysis (CAPD). Perit Dial Int 1989;9/1:61–64.
17 Luzar MA, Coles GA, Faller B, Slingeneyer A, Dah GD, Briat C, Wone C, Knefati Y, Kessler M, Peluso F: *Staphylococcus aureus* nasal carriage and infection in patients on continuous ambulatory peritoneal dialysis. N Engl J Med 1990;322/8:505–509.

18   Bernardini J, Piraino B, Holley J, Johnston JR, Lutes R: A randomized trial of *Staphylococcus aureus* prophylaxis in peritoneal dialysis patients: Mupirocin calcium ointment 2% applied to the exit site versus cyclic oral rifampin. Am J Kidney Dis 1996;27/5:695–700.

19   Prowant BF, Schmidt LM, Twardowski ZJ, Griebel CK, Burrows L, Ryan LP, Satalowich RJ: Peritoneal dialysis catheter exit site care. ANNA J 1988;15/4:219–222.

20   Twardowski ZJ, Nichols WK, Nolph KD, Khanna R: Swan neck presternal ('bath tub') catheter for peritoneal dialysis. Adv Perit Dial 1992;8:316–324.

21   Bertone AL: Management of exuberant granulation tissue. Vet Clin North Am Equine Pract 1989; 5/3:551–562.

22   Twardowski ZJ: Peritoneal catheter exit site infections: Prevention, diagnosis, treatment, and future directions. Semin Dial 1992;5/4:305–315.

23   Gokal R, Ash SR, Helfrich GB, Holmes CJ, Joffe P, Nichols WK, Oreopoulos DG, Riella MC, Slingeneyer A, Twardowski ZJ, Vas SI: Peritoneal catheters and exit-site practices: Toward optimum peritoneal access. Perit Dial Int 1993;13/1:29–39.

24   Strauss FG, Holmes D, Nortman DF, Friedman S: Hypertonic saline compresses: Therapy for complicated exit site infections; in Khanna R, et al (eds): Advances in Peritoneal Dialysis. Toronto, Peritoneal Dialysis Bulletin, 1993, vol 9, pp 248–250.

25   Scalamogna A, Castelnovo C, De Vecchi A, Ponticelli C: Exit-site and tunnel infections in continuous ambulatory peritoneal dialysis. Am J Kidney Dis 1991;18/6:674–677.

26   Piraino B, Bernardini J, Peitzman A, Sorkin M: Failure of peritoneal catheter cuff shaving to eradicate infection. Perit Dial Bull 1987;7/3:179–182.

27   Twardowski ZJ, Prowant BF, Pickett B, Nichols WK, Nolph KD, Khanna R: Four-year experience with swan neck presternal peritoneal dialysis catheter. Am J Kidney Dis 1996;27/1:99–105.

28   Prowant BF, Khanna R, Twardowski ZJ: Case reports for independent study. Perit Dial Int 1996; 16/3:S105–S114.

29   Twardowski ZJ, Nichols WK: Peritoneal dialysis access and exit site care including surgical aspects; in Gokal R, Khanna R, Krediet RT, Nolph KD (eds): Peritoneal Dialysis, ed 2. Dordrecht, Kluwer Academic Publishers, 2000, chap 9, pp 307–361.

30   Lok CE, Stanley KE, Hux JE, Richardson R, Tobe SW, Conly J: Hemodialysis infection prevention with polysporin ointment. J Am Soc Nephrol 2003;14/1:169–179.

Zbylut J. Twardowski, MD, PhD,
Professor Emeritus of Medicine,
University of Missouri, Dialysis Clinic, Inc.,
3300 LeMone Industrial Blvd., Columbia, MO 65201 (USA)
Tel. +1 573 443 1531, ext. 256, Fax +1 573 884 5506,
E-Mail twardowskiz@health.missouri.edu

Ronco C, Levin NW (eds): Hemodialysis Vascular Access and Peritoneal Dialysis Access.
Contrib Nephrol. Basel, Karger, 2004, vol 142, pp 435–446

....

Conditions Leading to Catheter Removal or Substitution

Roberto Dell'Aquila, Maria Pia Rodighiero, Monica Bonello, Claudio Ronco

Department of Nephrology, Dialysis and Transplantation,
Peritoneal Dialysis Unit, St. Bortolo Hospital, Vicenza, Italy

Introduction

A successful chronic peritoneal dialysis (PD) program requires a reliable peritoneal catheter allowing safe and permanent access to the peritoneal cavity. The problems related to the peritoneal catheter are known and they remain the major complications in CAPD and in APD treatments, despite a decrease in the incidence of peritonitis during the last years due to technological improvements, especially in the field of connectology.

The catheter-related complications make it necessary to suspend temporarily the PD and to treat the patients with hemodialysis. Sometimes the catheter-related problems lead to a definitive abandoning of PD treatments.

The ideal chronic peritoneal access should permit adequate peritoneal exchanges, high dialysate flow rates, should not have malfunctions and should prevent infection episodes. The key to have a safe and permanent access to the peritoneal cavity depends on many factors: (1) catheter design and its characteristics such as catheter size, intra- and extraperitoneal segments, and number of cuffs, (2) modality and techniques for catheter implantation including the exit site direction and tunnel length, and (3) careful approach of postoperative catheter care to minimize bacterial colonization, to prevent exit trauma, traction of the catheter cuffs and leakage due to excessive intra-abdominal pressure; for these reasons a break-in period of at least 15 days and very small intra-abdominal volumes of dialysate at the beginning of the peritoneal treatment are needed.

Concerning the causes of peritoneal catheter removal, there are two main categories: infectious problems and noninfectious problems/mechanical complications.

Infectious Problems

The most common complications related to PD access that lead to catheter removal and/or substitution are recurrent infections of the exit site, of the subcutaneous tunnel and peritonitis. Adequate care is required to prevent exit site and tunnel infections. Patient education and a dedicated clinical staff are of crucial importance. Efforts should be made to maintain a well-functioning peritoneal catheter access. The optimal frequency of exit site control has not been established, but a regular inspection, palpation and assessment of the exit and subcutaneous tunnel are mandatory.

As suggested by the DOQI guidelines [1], the catheter should be immobilized to avoid traumatic lesions and the exit site should be washed daily with liquid soap and water. Antibacterial soap could be used to keep the exit site clean and to diminish the resident bacteria. Some infections may be influenced by the characteristics of the catheter, by the tunnel configuration and by the implantation technique [2–4]. In fact the contamination and the bacteria penetration in the tissues depend on the bacterial species on the direction of the exit site, and the length and width of the subcutaneous tunnel.

Catheter-related infections are often caused by *Staphylococcus aureus* nasal carriage. Prevention is obtained by identifying carriers (patients and partners); all people positively screened for *S. aureus* should receive prophylactic treatment with intranasal mupirocin and the application of mupirocin to the exit site [5–9]. Some cases of mupirocin-resistant *S. aureus* have been reported [10]; in our PD unit we also observed this problem and switched nonresponder patients from mupirocin to tetracycline + sulfamethylthiazole nasal ointment with the eradication of the nasal *S. aureus*.

Generally, the removal of the peritoneal catheter is not necessary if the infection at the exit site occurs without other accompanying infections. In these circumstances an adequate antibiotic therapy depending on the bacterial species is enough to solve the problem.

Bacterial catheter-related infections (exit site, tunnel, inner cuff, biofilm and peritonitis) often cause the loss of the catheter and have been associated with significant morbidity. Catheter removal is necessary when the antibiotic therapy is not effective in solving the infection.

Some infections tend to recur as soon as the antibiotics are stopped. In this case a temporary catheter removal is also indicated. The new catheter should be placed only when the infection episode is completely solved waiting for at least 2 days after the suspension of antibiotic therapy, to exclude the recurrence of the infection.

In general the removal of peritoneal catheter is necessary when there is an inner catheter cuff infection with a high risk of peritonitis, even if there is no evidence of an infection of the sinus or of the external cuff. Removal may also be necessary when there is a permanent tunnel and/or exit site infection, especially if complicated by the presence of a suppurative exit site, but in this case the cuff-shaving technique offers the possibility to save the catheter. The external cuff can be completely removed with debridement of the area of cellulitis and revision of the tunnel; a subsequent peritonitis due to the same antimicrobial agent occurs in approximately 50% of the cases [11–13].

The simultaneous removal and replacement of the catheter is still a matter of controversy [14–16] but this option could prevent catheter loss and failure of the PD technique especially in patients with recurrent episodes of infection with the same bacterial species. However, in patients with fungal peritonitis or infections with *Pseudomonas* species and/or peritonitis [17, 18], the simultaneous removal and replacement of the catheter is not recommended. The best therapy is catheter removal and switching the patient to hemodialysis treatment for at least 6–8 weeks. Before a new peritoneal catheters is implanted it is necessary to evaluate the patient to assess the total absence of infection and its complete clinical resolution.

Bacterial peritonitis is often caused by external contamination due to a poor exchange technique of the patient or his partner. In these cases the removal of the catheter is not indicated since, generally, this kind of peritonitis is sensitive to antibiotic therapy. The kind and dose of antibiotics which are used depend on the etiology of the peritonitis. DOQI guidelines suggest different therapeutic schedules. Only when the bacterial peritonitis is recurrent and there is a resistance to the antibiotic therapy, is it necessary to suspend temporarily the PD treatment and remove the peritoneal access.

Another interesting situation is the sinus colonization by *Corynebacterium* JK: this kind of bacterium is embedded in a self-produced gel matrix sticking to the wall of the catheter and an antibiotic therapy may turn out to be ineffective. Thus the exteriorization of the external cuff might become necessary. If this treatment is not effective, catheter removal must be considered.

Fungal peritonitis is one of the most serious infectious complications with high morbidity and mortality. Its incidence varies from 1.5 to 10% [19] of all peritonitis episodes and frequently leads to the failure of the PD technique. The most important agents involved in fungal peritonitis are *Candida albicans*, *Candida parapsilosis*, *Candida glabrata* and *Aspergillus* spp. This kind of infection could be attributed to an immunocompromised situation of the patient, steroid therapy, underlying SLE (systemic lupus erythematosus), breach in the gastrointestinal tract and hospitalization, and abuse of antibiotics; antimicrobial therapy causes an alteration of fecal flora, transmigration into the peritoneal cavity and, particularly in the immunocompromised host, growth of fungi [19].

The fungi colonize the peritoneal catheter and they are embedded in the amorphous matrix on the surface of the catheter; thus, the antifungal therapy

Table 1. The most common noninfectious or mechanical complications leading to catheter removal and/or substitution

Leakage	Catheter obstruction
Bowel perforation	Catheter dislocation
Hernia	Broken catheter
Pleuroperitoneal communication	Sclerosant peritonitis
Peritoneal loss of function	Rare complication

and the instillation of antimycotics into the peritoneal catheter more often do not solve the infection. A rapid removal of catheter is required and the antifungal therapy must be continued for some weeks, even if the patient is treated with hemodialysis therapy. When antifungal therapy is unsuccessful, it is necessary to create a permanent vascular access in the patient that will be transferred – definitely – to a hemodialysis program.

Noninfectious Problems/Mechanical Complications

Mechanical problems may induce catheter dysfunction. The most common problems, listed in table 1, have an incidence that varies from 12 to 73% [20]. Surgical intervention and catheter replacement are often necessary to resolve these problems.

Leakage

This complication can occur immediately post-catheter implantation or later (>30 days). The early leakage appears at the catheter skin exit when the PD treatment starts soon after the implantation of the catheter (fig. 1). Normally, it is sufficient to suspend the PD treatment immediately and set up a prophylactic antibiotic therapy because of the risk of exit site or tunnel infection; catheter removal is not required.

Late leakage can occur after a long period of PD treatment and may be difficult to diagnose. Often a slow and insufficient drainage during the exchange procedures or a contraction of ultrafiltration may indicate a pericatheter leakage. A computerized tomography can help to identify the leakage site and its entity. This complication is frequent in diabetics, and obese and elderly patients.

Sometimes the leakage appears as a result of elevated intra-abdominal pressure due to the continuous presence of dialysate in the upright position of the patient. It has been assumed that female gender may be a risk factor

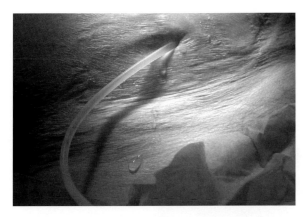

Fig. 1. Leakage in a 64-year-old obese woman.

involved in the development of late dialysis leaks [21]. Suspension of PD treatment for at least 1–2 weeks, reduction of dialysate volume during the exchanges, shift from CAPD to APD treatment with the patient in the supine position or surgical repair of the leakage site may be useful solutions. The removal of the catheter is only required when these corrective measures are ineffective.

Bowel Perforation

Bowel perforation is an uncommon complication and generally causes peritonitis with a wide spectrum of microorganisms especially gram-negative in association with gram-positive agents. It may be due to diverticular disease when diverticulitis is present [22]. Prophylaxis may be achieved with paromomycin sulfate and milk enzymes. Bowel perforation always calls for removal of the peritoneal catheter and immediate surgical resolution in the operating room.

Hernias

Hernias normally appear during the PD treatment due to an excessive volume of dialysate relative to the abdominal capacity in predisposed patients with abdominal tissue relaxation. This complication may appear in several sites determining different hernias as reported in table 2 (in the order of incidence). Frequently, hernia formation occurs in the inguinal or umbilical region, at the catheter implantation site or in relation to previous laparotomic incisions.

Catheter removal is not indicated. In case the reduction of exchange volumes and the option of a dry abdomen during the day are not effective, it is

Table 2. Different kinds of hernias complicating PD

Umbilical	Epigastric
Inguinal	Incisional
Catheter incision site	Cystocele
Ventral	Enterocele
Catheter exit site	Obturator

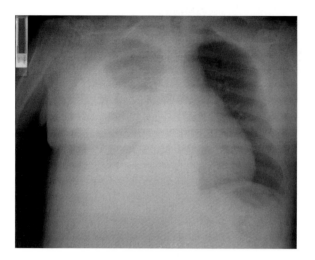

Fig. 2. Hydrothorax in a 65-year-old woman.

necessary to suspend the PD treatment and undertake surgical therapy. Generally, the PD treatment can restart 3–4 weeks after the surgery.

Pleuroperitoneal Communication

An increased intra-abdominal pressure may result in a leak of PD fluid from the peritoneal cavity, through the diaphragm, into the pleural space (fig. 2). The incidence of hydrothorax in PD patients is not known, but probably less than 5%, and frequently underestimated since patients are often asymptomatic. The pathogenesis probably depends on a localized absence of muscle fibers in the hemidiaphragm [23]. Thoracentesis is the immediate therapy of hydrothorax if respiration is compromised. Subsequent treatment depends on whether the patient decides to continue with PD or asks to change to hemodialysis, particularly if the occurrence of hydrothorax is highly distressing. If it is the patient's choice to continue with PD treatment there are different options: temporary hemodialysis (2–4 weeks) with a subsequent return to the PD

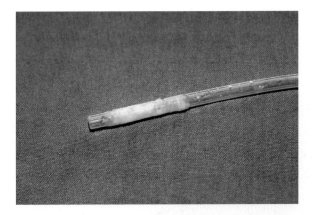

Fig. 3. Fibrin clot around the tip of the peritoneal catheter: half of the lateral holes are clotted.

program, temporary hemodialysis with a return to PD with lower intraperitoneal pressure, obliteration of the pleural space (pleurodesis), and operative repair by thoracotomy.

Peritoneal Loss of Function

Reduced solute clearance and loss of ultrafiltration represent a state of inadequate renal replacement by PD. If targets of adequacy and volume control cannot be achieved, a permanent transfer to hemodialysis is necessary in anuric patients, and thus the catheter should be removed.

Catheter Obstruction and Dislocation

Catheter malfunction is one of the most frequent complications of PD leading to the failure of the therapy. Common causes of catheter malfunction are malposition of the catheter, fibrous adhesions, omental wrapping, constipation and fibrin or blood clots. The one-way or two-way obstruction of the catheter should be differentiated in outflow obstruction, inflow obstruction or both. The outflow obstruction is characterized by a slow drainage flow making it impossible to drain the peritoneal cavity of the patient properly.

Intra- or extraluminal catheter obstruction may occur in the case of blood or fibrin clots (fig. 3).

Extraluminal catheter obstruction factors include the omental incarceration, stool-filled bowel due to constipation of the patient, catheter tip migration in fibrous adhesion pockets, particularly after a severe peritonitis episode and the dislocation of the catheter out of the pelvis (fig. 4–6); dynamic catheterography is essential in the early diagnosis of malfunction [24].

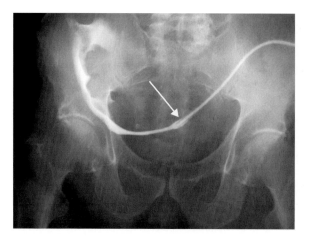

Fig. 4. Entrapment of the PD catheter in the bowel; arrow shows the tip of the device; only the central hole is open.

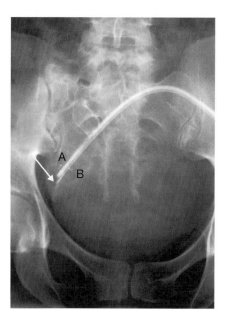

Fig. 5. Entrapment of the PD catheter in the bowel: arrow shows a fibrin clot at the tip of the catheter while letters A and B show the only two lateral holes which are open.

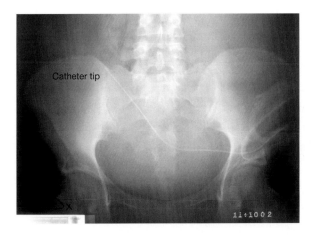

Fig. 6. Migration of the catheter tip in the perihepatic area.

The inflow obstruction occurs with a lower incidence than the outflow obstruction. Generally, this complication is due to intraluminal debris and to the important presence of blood or fibrin clots. The more common cause is the catheter kink along its course or relating to the exit site or subcutaneous tunnel.

Depending on the problems noninvasive therapies such as laxatives in the case of constipation, a change in the patient's body position, and treatment with heparin or urokinase (5,000 IU instilled into the catheter for 2–4 h) are recommended and the removal of the peritoneal catheter is not required except when the cause of the malfunctioning catheter is related to its position.

Sometimes a surgical approach like videolaparoscopic surgery or open surgery is useful to resolve the problem of catheter malposition or catheter migration [25]. These techniques permit the immediate surgical correction or the simultaneous catheter replacement. Nevertheless, the problems related to catheter malfunctions require the removal of the peritoneal catheter only after the other corrective actions and conservative measures have failed. Malfunction and migration of the catheter are often caused by the design of the device [26, 27].

Broken Catheter

In case of catheters broken as a result of accidental cuts with the scissors near the exit site or because of production defects in the catheter material, the surgical approach is recommended and the catheter removal is followed, after careful inspection of the peritoneal cavity, by the replacement of a new catheter. Moreover the barium sulfate used to render the catheter radiopaque makes the device brittle; silicone rubber catheters have been observed to stretch, crack or become brittle with age or after repeated exposure to Betadine® [28].

Sclerosant Peritonitis

The sclerosant peritonitis is a severe complication that leads to the failure of the peritoneal treatment. This kind of peritonitis makes the immediate removal of the catheter necessary. The main etiopathogenetic factor is the low biocompatibility of peritoneal solutions but other causes, in addition the PD fluids, are involved such as peritonitis, drugs (β-blockers) and disinfectants.

Rare Complications

Rare complications requiring the removal of the catheter may be listed as allergic reaction, hemoperitoneum, severe infusion/pressure pain, organ erosion, and no need for a peritoneal catheter.

Allergic reaction is an uncommon complication causing – in some cases – eosinophil peritonitis. It may be the result of many causes like some elements of PD solution, antibiotics or the proteinaceous biofilm that covered the Silastic tubing. In particularly sensitive patients this may determine the allergic problem. If the diagnosis confirms an allergic reaction to silicone rubber the removal of the catheter is recommended.

Intraperitoneal bleeding (hemoperitoneum) causes intense inflammatory reactions and extensive adhesions; this can lead to catheter failure requiring catheter removal.

The severe infusion/pressure pain is a problem that can occur when the catheter is stressed too much, leading to a possible 'jet effect' due to the high flow velocity of the dialysate during the exchange in the infusion phase.

This problem also depends on the type or the design of the catheter used. Catheters with a greater lumen and with a coiled intraperitoneal portion induce less abdominal pain because the major percentage of the solution flows with a shower effect and the poking force of the coiled catheter is less than a straight catheter. Normally, it is not necessary to remove the peritoneal catheter, but it is sufficient to regulate the speed of the flow of the solution, particularly during the first part of the infusion phase.

The organ erosion is an uncommon complication, but a severe one. It may appear as the result of a rubbing – light, but continuous – of the catheter tip. This complication damages the internal organs leading to intra-abdominal bleeding with or without peritonitis or peritoneal laceration or in few cases to some genital edema. The immediate removal of the peritoneal catheter is recommended.

The 'natural' definite removal of the peritoneal catheter is necessary when the patient is going to receive a different dialytic treatment, for example, after a renal transplant with the resumption of the renal function or for other reasons requiring a definitive end to PD treatment.

References

1 National Kidney Foundation-K/DOQI clinical practice guidelines for peritoneal dialysis adequacy, 2000. Am J Kidney Dis 2001;37(suppl 1):S65–S136.
2 Dasgupta MK: Moncrief-Popovich catheter and implantation technique: The AV fistula of peritoneal dialysis. Adv Ren Replace Ther 2002;9/2:116–124.
3 Twardowsky ZJ: Presternal peritoneal catheter. Adv Ren Replace Ther 2002;9/2:125–132.
4 Ash SR, Sutton JM, Mankus RA, Rossman J, de Ridder V, Nassvi MS, Ross J: Clinical trials of the T-fluted (Ash Advantage) peritoneal dialysis catheter. Adv Ren Replace Ther 2002;9/2:133–143.
5 Mupirocin Study Group: Nasal mupirocin prevents *Staphylococcus aureus* exit-site infection during peritoneal dialysis. J Am Soc Nephrol 1996;7:2403–2408.
6 Perez-Fontan M, Garcia-Falcon T, Rosales M, Rodrigues-Carmona A, Adeva M, Rodrigues-Lozana I, et al: Treatment of *Staphylococcus aureus* nasal carriages in CAPD with mupirocin: Long term results. Am J Kidney Dis 1993;22:708–712.
7 Thodis E, Bhaskaran S, Passadakis P, Bargman JM, Vas SI, Oreopoulos DG: Decrease in *Staphylococcus aureus* exit-site infection and peritonitis in CAPD patients by local application of mupirocin ointment at the catheter exit-site. Perit Dial Int 1998;18/3:261–270.
8 Thodis E, Passadakis P, Panagoutsos S, Bacheraki D, Euthimiadou A, Vargemezis V: The effectiveness of mupirocin preventing *Staphylococcus aureus* in catheter-related infections in peritoneal dialysis. Adv Perit Dial 2000;16:257–261.
9 Bernardini J, Piraino B, Holley J, Johnston JR, Lutes R: A randomized trial of *Staphylococcus aureus* prophylaxis in peritoneal dialysis patients: Mupirocin calcium ointment 2% applied to the exit-site versus cyclic oral rifampin. Am J Kidney Dis 1996;27:695–700.
10 Annigeri R, Conly J, Vas S, Dedier H, Prakashan KP, Bargman JM, Jassal V, Oreopoulos D: Emergence of mupirocin-resistant *Staphylococcus aureus* in chronic peritoneal dialysis patients using mupirocin prophylaxis to prevent exit-site infection. Perit Dial Int 2001;21:554–559.
11 Abraham G, Savin E, Ayiomamitis A, Izzat S, Vas SI, Mathews RB, et al: Natural history of exit-site infections in patients in CAPD. Perit Dial Int 1988;8:211–216.
12 Scalamogna A, Castelnovo C, De Vecchi A, Ponticelli C: Exit-site and tunnel infection in CAPD patients. Am J Kidney Dis 1991;18:674–677.
13 Piraino B: Peritoneal dialysis catheter replacement: Save the patient and not the catheter. Semin Dial 2003;16/1:72–75.
14 Swartz RD, Messana JM: Simultaneous catheter removal and replacement in peritoneal dialysis infections: Update and current recommendations. Adv Perit Dial 1999;15:205–208.
15 Singhal MK, Vas SI, Oreopoulos DG: Treatment of peritoneal dialysis catheter-related infections by simultaneous catheter removal and replacement. Is it safe? Perit Dial Int 1996;16:557–573.
16 Szeto CC, Chow KM, Leung CB, Wong TY, Wu AK, Wang AY, Lui SF, Li PK: Clinical course of peritonitis due to Pseudomonas species complicating peritoneal dialysis: A review of 104 cases. Kidney Int 2001;59:2309–2315.
17 Szabo T, Siccion Z, Izatt S, Vas SI, Bargman J, Oreopoulos DG: Outcome of *Pseudomonas aeruginosa* exit-site and tunnel infections: A single center's experience. Adv Perit Dial 1999;15: 209–212.
18 Saran R, Goel S, Khanna R: Fungal peritonitis in continuous ambulatory peritoneal dialysis. Int J Artif Organs 1996;19:441–445.
19 Bernardini J: Peritoneal dialysis catheter complications. Perit Dial Int 1996;16(suppl 1):S468–S471.
20 Albaz M, Kantaci G, Tuglular S, Tercuman N, Tetik G, Ozener C: Causes of late leaks in peritoneal dialysis patients. EDTNA ERCA J 2002;28/4:170–172.
21 Tranaeus A, Heimburger O, Granqvist S: Diverticular disease of the colon: A risk factor for peritonitis in continuous peritoneal dialysis. Nephrol Dial Transplant 1990;5/2:141–149.
22 Boeschoten EW, Krediet RT, Roos CM, Kloek JJ, Schipper MEI, Arisz L: Leakage of dialysate across the diaphragm: An important complication of continuous ambulatory peritoneal dialysis. Neth J Med 1986;29:242–246.
23 Scabardi M, Ronco C, Chiaramonte S, Feriani M, Agostini F, La Greca G: Dynamic catheterography in the early diagnosis of peritoneal catheter malfunction. Int J Artif Organs 1992;15:358–364.

24   Lee M, Donovan JF: Laparoscopic omentectomy for salvage of peritoneal dialysis catheter. J Endourol 2002;16/4:241–244.
25   Di Paolo N, Petrini G, Garosi G, Buoncristiani U, Brardi S, Monaci G: A new self-locating peritoneal catheter. Perit Dial Int 1996;16:623–627.
26   Gadallah MF, Mignone J, Torres C, Ramdeen G, Pervez A: The role of peritoneal dialysis catheter configuration in preventing catheter tip migration. Adv Perit Dial 2000;16:47–50.
27   Ward RA, Klein E, Wathen RL: Peritoneal catheters; in Investigation of the Risks and Hazards with Devices Associated with Peritoneal Dialysis and Sorbent Regenerated Dialysate Delivery Systems. Perit Dial Bull 1983;3(suppl 3):S9–S17.
28   Gadallah MF, Torres-Rivera C, Ramdeen G, Myrick S, Habashi S, Andrew G: Relationship between intraperitoneal bleeding, adhesions, and peritoneal dialysis catheter failure: A method of prevention. Adv Perit Dial 2001;17:127–179.

Roberto Dell'Aquila, MD,
Department of Nephrology, Dialysis and Transplantation,
Peritoneal Dialysis Unit, St. Bortolo Hospital,
Viale Rodolfi 27, IT–36100 Vicenza (Italy)
Tel. +39 044 4993650, Fax +39 044 4993973, E-Mail eagle@goldnet.it

Ronco C, Levin NW (eds): Hemodialysis Vascular Access and Peritoneal Dialysis Access.
Contrib Nephrol. Basel, Karger, 2004, vol 142, pp 447–461

....

New Catheter Design for Continuous Flow Peritoneal Dialysis

Claudio Ronco[a], *Angela Gloukhoff Wentling*[b], *Richard Amerling*[c],
Cosme Cruz[c], *Nathan W. Levin*[c]

[a] Department of Nephrology, St. Bortolo Hospital, Vicenza, Italy;
[b] Medcomp, Medical Components, Inc., Harleysville, Pa., and
[c] Renal Research Institute, Beth Israel Medical Center, New York, N.Y., USA

Introduction

Peritoneal dialysis (PD) is a well-established form of renal replacement therapy [1–5]. In recent years, different techniques of PD have been designed to meet the requirements of different patients [6–12]. The targets of adequacy for PD indicated by the DOQI document are, however, sometimes difficult to reach unless large amounts of fluid are utilized or nightly sessions are significantly prolonged [9–12]. Under such circumstances continuous flow peritoneal dialysis (CFPD) might represent a new option especially for patients with limited chances on standard CAPD or automated peritoneal dialysis (APD) schedules. Furthermore, CFPD makes it possible to explore the effects of high-dose treatment in PD with new potentially beneficial effects [13–20].

In CAPD, the relative efficiency can be improved to meet adequacy targets by increasing the volume exchanged and the number of exchanges. The same is true for APD while intermittent PD 3 times a week is inadequate practically in most cases in spite of all efforts. For CFPD, higher levels of efficiency can be reached but this assumes the utilization of large amounts of fluid per session (up to 100 liters). CFPD requires large amounts of fluid because of the high dialysate flows involved in the operational characteristics of the technique. However, the most important issue is that adequate peritoneal access must be available to make continuous inflow and outflow possible. In this paper we will describe the evolution of a catheter for CFPD from its initial design to its most updated configuration.

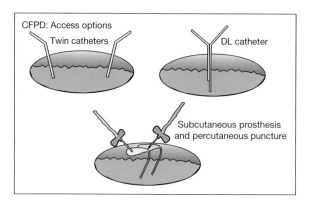

Fig. 1. Different options for peritoneal access in CFPD.

Peritoneal Access in CFPD

To perform CFPD, a two-way access must be available in order to allow for continuous inflow and outflow of the solution. This is most likely achieved with a double-lumen peritoneal catheter. Other options could be offered by two separate catheters or by two subcutaneous prosthetic devices (fig. 1). The double-lumen design does not necessarily increase the size of the tube or the discomfort of the patient. However, maximal care should be taken to obtain an optimized design and the real challenge is to minimize recirculation and mixing of the inflow and outflow dialysate. Possibly, the tips of the two lumens of the catheter must be in a position that maximizes exposure of the peritoneal surface during one single passage of the fluid from one lumen to another. Based on this concept, several catheters have been proposed but we have developed a newly conceived double-lumen catheter to be used for CFPD (Medcomp, Medical Components, Inc., Harleysville, Pa., USA).

The New CFPD Catheter

PD is a technique where dialysate solution is infused into the peritoneal cavity by gravity, and subsequently removed to be discarded. During PD, solutes and fluids are exchanged between the capillary blood and the intraperitoneal fluid through the peritoneum. 'Continuous flow peritoneal dialysis' relies on the continuous infusion of PD solution through one peritoneal access, and simultaneous drainage through another. This is achieved by using two catheters or a double-lumen catheter often in conjunction with an external system regenerating the spent

Table 1. CFPD: Access issues

Safety	Easy catheter insertion
	No adverse effects (compared to other PD
	catheters)
	Adequate biomaterials
Comfort	Tolerance and perfect wound sealing
	No mechanical disturbances
	No functional disturbances
Efficiency	High flow
	Low resistance
	Minimal recirculation
Exit Site	Minimal skin and subcutaneous damage
	One or two exit sites
	Possible substitution of external sections

dialysate. A constant intraperitoneal volume is maintained with high dialysate flow rates designed to maintain the highest solute concentration gradient between plasma and the solution.

CFPD provides many advantages as compared to regular PD, of which the most important are shorter sessions and better clearances to improve the quality of life for dialysis patients.

Advocated CFPD advantages are higher clearances, higher ultrafiltration, requiring lower glucose concentration, neutral pH of solution, improved host defenses, bicarbonate-based solution, reduction of advanced glycosilated end products (AGEs), reduction/elimination glucose degradation products (GDPs), fewer connections, lower rates of peritonitis, variable solute concentrations, reduced protein losses, shorter dialytic sessions and improved quality of life. The disadvantages are the unknown effect of high dialysate flow rates on peritoneal structures, the unknown effect of synthetic membranes (dialysate regeneration system) on peritoneal structures, the poor mixing of solution in the peritoneal cavity (recirculation), and cost.

The design of our new PD catheter attempts to eliminate some of the disadvantages of CFPD. The new catheter is intended to prevent the effects of high dialysate flow rates on the peritoneal membrane, and the poor mixing of solution in the peritoneal cavity. The requirements for a new CFPD catheter are in fact listed in table 1.

Reduction of Peritoneal Trauma and Discomfort

To reduce trauma to the peritoneal structure, we are using a low durometer silicone as the material of choice. Silicone is the most common material

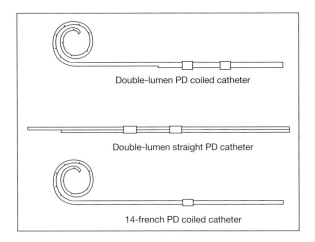

Double-lumen PD coiled catheter

Double-lumen straight PD catheter

14-french PD coiled catheter

Fig. 2. Different types of double-lumen PD catheter.

used for catheters due to its biocompatibility, softness, and flexibility in a large range of temperatures, and the fact that it does not contain clinically harmful leachable plasticizers. It is the ideal material to be used near the soft peritoneal structure. Special solutions are also being designed to prevent discomfort at the exit site or increased risk of infection.

Reduction of Intraperitoneal Dialysate Recirculation

High dialysate flow rates and consequent recirculation (due to channeling or poor mixing inside the peritoneal cavity) are other problems associated with CFPD. To eliminate these problems, we originally designed double-lumen catheters with one branch short and another long of a straight and of a spiral shape (fig. 2). Recently we have designed a novel catheter for CFPD equipped with a thin-walled silicone diffuser used to gently diffuse the inflow dialysate into the peritoneum (fig. 3). The holes on the round tapered diffuser are positioned to allow dialysate to perpendicularly exit 360° from the diffuser. The diffuser design and hole locations disperse the high-flow dialysate fluid at 360°, reducing trauma to the peritoneal walls and allowing the dialysate to mix into the peritoneum. The dispersed fluid infused into the peritoneal cavity is then drained through the second lumen whose tip is placed into the lower Douglas cavity. We designed several shapes for the diffuser from a disk to a bell shape (fig. 4). Finally, the diffuser was designed as a tear drop (fig. 5). Not only does the diffuser minimize recirculation, but it also reduces the possible pain or

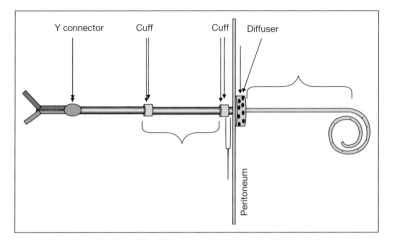

Fig. 3. The 'Ronco' catheter for CFPD.

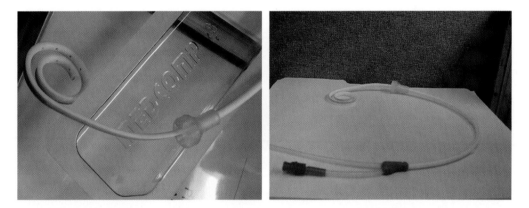

Fig. 4. The first version of the 'Ronco CFPD Cath' included a bell-shaped diffuser and a large hub that turned out to be impractical for subcutaneous tunneling.

discomfort derived from the high speed of fluid infusion in CFPD and it prevents jet lesions (fig. 6).

The next step was to create an adequate method for optimizing the subcutaneous tunnel and exit site. Different options were considered including a fixed hub with two separate exit sites. This, however, would have multiplied the risk of exit site infection and it was discarded. The second option was to design a soft and oval hub such that it could be passed through the skin. This, however, was still presenting a diameter that would have led to an excessively large skin hole (fig. 7). Finally we decided to design a removable hub that could be applied after

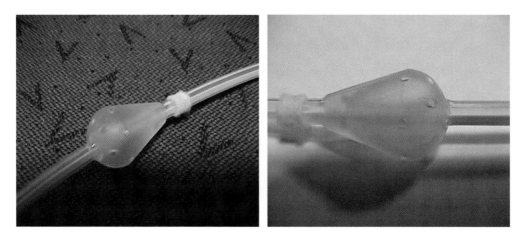

Fig. 5. The new version of the 'Ronco CFPD Cath' includes a softer, 'tear's drop'-shaped diffuser.

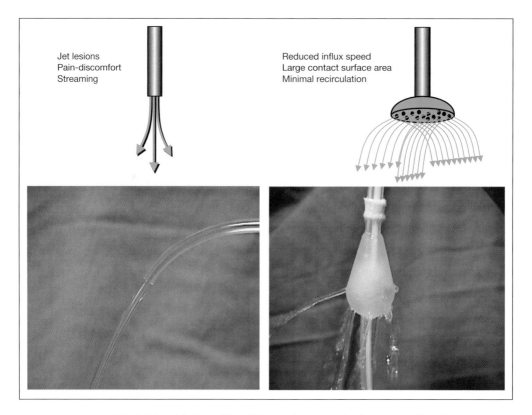

Jet lesions
Pain-discomfort
Streaming

Reduced influx speed
Large contact surface area
Minimal recirculation

Fig. 6. Pictorial view of the difference between a jet flow and a diffused flow.

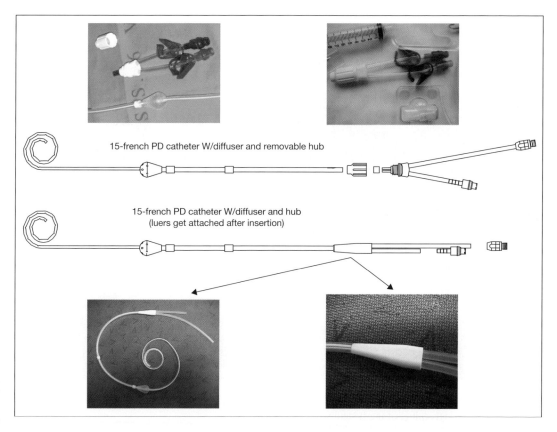

Fig. 7. In designing the hub for the new catheter two options were possible: (1) to generate a soft and thin hub (bottom) compressible in a way that it could be passed through the skin and (2) a removable hub (top) with two spikes enabling the passage of the cannula through the skin and connecting the y set subsequently.

the catheter had been extracted from the skin through a small adequate hole (fig. 7). To do this, a series of new tools including a new tunnelizer and a connector with two spikes to be adapted to the double-lumen cannula had to be designed and produced (fig. 8). Once the tray with all the necessary tools and accessories was put together (fig. 9), the insertion of the catheter became easy and safe.

CFPD Catheter Insertion

The insertion technique requires to insert the catheter lumen assembly first into the peritoneum and then to tunnel the catheter extension assembly through the subcutaneous skin layer. To achieve this goal adaptors/luers cannot be inserted onto the extensions prior to the insertion procedure. In making the

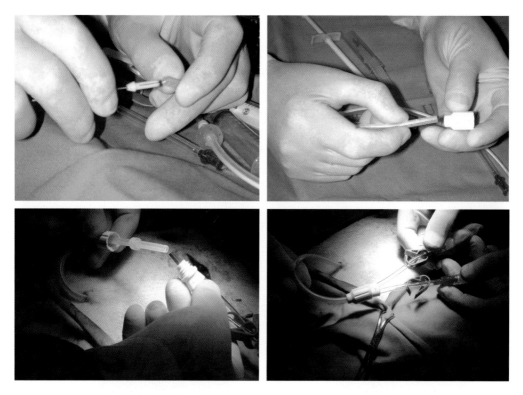

Fig. 8. Sequential view of the connection of the removable hub with the cannula and the final sealing of the system with a screw connector.

silicone diffuser thin walled, the diffuser is capable of being compressed and fitted into a sheath to be inserted into the peritoneum (fig. 10). Compression of the diffuser diminishes its volume, thus preventing the peritoneal surgical incision from being too large inducing possible subsequent problems of leakage. Once the catheter diffuser and coiled lumen are inserted into the peritoneum, the extension is tunneled through the subcutaneous tissue layer, and the removable hub is then connected to the two lumens through its special spikes (fig. 8).

The coiled design provides an increased bulk of tubing to separate the parietal and visceral layers of the peritoneum from obstructing the holes for outflow. This coiled design exists in other PD catheters. It is believed to be less traumatic to the viscera than the tip of a straight catheter.

Skin Exit Site and Catheter Care

The CFPD catheter contains two cuffs. The first cuff is attached onto the lumen 0.2 inch before the diffuser. The second cuff follows 3.94 inches after the

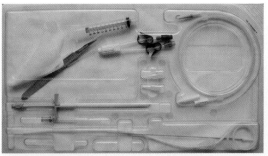
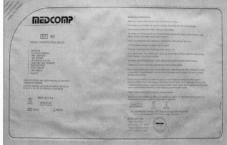
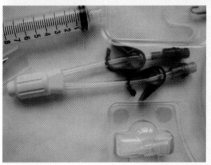
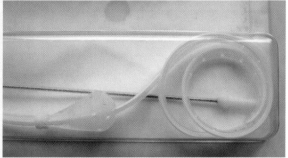

Fig. 9. Complete set for the catheter insertion prepared in a tray. The removable hub is clearly visible.

first cuff. The polyester cuffs are used for tissue in-growth to secure the catheters onto the subcutaneous tissue. As in other catheters the first cuff is placed just outside the sutured peritoneal parietal wall, while the second cuff is secured under the skin just before the exit hole. The removable hub guarantees that no larger skin hole is required to extract the catheter through the skin.

Flow versus Gravity, Recirculation, Flow versus Pressure in vitro Catheter Testing

The novel PD catheter with diffuser was tested against other catheters to determine whether the new design has improved 'flow versus gravity', 'recirculation', and 'flow versus pressure' characteristics. Examples of the graphs for the 14 french × 62 cm PD coiled catheter can be seen in figure 11. The gravity flow rate was determined by using the ISO 10555-3 procedure, 'Determination of Flow Rate through the Catheter'. To determine gravity flow a constant-level tank fitted with a delivery tube and a male luer fitting (capable when no test catheter is attached in providing 525 ± 25 ml/min, and having a hydrostatic head height of 1,000 ± 5 mm) was used as shown in figure 11. Deionized water

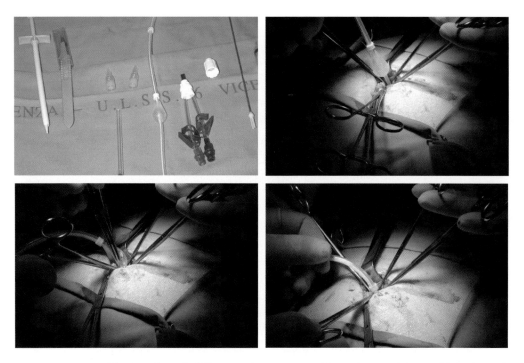

Fig. 10. The soft diffuser can be compressed by a clamp and inserted into the peritoneal cavity with no problem.

was allowed to flow through the catheter, and was collected at the distal end of the catheter for 1 min. The volume was recorded and plotted as shown.

The objective of recirculation testing is to determine the 'lumen to lumen' recirculation of the catheter. To do so, the catheter is inserted into a catheter insertion port with a water supply pipe flowing at 2.5 liters/min. Water conductivity is measured prior to testing and recorded. The PD catheter is connected to supply and withdraw lines. The withdraw line connects to the catheter lumen luer responsible for the outflow and the saline supply line connects to the inflow lumen luer. The rotary pump, which is connected to these lines, is turned on, up to 350 ml/min. The saline is supplied to the water pipe from the inflow line. From the outflow line, 200 ml of fluid is collected and then discarded. Then 300 ml of fluid is recollected from the outflow line. The pump is stopped and the supply line is clamped. The conductivity is measured from the 300 ml of fluid and recorded. To calculate the percentage of recirculation, the following formula is used:

$$\% \text{ recirculation} = \frac{(\text{outflow fluid, mS} - \text{water, mS})}{(\text{inflow fluid, mS})} \times 100$$

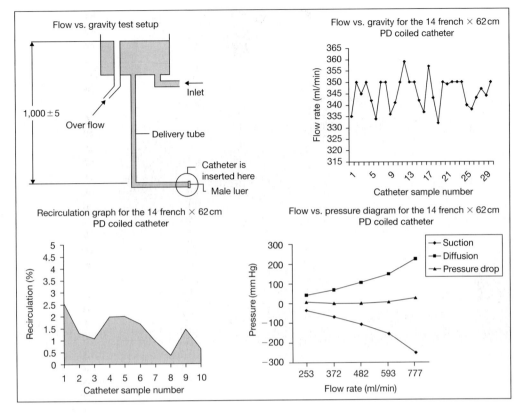

Fig. 11. Complete set of data collected in the in vitro study of the catheter. The system utilized is described in the top left panel while the flow pressure relationships are depicted in the graphs.

The data are then plotted on a graph (fig. 11).

Flow versus pressure testing is conducted to determine the pressure drop of the PD catheter. To achieve this, the catheter is connected to Medcomp's 'Flow vs Pressure' data acquisition machine, where the catheter suction and diffusion pressures and flow rates are recorded by pressure sensors and an ultrasonic flow meter. The tubing lines and supply tank are filled with Delflex PD solution with 4.25% and kept at a temperature of $37 \pm 2°C$. The catheter is then tested at five different flow rates at 1 min per flow rate. Flow rate and suction/diffusion pressure data are recorded each second via the 'Flow vs Pressure' data acquisition system. Once the testing is completed, the data acquisition system calculates the average flow rate and pressures. The data are retrieved and a graph, along with the calculated pressure drop of the suction and diffusion lumens, is drawn (fig. 11).

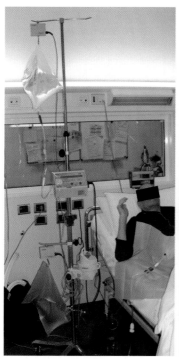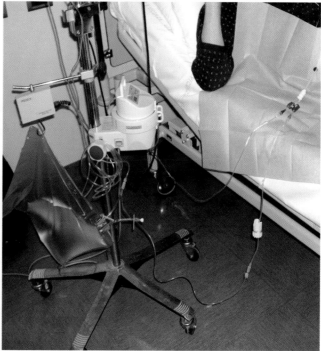

Fig. 12. A simple 'manual' system for CFPD utilizing the 'equaline device'. Inflow and outflow rates are regulated by load cells and smart clamps.

In vivo Experience

We have obtained the permission from the ethical committee of our department to perform the first implant of the catheter 1 year ago. The catheter was utilized for compassionate use in an 86-year-old man with end-stage kidney disease who could not be dialyzed because of the absence of vascular access and who needed high-dose PD due to poor dietary compliance and a high degree of catabolism.

The patient was treated with CFPD for 1 month with daily sessions of 30 liters using both manual and semiautomatic techniques. The set up was simple and utilized two load cells and a smart clamp in order to equalize the outflow to the inflow (fig. 12). Ultrafiltrate was drained at mid and end treatment. Different schedules with varying flows and tidal volumes were tested with encouraging results in terms of clearances as reported in figures 13 and 14. In particular, clearances for urea as high as 49 ml/min could be achieved.

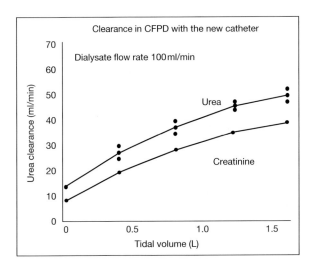

Fig. 13. Solute clearances measured with CFPD at fixed flow and variable tidal volume.

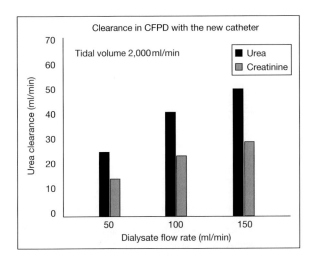

Fig. 14. Solute clearances measured with CFPD at fixed tidal volume and variable flows.

The patient could subsequently be treated with standard APD at a regime of 20 liters every night. The catheter has always been functioning perfectly and neither exit site infection nor peritonitis was observed. The hub was changed every 3 months.

The important point to draw attention to is the fact that the catheter after its use in CFPD could be easily and perfectly well used for APD utilizing only one of the two lumens. This suggests that such a catheter could theoretically be placed in every patient and be used for CFPD only when needed.

Conclusions

CFPD will probably represent one of the most exciting innovations in the field in the coming years. The availability of a suitable peritoneal access is the conditio sine qua non for a real development of the technique. It is our impression that our newly designed dual lumen catheter with the diffuser is the answer to many questions and problems relating to the technique.

References

1 Twardowski ZJ, Nolph KD, Khanna R, et al: Peritoneal equilibration test. Perit Dial Bull 1987;7: 138–147.
2 Diaz-Buxo JA, Youngblood BP, Torres AM: Delivered dialysis dose with PD Plus therapy: A multicenter study. Am J Nephrol 1998;18:520–524.
3 Durand PY, Freida P, Issad B, Chanliau J: How to reach optimal creatinine clearance in automated peritoneal dialysis. Perit Dial Int 1996;16(suppl 1):S167–S170.
4 Twardowski ZJ: Nightly peritoneal dialysis. Why, who, how and when. ASAIO Trans 1990;36: 8–16.
5 Amici G, Virga G, Da Rin G, Bocci C, Calconi G: Continuous tidal peritoneal dialysis (CTPD) prescription and adequacy targets. Adv Perit Dial 1998;14:64–67.
6 Holley JL, Piraino B: Careful patient selection and dialysis prescription are required for effective nightly intermittent peritoneal dialysis. Perit Dial Int 1994;14:155–158.
7 Friedlander MA, Rahman M, Tessman MJ, Hanslik TM, Ferrara KA, Newman LN: Variability in calculations of dialysis adequacy in patients using nightly intermittent peritoneal dialysis compared to CAPD. Adv Perit Dial 1995;11:93–96.
8 Durand PY, Slingeneyer A, Benevent D, Chanliau J: CAPD: Peritoneal clearances with a 5th nocturnal automated exchange (Baxter Quantum) (abstract). Perit Dial Int 1997;17(suppl 1):S15.
9 Piraino B, Bender F, Bernardini J: A comparison of clearances on tidal peritoneal dialysis and intermittent peritoneal dialysis. Perit Dial Int 1994;14/2:145–148.
10 Steinhauer HB, Keck I, Lubrich-Birkner I, Schollmeyer P: Increased dialysis efficiency in tidal peritoneal dialysis compared to intermittent peritoneal dialysis. Nephron 1991;58:500–501.
11 Flanigan MJ, Doyle C, Lim VS, Ullrich G: Tidal peritoneal dialysis: Preliminary experience. Perit Dial Int 1992;12:304–308.
12 Brandes JC, Packard WJ, Watters SK, Fritsche C: Optimization of dialysate flow and mass transfer during automated peritoneal dialysis. Am J Kidney Dis 1995;25:603–610.
13 Cruz C, Melendez A, Gotch F, Folden T, Levin NW, Crawford T, Diaz-Buxo JA: Continuous flow peritoneal dialysis (CFPD): Preliminary clinical experience. Perit Dial Int 2000;20(suppl 1):S6.
14 Raj DSC, Self M, Work J: Hybrid dialysis: Recirculation peritoneal dialysis revisited. Am J Kidney Dis 2000;36/1:58–67.
15 Mineshima M, Suzuki S, Sato Y, Ishimori I, Ishida K, Kaneko I, Agishi T: Solute removal characteristics of continuous recirculating peritoneal dialysis in experimental and clinical studies. ASAIO J 2000;46/1:95–98.

16   Diaz-Buxo JA: Continuous flow peritoneal dialysis. Nephrol News Issues 2001;15:18–21.
17   Ronco C, Diaz-Buxo JA: Automated peritoneal dialysis, revisitation of the past or beginning of a new PD era? Nephron 2001;87:1–7.
18   Gokal R: Peritoneal catheters and exit-site practices toward optimum peritoneal access: 1998 update. Perit Dial Int 1998;18:11–33.
19   Amerling R, Glezerman I, Savransky E, Dubrow A, Ronco C: Continuous flow peritoneal dialysis: Current perspectives. Contrib Nephrol 2003;140:294–304.
20   Ronco C, Gloukhoff A, Dell'Aquila R, Levin NW: Catheter design for continuous flow peritoneal dialysis. Blood Purif 2002;20:40–44.

Claudio Ronco, MD,
Department of Nephrology, St. Bortolo Hospital,
Viale Rodolfi, IT–36100 Vicenza (Italy)
Tel. +39 0444993869, Fax +39 0444993949, E-Mail cronco@goldnet.it

Author Index

Subject Index

Kidney Disease Outcomes Quality
  Initiative (continued)
  thrombolytic use
    catheter-based devices 38, 39
    grafts and fistulas 37, 38
  vascular access guidelines 30, 323, 351,
    352

LifeSite System
  clinical studies 185, 186, 211, 212
  complications
    care and maintenance-related
      complications 188, 189
    insertion-related complications 187,
      188
  features 180–182
  placement 182–184

Mahurkar catheter, features 132
Mesenteric bovine vein, graft utilization 6,
  7, 61, 62
Multimat sensor, vascular access
  recirculation measurement 261, 262

Nasal carriage, *Staphylococcus aureus*
  426, 427, 432, 436

Opti-Flow catheter
  comparative studies with other chronic
    central venous catheters 143–146
  design 132

Patient perspective, vascular access
  access preservation 369
  aseptic preparation 367
  communication
    information access 372, 373
    patients 372
    staff 371, 372
  importance 363, 364
  Medicare reimbursement 365
  pain 370, 371
  personal commentaries 364, 367–371
  recommendations 373, 374
  self-cannulation 366, 368, 369, 371
  standardized access care information
    368

technician preferences for grafts 368,
  369
temporary catheters 368
vascular surgeon differences 364, 365,
  368
Percutaneous intervention, *see* Stenosis;
  Thrombosis
Peritoneal dialysis catheters, *see also*
  Swan-neck catheters; Tenckhoff catheter
  bowel perforation 439, 440
  break-in period 410, 411
  continuous flow peritoneal dialysis
    adequacy targets 447
    advantages 448, 449
    double-lumen catheters
      care 454, 455
      clinical studies 458–460
      insertion 453, 454
      overview 393, 394
      peritoneal trauma and discomfort
        reduction 449, 450
      recirculation reduction 450, 451,
        453
      requirements 449
      testing in vitro 455–457
    peritoneal access options 448
  cuff extrusion management 416–418
  drainage time and breakpoint
    determination 419, 420
  exit site care
    appearance and healing 423, 424, 427,
      428
    bacterial colonization of catheter sinus
      426, 437
    early care 424, 425
    infection
      acute infection management 429,
        430
      appearance classification 427, 428
      chronic infection management 430
      equivocal exit management 431
      external cuff infection management
        431
      fungal infection 437, 438
      prevention 422, 423, 432
      removal and replacement of catheter
        436–438